Authentication of

Chinese Medicinal Materials by DNA Technology

Techniques and Applications

Second Edition

Authentication of Chinese Medicinal Materials by DNA Technology

Techniques and Applications

Second Edition

edited by

Pang-Chui SHAW
The Chinese University of Hong Kong, China

Hui CAO
Jinan University, China

Yat-Tung LO
The Chinese University of Hong Kong, China

World Scientific

NEW JERSEY • LONDON • SINGAPORE • BEIJING • SHANGHAI • HONG KONG • TAIPEI • CHENNAI • TOKYO

Published by

World Scientific Publishing Co. Pte. Ltd.
5 Toh Tuck Link, Singapore 596224
USA office: 27 Warren Street, Suite 401-402, Hackensack, NJ 07601
UK office: 57 Shelton Street, Covent Garden, London WC2H 9HE

British Library Cataloguing-in-Publication Data
A catalogue record for this book is available from the British Library.

AUTHENTICATION OF CHINESE MEDICINAL MATERIALS BY DNA TECHNOLOGY
Techniques and Applications
Second Edition

ISBN 978-981-126-153-4 (hardcover)
ISBN 978-981-126-154-1 (ebook for institutions)
ISBN 978-981-126-155-8 (ebook for individuals)

For any available supplementary material, please visit
https://www.worldscientific.com/worldscibooks/10.1142/13001#t=suppl

Contents

Preface ix
Contributing Authors xiii

Part I Introduction **1**

Chapter 1 General Introduction 3

Part II General Methodology and Techniques for Molecular Authentication **27**

Chapter 2 DNA Extraction for Medicinal Materials 29
Hoi-Yan Wu, Forrest Chung-Fai Yau & Fai-Ngor Ngan

Chapter 3 General Methodology 67
Mavis Hong-Yu Yik

Chapter 4 Bioinformatics for DNA Sequencing Data Analysis 89
Yat-Tung Lo

Part III DNA Fingerprinting-based Techniques for Molecular Authentication **127**

Chapter 5 Authentication of Medicinal Materials and Their Formula by Randomly Primed Polymerase Chain Reaction 129
Hui Cao, Ying Zhang, Kur-Ta Cheng & Pang-Chui Shaw

Chapter 6 Authentication of Medicinal Materials by Amplified Fragment Length Polymorphism 153
Hui Cao, Ying Zhang & Pang-Chui Shaw

Chapter 7 Authentication of Medicinal Materials by Polymerase Chain Reaction–Restriction Fragment Length Polymorphism 171
Hui Cao, Ying Zhang, Ping Li & Katsuko Komatsu

Chapter 8 Authentication of Medicinal Materials by Sequence Characterised Amplified Region 199
Grace Wing-Chiu But, Jun Wang, Wai-Yan Ha, Forrest Chung-Fai Yau, Paul Pui-Hay But & Pang-Chui Shaw

Chapter 9 Authentication of Medicinal Materials by Multiplex Polymerase Chain Reaction 219
Zheng-Fei Lu

Part IV DNA Sequencing-based Techniques for Molecular Authentication 267

Chapter 10 Identification of Medicinal Materials Using Forensically Informative Nucleotide Sequencing 269
Ming Li

Chapter 11 DNA Barcoding as a Standard Molecular Authentication Technique 305
Hui Yao, Jian-Ping Han, Xiaohui Pang, Lin-Chun Shi, Li Xiang, Xi-Wen Li, Chao Xiong, Jing-Yuan Song & Shi-Lin Chen

Chapter 12 Authentication of Medicinal Products by Adaptor Ligation-Mediated Polymerase Chain Reaction and Metabarcoding 333
Yat-Tung Lo, Mavis Hong-Yu Yik & Xiao Lin

Chapter 13 Super-Barcoding of Medicinal Materials Based on Complete Plastid Genomes and Nuclear Ribosomal DNA 363
Hyun-Seung Park, Padmanaban Mohanan & Tae-Jin Yang

Part V Advanced Applications and Outlook of Molecular Authentication Techniques 391

Chapter 14 Rapid Detection of CITES-Listed Shark Species Using Loop-Mediated Isothermal Amplification 393
Grace Wing-Chiu But, Hoi-Yan Wu, Kwang-Tsao Shao & Pang-Chui Shaw

Chapter 15 Rapid Identification of Medicinal Materials by Lateral Flow Dipstick Diagnosis 437
Grace Wing-Chiu But, Ka-Lok Wong & Pang-Chui Shaw

Chapter 16 Barcoding High-Resolutions Melting Analysis 457
Suchada Sukrong, Kannika Thongkhao, Chayapol Tungphatthong & Thatree Phadungcharoen

Chapter 17 Setting Up a DNA Laboratory for Molecular Authentication 483
Ka-Lok Wong & Wai-Yan Ha

Chapter 18 Concluding Remarks 501

Index 509

Preface

For centuries, Chinese medicinal materials have been used for therapeutic purposes to cure and prevent diseases. In recent years, scientific research has confirmed the pharmacological efficacies of many of these materials. The trade of medicinal materials and derived dietary supplements brings great revenue. However, the confusion and adulteration due to the lack of proper quality control deters their wider application. Both in the marketplace and in literature, it is not uncommon to find that a given material is assigned with different names and that different materials may share a same common name. The challenge of correct identification is compounded by substitutions and unscrupulous adulterations, in some instances leading to poisoning.

To establish a healthy system for the application of traditional Chinese medicine, it is essential to properly authenticate raw materials and finished products. To this end, many countries have begun implementing standards for quality assurance of Chinese medicinal materials, particularly for those that are expensive and imported. With the advancement of DNA technology, molecular approach has become an important tool to complement organoleptic, morphological, anatomical and chemical techniques for the authentication and quality assurance of Chinese medicinal materials. As compared to these phenotypic markers, molecular markers are more consistent and are definitive of a specific taxon. The wide array of sequences and patterns in the genomic, chloroplast and mitochondrial DNA offers numerous physical markers for characterising a species.

In 2002, we published 'Authentication of Chinese Medicinal Materials by DNA Technology', which is the first international reference in this field. After 20 years, this new edition updates the various useful techniques and describes the new techniques developed for molecular authentication. The procedures of each DNA technique are provided in detail for 'step-by-step' experiments. We hope that this book will stimulate wider application of molecular techniques in the authentication of medicinal materials and facilitate the advancement of this promising field.

This book is divided into five parts with 18 chapters. Part I (Chapter 1) reviews the status of the authentication of Chinese medicinal materials and introduces a wide range of the DNA techniques. Part II (Chapters 2 to 4) lists the experimental procedures, equipment and reagents for DNA extraction (Chapter 2), general molecular procedures (Chapter 3) and common bioinformatics tools (Chapter 4). For some procedures, precautions to be taken are also noted. Part III (Chapters 5 to 9) describes the DNA fingerprinting-based techniques that apply polymerase chain reaction (PCR) at various levels of relaxed stringency to reveal the differences in genomes. These techniques, including Random Amplified Polymorphic DNA (RAPD; Chapter 5), Amplified Fragment Length Polymorphism (AFLP; Chapter 6) and PCR-Restriction Fragment Length Polymorphism (PCR-RFLP; Chapter 7), do not require any prior knowledge of the DNA sequence of an organism. The fingerprint pattern isolated from RAPD can further be used to generate DNA sequences for Sequence Characterised Amplification Region (SCAR; Chapter 8). Multiplex PCR (Chapter 9) utilises multiple sets of primers to generate a series of amplicons in one reaction system, allowing cost-effective authentication in terms of time and labour. Part IV (Chapters 10 to 13) describes the use of DNA sequencing-based techniques such as Forensically

Informative Nucleotide Sequencing (FINS; Chapter 10) and popular DNA barcoding (Chapter 11) for effective authentication. With the development of high-throughput sequencing, application on metabarcoding (Chapter 12) and super-barcoding (Chapter 13) are also discussed. Part V (Chapters 14 to 18) shows the recent advancement in molecular authentication, such as isothermal amplification (Chapter 14) and lateral flow dipstick diagnosis (Chapter 15), which may be developed into on-site detection tools, and Barcoding High-Resolution Melting (Barcoding HRM; Chapter 16), which allows differentiation between closely related substitutes. Guidelines for setting up a good DNA laboratory to avoid possible contamination (Chapter 17) and concluding remarks on the outlook of molecular authentication (Chapter 18) are also given in this final part.

We would like to thank all the contributors for providing their first-hand experience in molecular authentication. We are also grateful to Ms. Sook-Cheng Lim of World Scientific Publishing Pte Ltd. for co-ordinating the project. Last but not least, we thank the Li Dak Sum Yip Yio Chin R&D Centre for Chinese Medicine, The Chinese University of Hong Kong, for providing financial support for the publication of this book.

Pang-Chui Shaw
Hui Cao
Yat-Tung Lo

Contributing Authors

But, Paul Pui-Hay	School of Life Sciences, The Chinese University of Hong Kong, Hong Kong, China
But, Grace Wing-Chiu	School of Life Sciences, The Chinese University of Hong Kong, Hong Kong, China
Cao, Hui	College of Pharmacy, Jinan University, Guangzhou, Guangdong, China
Chen, Shi-Lin	Institute of Chinese Materia Medica, China Academy of Chinese Medical Sciences, Beijing, China
Cheng, Kur-Ta	Faculty of Medicine, Taipei Medical University, Taipei, Taiwan
Ha, Wai-Yan	Government Chinese Medicines Testing Institute, Chinese Medicine Regulatory Office, Department of Health, The Government of the Hong Kong Special Administrative Region of the People's Republic of China
Han, Jian-Ping	Engineering Research Centre of Chinese Medicine Resource, Ministry of Education, Institute of Medicinal Plant Development, Chinese

	Academy of Medical Sciences and Peking Union Medical College, Beijing, China
Komatsu, Katsuko	Institute of Natural Medicine, Toyama University, Toyama, Japan
Li, Ming	Institute of Chinese Medicine & Office of University General Education, The Chinese University of Hong Kong, Hong Kong, China
Li, Ping	School of Traditional Chinese Pharmacy, The China Pharmaceutical University, Nanjing, Jiangsu, China
Li, Xi-Wen	Institute of Chinese Materia Medica, China Academy of Chinese Medical Sciences, Beijing, China
Lin, Xiao	Centre for Soybean Research of the State Key Laboratory of Agrobiotechnology, The Chinese University of Hong Kong, Hong Kong, China
Lo, Yat-Tung	Institute of Chinese Medicine, The Chinese University of Hong Kong, Hong Kong, China
Lu, Zheng-Fei	Herbalife International of America, Inc., Los Angeles, United States of America
Mohanan, Padmanaban	Department of Agriculture, Forestry and Bioresources, Research Institute of Agriculture and Life

Sciences, and Plant Genomics and Breeding Institute, College of Agriculture and Life Sciences, Seoul National University, Seoul, Republic of Korea

Ngan, Fai-Ngor	Institute of Chinese Medicine, The Chinese University of Hong Kong, Hong Kong, China
Pang, Xiaohui	Engineering Research Center of Chinese Medicine Resource, Ministry of Education, Institute of Medicinal Plant Development, Chinese Academy of Medical Sciences and Peking Union Medical College, Beijing, China
Park, Hyun-Seung	Department of Integrative Biological Sciences and Industry, Sejong University, Seoul, Republic of Korea
Phadungcharoen, Thatree	Center of Excellence in DNA Barcoding of Thai Medicinal Plants, Department of Pharmacognosy and Pharmaceutical Botany, Faculty of Pharmaceutical Sciences, Chulalongkorn University, Bangkok, Thailand
Shao, Kwang-Tsao	Systematics and Biodiversity Information Division, Biodiversity Research Centre, Academia Sinica, Taipei, Taiwan

Shaw, Pang-Chui	Li Dak Sum Yip Yio Chin R&D Centre for Chinese Medicine, School of Life Sciences, State Key Laboratory of Research on Bioactivities and Clinical Applications of Medicinal Plants and Institute of Chinese Medicine, The Chinese University of Hong Kong, Hong Kong, China
Shi, Lin-Chun	Engineering Research Centre of Chinese Medicine Resource, Ministry of Education, Institute of Medicinal Plant Development, Chinese Academy of Medical Sciences and Peking Union Medical College, Beijing, China
Song, Jing-Yuan	Key Lab of Chinese Medicine Resources Conservation, State Administration of Traditional Chinese Medicine of the People's Republic of China, Institute of Medicinal Plant Development, Chinese Academy of Medical Sciences and Peking Union Medical College, Beijing, China
Sukrong, Suchada	Center of Excellence in DNA Barcoding of Thai Medicinal Plants, Department of Pharmacognosy and Pharmaceutical Botany, Faculty of Pharmaceutical Sciences, Chulalongkorn University, Bangkok, Thailand

Thongkhao, Kannika	Center of Excellence in DNA Barcoding of Thai Medicinal Plants, Department of Pharmacognosy and Pharmaceutical Botany, Faculty of Pharmaceutical Sciences, Chulalongkorn University, Bangkok, Thailand
Tungphatthong, Chayapol	Center of Excellence in DNA Barcoding of Thai Medicinal Plants, Department of Pharmacognosy and Pharmaceutical Botany, Faculty of Pharmaceutical Sciences, Chulalongkorn University, Bangkok, Thailand
Xiang, Li	Institute of Chinese Materia Medica, China Academy of Chinese Medical Sciences, Beijing, China
Xiong, Chao	Institute of Chinese Materia Medica, China Academy of Chinese Medical Sciences, Beijing, China
Wang, Jun	School of Life Sciences, The Chinese University of Hong Kong, Hong Kong, China
Wong, Ka-Lok	Government Chinese Medicines Testing Institute, Chinese Medicine Regulatory Office, Department of Health, The Government of the Hong Kong Special Administrative Region of the People's Republic of China

Wu, Hoi-Yan	Li Dak Sum Yip Yio Chin R&D Centre for Chinese Medicine, The Chinese University of Hong Kong, Hong Kong, China
Yang, Tae-Jin	Department of Agriculture, Forestry and Bioresources, Research Institute of Agriculture and Life Sciences, and Plant Genomics and Breeding Institute, College of Agriculture and Life Sciences, Seoul National University, Seoul, Republic of Korea
Yao, Hui	Engineering Research Centre of Chinese Medicine Resource, Ministry of Education, Institute of Medicinal Plant Development, Chinese Academy of Medical Sciences and Peking Union Medical College, Beijing, China
Yau, Forrest Chung-Fai	Institute of Chinese Medicine, The Chinese University of Hong Kong, Hong Kong, China
Yik, Mavis Hong-Yu	Li Dak Sum Yip Yio Chin R&D Centre for Chinese Medicine, The Chinese University of Hong Kong, Hong Kong, China
Zhang, Ying	College of Pharmacy, Jinan University, Guangzhou, Guangdong, China

Part I
Introduction

Chapter 1

General Introduction

1.1 Introduction

According to the statistical studies from World Health Organization, more than 80% of the world population use traditional medicine for treating diseases (World Health Organization, 2019). The use of traditional Chinese medicine (TCM) for therapeutic purpose has been practised for centuries in China and Asia. Recently, various forms of medicinal products such as capsules, granules and pills are available for easy medicine consumption to meet the contemporary trend of 'back to nature'. More than 2,700 types of medicinal materials, such as extracts and processed medicinal products of Chinese medicinal materials, are listed in the 2020 edition of the *Chinese Pharmacopoeia*. With the use of traditional medicine for healthcare or therapeutic purpose in the world population and the emergence of various dietary supplements made from natural products, the trade of medicinal materials brings great revenue. For instance, 57% of complementary medicine was spent on natural products in the United Kingdom with a sale of around GBP 115 million (Barnes, 2003). In Germany, 33% of its people frequently use natural products for treating inflammatory bowel disease (Joos *et al.*, 2006). In Australia, 26% of the population use natural products with a AUD 2.3 billion expenditure (MacLennan, Wilson &

Taylor, 2002). In Hong Kong, import and export trade of Chinese medicinal materials bring HKD 2.35 billion and HKD 0.95 billion in year 2011, respectively (Cheung, Buckley & Watanabe, 2017).

Substitutes and adulterants of medicinal materials are often introduced intentionally or accidentally. Owing to the geographical difference in China with distinct climates, the species of medicinal materials used among various provinces are diverse. Synonyms (different species sharing the same nomenclature) and homonyms (same species with different nomenclatures) of medicinal materials and their adulterants are frequently found. In addition, the morphological characteristics and tissue histology are highly similar for closely related species, especially when the medicinal materials are in the form of prepared slices, granules and other forms of processed products, which lead to difficulties in differentiation. Some dishonest merchants may substitute the original product with cheaper versions in order to reduce the production costs. The problem of adulteration is not only wasting the customer's money, but also seriously interfering with the therapeutic effects, even leading to life-threatening toxicity (Ma, Zhu, Li, Dong & Tsim, 2001), cancer (Efferth, 2005) or even death (Yip, Chau, Mak & Kwan, 2007). In order to ensure that genuine medicinal materials are used, various authentication techniques have been established and recorded as statutory guidelines by regulatory agencies.

1.2 Existing Tools in the Authentication of Medicinal Materials

Traditional means for authentication mainly depend on morphological and histological characteristics. Morphological identification includes the inspection of organoleptic markers such as shape, colour, texture and odour of the medicinal materials. This method is simple and direct, but its accuracy heavily depends on the examiner's experience and judgement. It is also difficult to identify processed medicinal materials when they are in powdered form or in shredded pieces. With the advancement of analytical technologies, chromatographic, biochemical and molecular approaches have been applied for authentication work and facilitating the standardisation, modernisation and internationalisation of manufacturing industry. A general comparison of different authentication methods is shown in Table 1.1.

Table 1.1 Comparison of Technical Skill Level, Cost Required and Differentiation Power for Major Authentication Methods

Authentication method	Technical skill	Cost required	Differentiation power
1. Organoleptic inspection	++++	+	++
2. Microscopic analysis	++++	+	++
3. Thin-layer chromatography (TLC)	++	++	+++
4. High-performance liquid chromatography (HPLC)/gas chromatography (GC)/mass spectrometry (MS)	+++++	+++++	++++
5. Allozymes, isozymes	+++	+++	+++
6. Antibodies	++	+++++	++++
7. DNA fingerprinting	+++	+++	++++
8. DNA sequencing	+++	+++	+++++

'+++++' indicates the highest degree, '+' indicates the least degree.

1.2.1 Organoleptic and Histological Analysis

Morphological and organoleptic identification by assessing the physical shape, size, colour, odour and texture of medicinal materials have been practised over a long history. The characteristics of a sample is compared with voucher specimens and literatures such as Compendium of Materia Medica (In Chinese: Bencao Gangmu) (Zhang, Shaw, Sze, Wang & Tong, 2007; Zhao *et al.*, 2006; Zhao, Xiao, Xiao & Yuen, 2007). This approach is simple, convenient and non-destructive, yet the accuracy heavily depends on the examiner's experience and judgement (Plutowska & Wardencki, 2007; Xiong *et al.*, 2014; Zou *et al.*, 2015).

Microscopic examination is frequently used to reveal the characteristic cell components or tissues. However, related species may have similar microscopic characteristics. Other factors including geographical environment, growth period and the storage condition may affect the fine structure of the material. Moreover, highly processed material may cause severe damage of the macroscopic and microscopic features.

1.2.2 Chemical Analysis

Chemical constituents such as active ingredients and characteristic compounds may be used as markers for authentication. Thin-layer chromatography (TLC) and high-performance liquid chromatography (HPLC) are the two golden tools in the authentication of medicinal materials. Recent advancements of analytical technologies such as high-performance thin-layer chromatography (HPTLC), capillary electrophoresis (CE), ultra-high-pressure liquid chromatography (UHPLC) and multidimensional chromatography bring increased accuracy and precision. Increased sensitivity can be achieved by coupling chromatography with mass spectrometry (MS) for detection. For example, in the HPTLC and HPLC analysis of the *Panax* species, several ginsenosides have been used as markers. Rf is the ginsenoside uniquely present in *Panax ginseng* but not *P. quinquefolius* nor *P. notoginseng* (Li *et al.*, 2000). Ginsenoside Rb2 is detected in abundance in

P. ginseng, but in trace amount in the other two ginsengs (Wan, Li, Chen & Wang, 2007). Notoginsenoside R1 is the characteristic marker compound in *P. notoginseng*. Pseudoginsenoside F11 is a marker compound in *P. quinquefolius* (Chan *et al.*, 2000). Increased sensitivity and resolution have been achieved by HPLC-MS (Li, Luo, Liang, Hu & Wang, 2010) and HPLC-evaporative light scattering detection (ELSD) (Li & Fitzloff, 2002) to separate F11 from Rf, which have similar retention times under most HPLC conditions (Chan *et al.*, 2000). A UHPLC/Q-TOF-MS was developed for 2-minute analyses of Rf and F11 in Asian ginseng adulterated with American ginseng (Li *et al.*, 2010). Other spectrometric methods such as two-dimensional (2D) correlation Fourier transform infrared (FTIR) spectroscopy (Lu *et al.*, 2008) and 2D nuclear magnetic resonance (NMR) spectroscopy (Yang *et al.*, 2006) have been reported for effective differentiation.

On the contrary, there are limitations in chemical analysis. Contents of the chemical components may be affected by physiological conditions, harvesting period and storage conditions. Moreover, it is difficult to distinguish between closely related species, as many contain similar chemicals. In addition, instruments such as HPLC, CE, MS and NMR are expensive and need well-trained personnel to operate. They may not be affordable in many analytical laboratories.

1.2.3 Biochemical Analysis

Since the 1960's, biochemical markers such as allozymes (different allelic form of enzymes encoded by a single locus gene) and isozymes (enzymes encoded by alleles at more than one locus) have been used for characterising and identifying genotypes and varieties of crop plants and animals, studying population genetics, examining geographical patterns of variation and linkage mapping. They are also used to identify medicinal materials as well. For example, isoelectric focusing in thin-layer polyacrylamide slab gels showed eight enzyme systems, i.e., glucose-6-phosphate isomerase (*GPI*, E.C.5.3.1.9), phosphoglucomutase (*PGM*, E.C.2.7.5.1), malate dehydrogenase (*MDH*, E.C. 1.1.1.37), esterase (*EST*, E.C.3.1.1.7), diaphorase (*DIA*, E.C.1.6.2.2), α-amylase (α-*AMY*, E.C.3.2.1.1), phosphogluconate dehydrogenase (*PGD*, E.C. 1.1.1.44) and acid phosphatase (*ACP*, E.C.3.1.3.2), with good resolution and differentiation power for analysing genetic diversity and population structure in both intraspecific and interspecific levels between three medicinal *Epimedium* species distributed in 11 natural populations in the western Hubei Province in China (Xu, Li, Wang & Huang, 2007).

There are limitations in isozyme polymorphism. It is of no surprise that some species, even with apparent differences in morphological traits and genetic features, are monomorphic for most isozymes (Sunnucks, 2000). A further limitation is that the level of isozymes is affected by the temporal and spatial regulation of gene expression and by environmental factors. It is evident in the *Ganoderma* species that the isozyme profile is variable, depending upon the stage of plant development (Kumar, Sharma, Kumar & Ramchiary, 2015). Moreover, protein is prone to degradation after harvesting and prolonged storage; thus, good preservation is required before the analysis.

Immunological analysis using antibodies is a very powerful and highly reproducible authentication tool. It can distinguish isozymes as well as other proteins. A single difference in amino acid sequences may change the epitope of the protein, which is recognised by a specific antibody. Accordingly, antibodies can differentiate polymorphic proteins and species-specific proteins from different organisms. For instance, monoclonal antibodies have been prepared against ginsenoside Rf (Nah *et al*., 2000), Rb1 (Zhao, Hou, Qian, Xu & Sun, 2007), Rh1 and Rg2 (Qu *et al*., 2015), Rg1 (Fukuda, Tanaka & Shoyama, 2000), Rg3 (Joo, Ha, Shin, Son & Kim, 2009) and Gintonin (Lee *et al*., 2015). The monoclonal antibodies raised were then used for enzyme-linked immunosorbent assay (ELISA) or enzyme immunoassay (EIA) for quantification of various ginseng preparations, including crude ginseng fractions, commercial ginseng products and body fluids. Although antibodies may also be developed into a diagnostic kit for rapid testing, tremendous effort is required for screening a suitable antigen and for generating the antibody.

1.3 Molecular Marker Technologies

DNA carries all the genetic instructions for the development, functioning, growth and reproduction of an organism. It has been used in various applications such as forensic science (Alonso *et al*., 2006; Melton & Holland, 2007), archaeology (Vural & Tirpan, 2010), paleogenomics (Burger, Hummel & Herrmann, 2000) and food quality control (Bottero & Dalmasso, 2011; Mafra, Ferreira & Oliveira, 2008; Rodriguez-Ramirez, Gonzalez-Cordova & Vallejo-Cordoba, 2011). Since the early 1990's, with the advance of molecular cloning, polymerase chain reaction (PCR) and DNA sequencing technologies, our team has introduced molecular techniques to identify plant and animal medicinal materials. From the 2010 edition of the Chinese Pharmacopeia, molecular authentication has been officially adopted and used to authenticate Agkistrodon, Bungarus Parvus, Dendrobii Caulis, Fritillariae Cirrhosae Bulbus and Zaocys. Molecular techniques have also been included in the British Pharmacopoeia (British Pharmacopoeia Commission, 2018) and is planned to be included in the US Pharmacopoeia for the identification of medicinal materials. We anticipate that more molecular authentication protocols will be published in more pharmacopoeias.

DNA-based marker is based on a genotype that is less affected by age, physiological condition of samples and environmental factors. They are not tissue-specific and can be detected at any phase of organism development. Only a trace amount of a sample is enough for analysis and the physical form of the sample does not restrict the detection. These features are particularly suitable for the authentication of medicinal materials that are expensive or in limited supply. The power of discrimination, accuracy and repeatability of DNA-based markers is so high that adulterants, substitutes, closely related varieties and species from different geographic cultivars may be differentiated (Li, Jiang, But, Shaw & Yuan, 2019; Zhang *et al.*, 2007). The technical skills required for some molecular techniques are comparatively simple, and the setup cost for equipment such as a PCR thermocycler and electrophoretic apparatus are now more affordable, thus lowering the operation costs for the laboratory. In addition, by studying the phylogenetic relationships between species, it may also facilitate the discovery of related chemicals in substitutes, which may lead to the reduced use of endangered species (Luo *et al.*, 2013).

A diverse array of DNA-based marker technologies has been established to explore various DNA polymorphism. They can be classified into three broad types: hybridization-based, PCR-based and DNA sequencing-based. A general comparison of the commonly available molecular markers for the authentication of medicinal materials is presented in Table 1.2. In the following, we provide a general account of representative molecular marker

Table 1.2 Commonly Available Molecular Authentication Markers for Medicinal Materials

Molecular marker	Principle in brief	Abundance of marker	Genomic DNA required	Primers/ probes	Reproducibility	Cost	References
Randomly amplified polymorphic DNA (RAPD)	A single primer of arbitrary selected nucleotide sequence is used to amplify the template DNA at various specific sites and generate species-specific DNA fingerprints	Very high	<50 ng	Random	Low	Low	(Chatti *et al.*, 2010; Li & Ding, 2010; Lim, Mudge & Weston, 2007)
Inter-simple sequence repeat (ISSR)	Short tandem repetitive DNA sequences are PCR amplified and the polymorphism in the length and number of repeats are detected	Medium	<50 ng	Specific to repeats	Medium	Medium	(Hu *et al.*, 2007; Kojoma, Iida, Makino, Sekita & Satake, 2002; Shi, Wang, Wang, Tu & Li, 2009; Song, Li, Wang & Wang, 2010)

(Continued)

Table 1.2 (*Continued*)

Molecular marker	Principle in brief	Abundance of marker	Genomic DNA required	Primers/ probes	Reproducibility	Cost	References
Sequence characterised amplified region (SCAR)	Species-specific diagnostic primers are used to amplify the genomic DNA under stringent condition for species differentiation	High	<50 ng	Specific	Very high	Medium	(Dnyaneshwar, Preeti, Kalpana & Bhushan, 2006; M. Y. Lee *et al.*, 2006; Sze *et al.*, 2008; Wang, Ha, Ngan, But & Shaw, 2001; Yau, Wong, Wang, But & Shaw, 2002)
Amplified fragment length polymorphism (AFLP)	The genomic DNA is first digested by restriction enzymes, followed by ligation with synthetic adaptors and PCR amplification. The amplified fragments are then separated on a highly resolving sequencing gel to generate fingerprints	Very high	200–300 ng	Specific to adaptor sequence	High	High	(Datwyler & Weiblen, 2006; Ha, Shaw, Liu, Yau & Wang, 2002; Passinho-Soares, Felix, Kaplan, Margis-Pinheiro & Margis, 2006)

Restriction fragment length polymorphism (RFLP)/ PCR-RFLP	The genomic DNA is cleaved with restriction enzymes, followed by gel electrophoresis and blotting procedures. DNA fragments may be directly visualised or detected by labelled probes. When combined with PCR, PCR-RFLP allows analysis of genomic DNA in minute amount	High	2,000–5,000 ng (RFLP) <50 ng (PCR-RFLP)	Specific	High	High	(Gong, Fu, Luo & Qiu, 2006; J. H. Lee, Lee, Sung, Bang & Moon, 2009; Li *et al.*, 2007)
DNA barcoding	DNA barcoding region is obtained by PCR and sequenced. The obtained DNA sequences are then aligned and compared with a DNA barcode database to find out the best matched species	High	<50 ng	Specific	Very high	Medium	(de Vere, Rich, Trinder & Long, 2015; Kress & Erickson, 2012; Li, Cao, But & Shaw, 2011; Li *et al.*, 2012; Wong, But & Shaw, 2013; J. Xu, 2016)

techniques, which will be further elaborated in Parts III and IV of this book.

1.3.1 Hybridisation-based Markers

Hybridisation-based marker technologies use complementary DNA (cDNA), cloned DNA elements or synthetic oligonucleotides as probes, which are labelled with radioisotopes or conjugated enzymes that catalyse a coloured reaction, to hybridise target DNA. Restriction fragment length polymorphism (RFLP) is the representative technique and is the most widely applied in genome mapping, marker-aided breeding, systematics and evolution studies. In RFLP, the template DNA is first cleaved with restriction enzymes. Because of restriction length polymorphism, the number and size of resultant DNA fragments produced by restriction enzymes are different between genuine and its adulterant. The restriction enzyme-digested DNA from the examined subject is then separated by electrophoresis, transferred to a solid support matrix for fixation and hybridised with a labelled probe for species identification. The polymorphism occurs because mutations remove a restriction site or create a new restriction site. These alterations are then detected by using a hybridisation probe, which is a repetitive DNA sequence with lower C_0t value. As a result, a specific labelled DNA fingerprint is displayed (Figure 1.1). In RFLP, the choice of the DNA probe/restriction enzyme is crucial for data analysis.

Because of restriction length polymorphism, the number and size of resultant DNA fragments produced by restriction enzymes are different between genuine and its adulterant. After electrophoresis, the products are transferred to a solid matrix and hybridised with a labelled probe for species identification.

DNA probes for detecting repeated DNA sequences can be divided into two types: (1) tandem repeats, which are present as

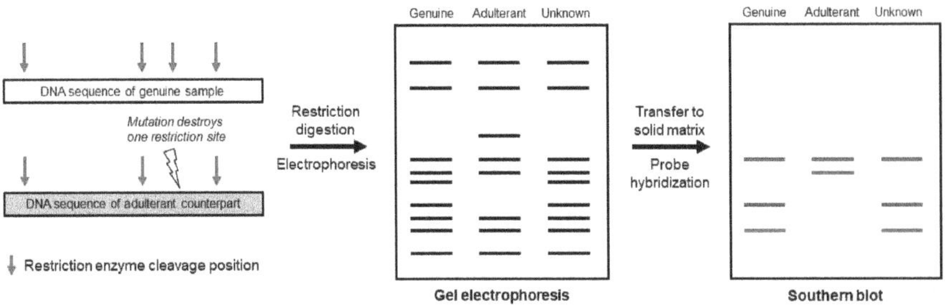

Fig. 1.1 Schematic diagram of restriction fragment length polymorphism (RFLP).

clusters in chromosomes and (2) dispersed repeats, which are distributed over all the chromosomes. Shorter repeating sequences, which are generally <6 bp in length and are repeated from a few to many thousands of times, are designated as 'microsatellites' or simple sequence repeat (SSR). The regions flanking the microsatellite loci can be amplified by PCR, thus providing co-dominant sequence-tagged sites (STS) or a repetitive sequence to act as a probe to generate DNA fingerprints such as in the differentiation of *P. ginseng* and *P. quinquefolius* (Ho & Leung, 2002). The abundance and ubiquitous distribution of microsatellites make them valuable in linkage mapping, identification of quantitative traits loci and forensic cases. Additionally, primers developed in one species can be used in related taxa. However, RFLP is not commonly used for the authentication of medicinal products with extensive processing and storage, since a large amount of intact DNA is a prerequisite for generating valid fingerprints.

1.3.2 PCR-based Markers

PCR is an in vitro technique to amplify a defined region of the template DNA enzymatically into millions of copies. The specific multiplication is attributed to the presence of primers, which are single-stranded polynucleotides that recognise and bind to the complementary DNA sequence on the template DNA. The amplification process starts with denaturation of the double-stranded template DNA to single-stranded DNA under high temperature, usually between 90°C and 95°C, followed by the specific annealing of the primers to allow complementary binding of primers to the single-stranded template DNA at a lower temperature. The annealed primers are then extended according to the template DNA sequence by a thermostable DNA polymerase. Repeating the denaturation-annealing-extension cycle leads to an exponential accumulation of the DNA fragment of the defined sequence (Figure 1.2). The amplified products are then fractionated on agarose, polyacrylamide or other gel matrix and visualised by ethidium bromide (EtBr) or fluorescence dyes (e.g., SYBR Safe), autoradiography (using an isotope-labelled primer) or fluorescence (using a fluorescence-labelled primer). The distance of the amplified region is usually from 100 bp to a few kilobases (kb), although 'long distance PCR' allows amplification of 30 kb or beyond (Jia, Guo, Zhao & Wang, 2014). PCR amplification of most of the region of a DNA sample is possible, providing their flanking sequences

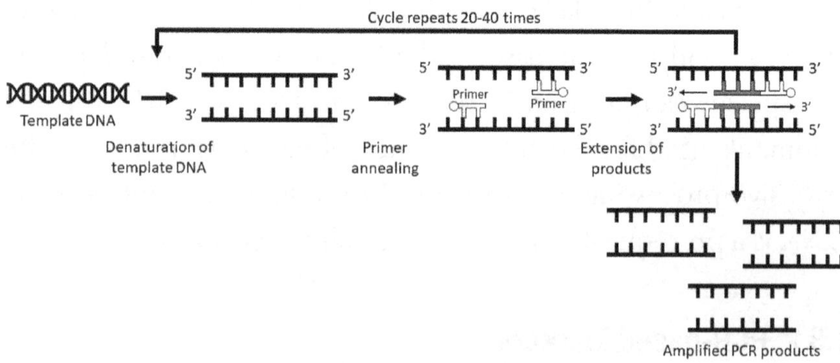

Fig. 1.2 Schematic diagram of polymerase chain reaction (PCR). The double-stranded DNA is separated during the denaturation step; specific primers are bound to single-stranded DNA template during the annealing step; and flanked regions are then amplified by DNA polymerase during the extension step. The cycles are repeated 20–40 times to produce millions of DNA copies for downstream analysis.

are known, as these are needed for designing primers. Owing to the sensitivity and ability to amplify DNA from a small amount of material, a variety of PCR-derived methods such as RAPD, ISSR, SCAR, AFLP and PCR-RFLP have been established, which will be further discussed in Chapters 5–8, and used for the authentication of various medicinal materials.

1.3.3 DNA Sequencing-Based Markers

DNA sequencing is the most definitive means for identifying medicinal material, as maximum genetic information can be obtained from an amplified DNA fragment. Genetic variations such as transversion, transition, insertion, deletion or single nucleotide polymorphism (SNP) between species can be assessed directly. In general, sequence homology within the same species is high, whereas it is low between different species or families; their relationship can thus be estimated by constructing the phylogenetic tree. A representative example of DNA sequencing is DNA barcoding that uses a recognised, standard and short DNA region for accurate and quick authentication. Proposed by Paul Hebert and colleagues in 2003 (Hebert, Cywinska, Ball & deWaard, 2003), DNA barcoding gains wide interest and acts as routine practice for species identification nowadays (de Vere, Rich, Trinder & Long, 2015; Marshall, 2005; Miller, 2007; Schindel & Miller, 2005; Xu, 2016). DNA sequence data obtained are usually deposited in a DNA database, which is publicly available for searching and comparison using bioinformatics tools. A general workflow for identifying unknown samples using DNA sequencing is illustrated in Figure 1.3.

Chapters 10 and 11 in this book are devoted to the use of DNA sequencing and DNA barcoding as a means for authenticating medicinal materials. Currently, a laboratory can easily

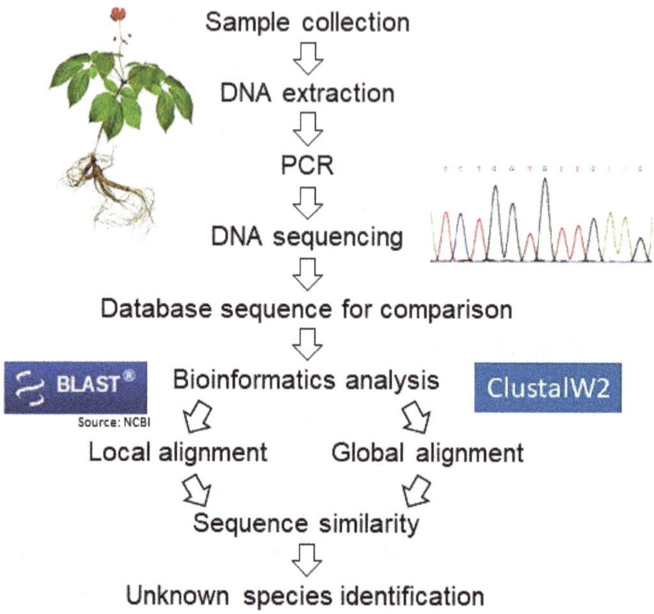

Fig. 1.3 General workflow and steps involved for identifying unknown samples using DNA sequencing.

generate many thousands of base pairs of DNA sequences within a day using an automatic DNA sequencing machine. Coupled with the decline in prices of consumables and equipment, DNA sequencing has become a common means for the authentication of medicinal materials.

1.3.4 Emerging DNA Techniques

Conventional DNA sequencing (i.e., Sanger sequencing) is not applicable to DNA from a mixed product because of overlapping sequencing chromatograms. Next-generation sequencing (NGS) techniques give massive parallelisation of sequencing reactions to generate multiple reads with various read lengths, thus different components in medicinal products can be identified. NGS also facilitates the determination of contaminants, which is essential for the quality control regulation in a Good Manufacturing Practice

(GMP) factory. In NGS analysis workflow, the constructed library is first sequenced to obtain a pool of genomic data, followed by bioinformatics analysis and comparison, with reference to the DNA database. Currently, second-generation sequencing such as Illumina Sequencing and Ion Torrent Sequencing, and third-generation sequencing such as PacBio Sequencing and Nanopore Sequencing are representative NGS platforms. Chapters 12 and 13 provide case studies on using DNA metabarcoding for authentication and quality control of medicinal products, and discuss the key technological challenges with future directions.

1.4 Conclusion

Molecular technology provides an independent approach for the authentication of medicinal materials. Various applications such as quality control of the medicinal materials, detection of transgene, discovery of substitutes and adulterants, and protection of endangered species have been known. With the increase in global trading of medicinal materials and dietary supplements, accurate and speedy authentication is essential for correct labelling to ensure food safety. Molecular authentication has become a standard tool.

References

Alonso, A., Albarran, C., Martin, P., Garcia, P., Capilla, J., Garcia, O., de la Rua, C., Izaguirre, N., Pereira, F., Pereira, L., Amorim, A., & Sancho, M. (2006). Usefulness of microchip electrophoresis for the analysis of mitochondrial DNA in forensic and ancient DNA studies. *Electrophoresis, 27*(24), 5101–5109. doi:10.1002/elps.200600331

Barnes, J. (2003). Quality, efficacy and safety of complementary medicines: Fashions, facts and the future. Part I. Regulation and quality. *Br J Clin Pharmacol, 55*(3), 226–233. doi:10.1046/j.1365-2125.2003.01810.x

Bottero, M. T., & Dalmasso, A. (2011). Animal species identification in food products: Evolution of biomolecular methods. *Vet J, 190*(1), 34–38. doi:10.1016/j.tvjl.2010.09.024

British Pharmacopoeia Commission. (2018). DNA barcoding as a tool for botanical identification of herbal drugs. In *British Pharmacopoeia Supplementary Chapter SC VII D*. London, UK: TSO.

Burger, J., Hummel, S., & Herrmann, B. (2000). Palaeogenetics and cultural heritage. Species determination and STR-genotyping from ancient DNA in art and artefacts. *Thermochim Acta, 365*(1), 141–146. doi:10.1016/S0040-6031(00)00621-3

Chan, T. W., But, P. P., Cheng, S. W., Kwok, I. M., Lau, F. W., & Xu, H. X. (2000). Differentiation and authentication of Panax ginseng, Panax quinquefolius, and ginseng products by using HPLC/MS. *Anal Chem, 72*(6), 1281–1287. doi:10.1021/ac990819z

Chatti, K., Baraket, G., Ben Abdelkrim, A., Saddoud, O., Mars, M., Trifi, M., & Salhi Hannachi, A. (2010). Development of molecular tools for characterization and genetic diversity analysis in Tunisian fig (Ficus carica) cultivars. *Biochem Genet, 48*(9–10), 789–806. doi:10.1007/s10528-010-9360-1

Cheung, K. L. C., Buckley, E. R., & Watanabe, K. (2017). Traditional Chinese medicine market in Hong Kong. *J Complement Med Altern Health, 4*(1), 555630. doi:10.19080/JCMAH.2017.04.555630

Datwyler, S. L., & Weiblen, G. D. (2006). Genetic variation in hemp and marijuana (Cannabis sativa L.) according to amplified fragment length polymorphisms. *J Forensic Sci, 51*(2), 371–375. doi:10.1111/j.1556-4029.2006.00061.x

de Vere, N., Rich, T. C., Trinder, S. A., & Long, C. (2015). DNA barcoding for plants. *Methods Mol Biol, 1245*, 101–118. doi:10.1007/978-1-4939-1966-6_8

Dnyaneshwar, W., Preeti, C., Kalpana, J., & Bhushan, P. (2006). Development and application of RAPD-SCAR marker for identification of Phyllanthus emblica LINN. *Biol Pharm Bull, 29*(11), 2313–2316. doi:10.1248/bpb.29.2313

Efferth, T. (2005). Microarray-based prediction of cytotoxicity of tumor cells to cantharidin. *Oncol Rep, 13*(3), 459–463. Retrieved from https://www.ncbi.nlm.nih.gov/pubmed/15706417

Fukuda, N., Tanaka, H., & Shoyama, Y. (2000). Formation of monoclonal antibody against a major ginseng component, ginsenoside Rg1 and its characterization. Monoclonal antibody for a ginseng saponin. *Cytotechnology, 34*(3), 197–204. doi:10.1023/A:1008162703957

Gong, W., Fu, C. X., Luo, Y. P., & Qiu, Y. X. (2006). Molecular identification of Sinopodophyllum hexandrum and Dysosma species using cpDNA sequences and PCR-RFLP markers. *Planta Med, 72*(7), 650–652. doi:10.1055/s-2006-931535

Ha, W. Y., Shaw, P. C., Liu, J., Yau, F. C., & Wang, J. (2002). Authentication of Panax ginseng and Panax quinquefolius using amplified fragment length polymorphism (AFLP) and directed amplification of minisatellite region DNA (DAMD). *J Agric Food Chem, 50*(7), 1871–1875. doi:10.1021/jf011365l

Hebert, P. D., Cywinska, A., Ball, S. L., & deWaard, J. R. (2003). Biological identifications through DNA barcodes. *Proc Royal Soc B Biol Sci, 270*(1512), 313–321. doi:10.1098/rspb.2002.2218

Ho, I. S., & Leung, F. C. (2002). Isolation and characterization of repetitive DNA sequences from Panax ginseng. *Mol Genet Genom, 266*(6), 951–961. doi:10.1007/s00438-001-0617-6

Hu, Y., Zhang, Q., Xin, H., Qin, L. P., Lu, B. R., Rahman, K., & Zheng, H. (2007). Association between chemical and genetic variation of Vitex rotundifolia populations from different locations in China: Its implication for quality control of medicinal plants. *Biomed Chromatogr, 21*(9), 967–975. doi:10.1002/bmc.841

Jia, H., Guo, Y., Zhao, W., & Wang, K. (2014). Long-range PCR in next-generation sequencing: Comparison of six enzymes and evaluation on the MiSeq sequencer. *Sci Rep, 4*, 5737. doi:10.1038/srep05737

Joo, E. J., Ha, Y. W., Shin, H., Son, S. H., & Kim, Y. S. (2009). Generation and characterization of monoclonal antibody to ginsenoside Rg3. *Biol Pharm Bull, 32*(4), 548–552. doi:10.1248/bpb.32.548

Joos, S., Rosemann, T., Szecsenyi, J., Hahn, E. G., Willich, S. N., & Brinkhaus, B. (2006). Use of complementary and alternative medicine in Germany — a survey of patients with inflammatory bowel disease. *BMC Complement Altern Med, 6*, 19. doi:10.1186/1472-6882-6-19

Kojoma, M., Iida, O., Makino, Y., Sekita, S., & Satake, M. (2002). DNA fingerprinting of Cannabis sativa using inter-simple sequence repeat (ISSR) amplification. *Planta Med, 68*(1), 60–63. doi:10.1055/s-2002-19875

Kress, W. J., & Erickson, D. L. (2012). DNA barcodes: Methods and protocols. *Methods Mol Biol, 858*, 3–8. doi:10.1007/978-1-61779-591-6_1

Kumar, A., Sharma, K. K., Kumar, P., & Ramchiary, N. (2015). Laccase isozymes from Ganoderma lucidum MDU-7: Isolation, characterization, catalytic properties and differential role during oxidative stress. *J Mol Catal B Enzym, 113*, 68–75. doi:10.1016/j.molcatb.2015.01.010

Lee, B. H., Choi, S. H., Kim, H. J., Jung, S. W., Kim, H., Shin, H. C., Lee, J-H., Hwang, S. H., Kim, H. C., & Nah, S. Y. (2015). Preparation of a monoclonal antibody against gintonin and its use in an enzyme immunoassay. *Biol Pharm Bull, 38*(10), 1631–1637. doi:10.1248/bpb.b15-00171

Lee, J. H., Lee, J. W., Sung, J. S., Bang, K. H., & Moon, S. G. (2009). Molecular authentication of 21 Korean artemisia species (Compositae) by polymerase chain reaction-restriction fragment length polymorphism based on trnL-F region of chloroplast DNA. *Biol Pharm Bull, 32*(11), 1912–1916. doi:10.1248/bpb.32.1912

Lee, M. Y., Doh, E. J., Park, C. H., Kim, Y. H., Kim, E. S., Ko, B. S., & Oh, S. E. (2006). Development of SCAR marker for discrimination of Artemisia princeps and A. argyi from other Artemisia herbs. *Biol Pharm Bull, 29*(4), 629–633. doi:10.1248/bpb.29.629

Li, L., Luo, G. A., Liang, Q. L., Hu, P., & Wang, Y. M. (2010). Rapid qualitative and quantitative analyses of Asian ginseng in adulterated American ginseng preparations by UPLC/Q-TOF-MS. *J Pharm Biomed Anal, 52*(1), 66–72. doi:10.1016/j.jpba.2009.12.017

Li, M., Cao, H., But, P. P. H., & Shaw, P. C. (2011). Identification of herbal medicinal materials using DNA barcodes. *J Syst Evol, 49*(3), 271–283. doi:10.1111/j.1759-6831.2011.00132.x

Li, M., Jiang, C., But, P. H. P., Shaw, P. C., & Yuan, Y. (2019). Molecular identification of traditional medicinal materials. In L. Q. Huang (Ed.), *Molecular Pharmacognosy* (pp. 13–39). Singapore: Springer Singapore.

Li, M., Wong, K. L., Chan, W. H., Li, J. X., But, P. P. H., Cao, H., & Shaw, P. C. (2012). Establishment of DNA barcodes for the identification of the botanical sources of the Chinese 'cooling' beverage. *Food Control, 25*(2), 758–766. doi:10.1016/j.foodcont.2011.12.008

Li, W., & Fitzloff, J. F. (2002). HPLC with evaporative light scattering detection as a tool to distinguish asian ginseng (*Panax ginseng*) and North American ginseng (*Panax quinquefolius*). *J Liq Chromatogr Relat Technol, 25*(1), 17–27. doi:10.1081/JLC-100108536

Li, W., Gu, C., Zhang, H., Awang, D. V., Fitzloff, J. F., Fong, H. H., & van Breemen, R. B. (2000). Use of high-performance liquid chromatography-tandem mass spectrometry to distinguish Panax ginseng C. A. Meyer (Asian ginseng) and Panax quinquefolius L. (North American ginseng). *Anal Chem, 72*(21), 5417–5422. doi:10.1021/ac000650l

Li, X., Ding, X., Chu, B., Ding, G., Gu, S., Qian, L., Wang, Y., & Zhou, Q. (2007). Molecular authentication of Alisma orientale by PCR-RFLP and ARMS. *Planta Med, 73*(1), 67–70. doi:10.1055/s-2006-951746

Li, Y., & Ding, W. L. (2010). Genetic diversity assessment of Trollius accessions in China by RAPD markers. *Biochem Genet, 48*(1–2), 34–43. doi:10.1007/s10528-009-9290-y

Lim, W., Mudge, K. W., & Weston, L. A. (2007). Utilization of RAPD markers to assess genetic diversity of wild populations of North American ginseng (Panax quinquefolium). *Planta Med, 73*(1), 71–76. doi:10.1055/s-2006-951768

Lu, G. H., Zhou, Q., Sun, S. Q., Leung, K. S. Y., Zhang, H., & Zhao, Z. Z. (2008). Differentiation of Asian ginseng, American ginseng and Notoginseng by Fourier transform infrared spectroscopy combined with two-dimensional correlation infrared spectroscopy. *J Mol Struct, 883–884*, 91–98. doi10.1016/j.molstruc.2007.12.008

Luo, J. Y., Yan, D., Song, J. Y., Zhang, D., Xing, X. Y., Han, Y. M., Yang, M. H., Dong, X. P., Peng, C., Chen, S. L., & Xiao, X. H. (2013). A strategy for trade monitoring and substitution of the organs of threatened animals. *Sci Rep, 3*, 3108. doi:10.1038/srep03108

Ma, X. Q., Zhu, D. Y., Li, S. P., Dong, T. T., & Tsim, K. W. (2001). Authentic identification of stigma Croci (stigma of Crocus sativus) from its adulterants by molecular genetic analysis. *Planta Med, 67*(2), 183–186. doi:10.1055/s-2001-11533

MacLennan, A. H., Wilson, D. H., & Taylor, A. W. (2002). The escalating cost and prevalence of alternative medicine. *Prev Med, 35*(2), 166–173. doi:10.1006/pmed.2002.1057

Mafra, I., Ferreira, I. M. P. L. V. O., & Oliveira, M. B. P. P. (2008). Food authentication by PCR-based methods. *Eur Food Res Technol, 227*(3), 649–665. doi:10.1007/s00217-007-0782-x

Marshall, E. (2005). Taxonomy. Will DNA bar codes breathe life into classification? *Science, 307*(5712), 1037. doi:10.1126/science.307.5712.1037

Melton, T., & Holland, C. (2007). Routine forensic use of the mitochondrial 12S ribosomal RNA gene for species identification. *J Forensic Sci, 52*(6), 1305–1307. doi:10.1111/j.1556-4029.2007.00553.x

Miller, S. E. (2007). DNA barcoding and the renaissance of taxonomy. *Proc Nat Acad Sci USA, 104*(12), 4775–4776. doi:10.1073/pnas.0700466104

Nah, J. J., Song, J. Y., Choi, S., Kim, S. C., Rhim, H. W., Oh, T. H., Lee, S. M., & Nah, S. Y. (2000). Preparation of monoclonal antibody against ginsenoside Rf and its enzyme immunoassay. *Biol Pharm Bull, 23*(5), 523–526. doi:10.1248/bpb.23.523

Passinho-Soares, H., Felix, D., Kaplan, M. A., Margis-Pinheiro, M., & Margis, R. (2006). Authentication of medicinal plant botanical identity by amplified fragmented length polymorphism dominant DNA marker: Inferences from the Plectranthus genus. *Planta Med, 72*(10), 929–931. doi:10.1055/s-2006-946673

Plutowska, B., & Wardencki, W. (2007). Aromagrams — Aromatic profiles in the appreciation of food quality. *Food Chem, 101*(2), 845–872. doi:10.1016/j.foodchem.2005.12.028

Qu, H., Wang, Y., Shan, W., Zhang, Y., Feng, H., Sai, J., Wang, Q. G., & Zhao, Y. (2015). Development of ELISA for detection of Rh1 and Rg2 and potential method of immunoaffinity chromatography for separation of epimers. *J Chromatogr B, 985*, 197–205. doi10.1016/j.jchromb.2015.01.037

Rodriguez-Ramirez, R., Gonzalez-Cordova, A. F., & Vallejo-Cordoba, B. (2011). Review: Authentication and traceability of foods from animal origin by polymerase chain reaction-based capillary electrophoresis. *Anal Chim Acta, 685*(2), 120–126. doi:10.1016/j.aca.2010.11.021

Schindel, D. E., & Miller, S. E. (2005). DNA barcoding a useful tool for taxonomists. *Nature, 435*(7038), 17. doi:10.1038/435017b

Shi, H. M., Wang, J., Wang, M. Y., Tu, P. F., & Li, X. B. (2009). Identification of Cistanche species by chemical and inter-simple sequence repeat fingerprinting. *Biol Pharm Bull, 32*(1), 142–146. doi:10.1248/bpb.32.142

Song, Z., Li, X., Wang, H., & Wang, J. (2010). Genetic diversity and population structure of Salvia miltiorrhiza Bge in China revealed by ISSR and SRAP. *Genetica, 138*(2), 241–249. doi:10.1007/s10709-009-9416-5

Sunnucks, P. (2000). Efficient genetic markers for population biology. *Trends Ecol Evol, 15*(5), 199–203. doi:10.1016/S0169-5347(00)01825-5

Sze, S. C., Song, J. X., Wong, R. N., Feng, Y. B., Ng, T. B., Tong, Y., & Zhang, K. Y. (2008). Application of SCAR (sequence characterized amplified region) analysis to authenticate Lycium barbarum (wolfberry) and its adulterants. *Biotechnol Appl Biochem, 51*(Pt 1), 15–21. doi:10.1042/BA20070096

Vural, H. C., & Tirpan, A. A. (2010). Species determination of ancient bone DNA from fossil skeletal remains of Turkey using molecular techniques. *Sci Res Essays, 5*(16), 2250–2256.

Wan, J. B., Li, S. P., Chen, J. M., & Wang, Y. T. (2007). Chemical characteristics of three medicinal plants of the Panax genus determined by HPLC-ELSD. *J Sep Sci, 30*(6), 825–832. doi:10.1002/jssc.200600359

Wang, J., Ha, W. Y., Ngan, F. N., But, P. P., & Shaw, P. C. (2001). Application of sequence characterized amplified region (SCAR) analysis to authenticate Panax species and their adulterants. *Planta Med, 67*(8), 781–783. doi:10.1055/s-2001-18340

Wong, K. L., But, P. P., & Shaw, P. C. (2013). Evaluation of seven DNA barcodes for differentiating closely related medicinal Gentiana species and their adulterants. *Chin Med, 8*(1), 16. doi:10.1186/1749-8546-8-16

World Health Organization. (2019). *WHO Global Report on Traditional and Complementary Medicine 2019*. World Health Organization.

Xiong, Y., Xiao, X., Yang, X., Yan, D., Zhang, C., Zou, H., Hui Lin, Lian Peng, Xiao Xiao, & Yan, Y. (2014). Quality control of Lonicera japonica stored for different months by electronic nose. *J Pharm Biomed Anal, 91*, 68–72. doi:10.1016/j.jpba.2013.12.016

Xu, J. (2016). Fungal DNA barcoding. *Genome, 59*(11), 913–932. doi:10.1139/gen-2016-0046

Xu, Y., Li, Z., Wang, Y., & Huang, H. (2007). Allozyme diversity and population genetic structure of three medicinal epimedium species from Hubei. *J Genet Genom, 34*(1), 56–71. doi:10.1016/S1673-8527(07)60007-1

Yang, S. Y., Kim, H. K., Lefeber, A. W., Erkelens, C., Angelova, N., Choi, Y. H., & Verpoorte, R. (2006). Application of two-dimensional nuclear magnetic resonance spectroscopy to quality control of ginseng commercial products. *Planta Med, 72*(4), 364–369. doi:10.1055/s-2005-916240

Yau, F. C., Wong, K. L., Wang, J., But, P. P., & Shaw, P. C. (2002). Generation of a sequence characterized amplified region probe for authentication of crocodilian species. *J Exp Zool, 294*(4), 382–386. doi:10.1002/jez.10199

Yip, P. Y., Chau, C. F., Mak, C. Y., & Kwan, H. S. (2007). DNA methods for identification of Chinese medicinal materials. *Chin Med, 2*, 9. doi:10.1186/1749-8546-2-9

Zhang, Y. B., Shaw, P. C., Sze, C. W., Wang, Z. T., & Tong, Y. (2007). Molecular authentication of Chinese herbal materials. *J Food Drug Anal, 15*(1), 1. Retrieved from http http://hub.hku.hk/bitstream/10722/89657/1/re01.htm

Zhao, S. J., Hou, C. X., Qian, Y. C., Xu, L. X., & Sun, L. L. (2007). Preparation and identification of monoclonal antibody against Ginsenoside Rb1. [Preparation and Identification of Monoclonal Antibody against Ginsenoside Rb1]. *J Jilin Univ (Eng Technol Ed), 37*(1), 245–248. Retrieved from https://www.AiritiLibrary.com/Publication/Index/16715497-200701-37-1-245-248-a

Zhao, Z., Hu, Y., Liang, Z., Yuen, J. P., Jiang, Z., & Leung, K. S. (2006). Authentication is fundamental for standardization of Chinese medicines. *Planta Med, 72*(10), 865–874. doi:10.1055/s-2006-947209

Zhao, Z., Xiao, P., Xiao, Y., & Yuen, J. P. S. (2007). Quality assurance of Chinese Herbal Medicines (CHMs). *J Food Drug Anal, 15*(4), 337–346.

Zou, H. Q., Lu, G., Liu, Y., Bauer, R., Tao, O., Gong, J. T., Zhao, L. Y., Li, J. H., Ren, Z. Y., & Yan, Y. H. (2015). Is it possible to rapidly and non-invasively identify different plants from Asteraceae using electronic nose with multiple mathematical algorithms? *J Food Drug Anal, 23*(4), 788–794. doi:10.1016/j.jfda.2015.07.001

Part II
General Methodology and Techniques for Molecular Authentication

Chapter 2

DNA Extraction for Medicinal Materials

Hoi-Yan Wu, Forrest Chung-Fai Yau & Fai-Ngor Ngan

2.1 Introduction

Chinese Materia Medica (CMM) is a diverse group of materials that can be roughly categorised into plant-derived CMMs, animal-derived CMMs and mineral-derived CMMs, based on the source. Plant-derived CMMs usually have a rigid polysaccharide cell wall and contain polysaccharides, pigments and secondary metabolites that, if not removed, would inhibit polymerase chain reaction (PCR) and subsequent experiments. The medicinally used materials are collected from different parts of the plants. It is generally easier to isolate DNA from leaves and flowers, which contain more living cells before being harvested, than from woody roots and barks, which contain more compressed cells and are sometimes regarded as recalcitrant materials (Bahnweg *et al.*, 1998). Decoction slices of CMMs are mostly dried, some of them have been further processed by soaking, steaming, roasting or frying with salt, honey or wine. These processes would affect the quality and quantity of the DNA isolated. Animal-derived CMMs generally contain less PCR inhibitors and are less challenging in DNA extraction. The successful development and applicability of DNA-based identification methods rely on the efficient isolation of high-quality DNA from the sample. The origin, nature and composition of the sample governs the difficulty in extracting amplifiable DNA.

Traditional DNA isolation method involves ethanol precipitation of DNA, which could be co-precipitated with contaminants like polysaccharides and polyphenols in the extraction buffer. The use of cetyl trimethyl ammonium bromide (CTAB) under high salt concentrations in the extraction buffer could increase the solubility of polysaccharides and prevent them from co-precipitating with DNA (Grazina, Amaral, & Mafra, 2020; Porebski, Bailey, & Baum, 1997). However, these classical methods often involve the use of toxic solvents like phenol and chloroform. Moreover, precipitated DNA needs to be dried with the tube open, making it prone to environmental and cross-contamination. The procedures of both traditional CTAB extraction and potassium acetate/SDS precipitation are included in Sections 2.2.1–2.2.2 for reference. Silica column-based extraction methods are more popular nowadays and have been adopted in various commercial kits. Among the numerous methods or commercial kits available, there is one optimised method that was shown to work on both plant and animal samples. The method was firstly published by Ivanova (Ivanova, Dewaard, & Hebert, 2006) and released as CCDB Protocol by the Canadian Centre for DNA Barcoding (https://ccdb.ca/site/wp-content/uploads/2016/09/CCDB_DNA_Extraction.pdf). This method has been optimised and further validated by the Government Chinese Medicines Testing Institute (GCMTI) of Department of Health in Hong Kong (https://www.cmro.gov.hk/files/gcmti/research/testing_methods/GCMTI_RD_5_2020.pdf and https://www.cmro.gov.hk/files/gcmti/research/testing_methods/GCMTI_RD_6_2020.pdf). In this chapter, we show the applicability of this method on both plant- and animal-derived CMMs. Two commercial extraction kits that are well-known for the isolation of DNA from highly processed materials were also carried out on the same samples. For fair comparison, the silica columns used in the CCDB/GCMTI methods are the same as those provided in the commercial kits.

2.2 Classical Extraction Methods

2.2.1 CTAB Extraction [modified from (Draper & Scott, 1988)]

Equipment

- Benchtop centrifuge

Reagents

- Chloroform/isoamyl alcohol (24:1)
- CTAB, 10%
    - 10% (w/v) CTAB
    - 0.7 M NaCl
- CTAB extraction buffer
    - 1% (w/v) CTAB
    - 10 mM ethylenediaminetetraacetic acid (EDTA)
    - 20 mM 2-Mercaptoethanol
    - 0.7 M NaCl
    - 50 mM Tris-HCI (pH 8.0)
- CTAB precipitation buffer
    - 1% (w/v) CTAB
    - 10 mM EDTA
    - 50 mM Tris-HCI (pH 8.0)
- Ethanol, 70%
- Ethanol, 100%
- NaCl, 1 M
- TE buffer, pH 8.0
    - 1 mM EDTA, pH 8.0
    - 10 mM Tris-HCl, pH 8.0

Procedures

1. Add 2-Mercaptoethanol to the CTAB extraction buffer to give a final concentration of 20 mM and then pre-warm it to 56°C.
2. Weigh out 0.1–0.2 g ground sample powder and place it in a microcentrifuge tube.
3. Add 600 μL of the pre-warmed buffer to the sample and incubate in a 56°C water bath for 30 min, with occasional shaking.
4. Allow the mixture to cool at room temperature and extract with an equal volume of chloroform/isoamyl alcohol. Emulsify by gentle inversions and centrifuge at 13,000 × g for 10 min. Transfer the top phase to a clean microcentrifuge tube.
   Note: Do not vortex the sample vigorously. It will shear genomic DNA.
5. Wash the protein interface in the original tube with 100 μL of 1 × CTAB extraction buffer. Centrifuge to remove the top phase and pool it with the top phase collected at Step 4.
6. Add 0.1-fold volume of 10% CTAB into the aqueous phase. Mix and repeat chloroform/isoamyl alcohol extraction.
   Note: 10% CTAB is very viscous, pre-warm at 56°C before use.
7. Transfer the aqueous phase to a clean tube and add an equal volume of 1 × CTAB precipitation buffer. Leave it at room temperature for 1 h.
   Note: i) The precipitation time may be longer, even overnight, while temperature is maintained above 20°C.
   ii) White precipitate should form after adding CTAB precipitation buffer. If not, add more buffer or precipitate by adding a 2.5-fold volume of cold ethanol.
8. Centrifuge the solution at 13,000 × g for 15 min. Pour off the supernatant and drain the pellet.

Note: i) The CTAB-nucleic acids are quite stable, and the procedure can be stopped at this stage.
ii) The pellet should be whitish; if not, after redissolving, extract with phenol to remove impurities.

9. Redissolve the pellet in 400 μL of 1 M NaCl. Add 2-fold volume of cool absolute ethanol to precipitate nucleic acids, mix and place at –20°C overnight or 70°C for 30 min to 1 h.
   Note: Make sure the pellet is completely dissolved before adding ethanol. To facilitate the process, incubate at 60°C for 30 min.
10. Centrifuge the suspension at 13,000 × g for 10 min and wash the pellet twice with 70% ethanol. Air-dry the pellet and resuspend it in 50 μL TE buffer or double-distilled water.
    Note: Disperse the pellet during ethanol washes, which helps to remove any remaining CTAB.
11. Check DNA purity and concentration.
    Note: i) If the DNA solution is required to be RNA-free, follow Section 2.2.3.
    ii) Do not over-dry the pellet as it may be difficult to resuspend the DNA in TE or distilled water.
    iii) The DNA preparation can be stored at 4°C for 6 months, or at –20°C for a longer period of time.
    iv) Avoid repeated freeze-thaw cycles, which tend to break down high molecular weight DNA.

2.2.2 Potassium Acetate/SDS Precipitation Method [modified from (Dellaporta, Wood, & Hicks, 1983)]

Equipment

- Beckman centrifuge
- Beckman JA-20 rotor

Reagents

- 2-Mercaptoethanol
- Chloroform/isoamyl alcohol (24:1)
- Extraction buffer
  - 10 mM 2-Mercaptoethanol
  - 50 mM EDTA pH 8.0
  - 500 mM NaCl
  - 100 mM Tris HCl pH 8.0
- Isopropanol
- Phenol/chloroform/isoamyl alcohol (25:24:1)
- Potassium acetate, 5 M
- Sodium acetate, 3 M, pH 5.2
- SDS, 20%
- TE buffer, pH 8.0
  - 1 mM EDTA, pH 8.0
  - 10 mM Tris-HCl, pH 8.0

Procedures

1. Transfer 0.5–1 g ground sample powder into a 50-mL centrifuge tube containing 15 mL pre-warmed extraction buffer.
2. Add fresh 2-Mercaptoethanol to a final concentration of 10 mM.
3. Mix thoroughly with 1 mL 20% SDS by vigorous shaking.
4. Incubate the tube at 56°C for 45 min with occasional shaking.
5. Add 5 mL 5 M potassium acetate, shake vigorously and chill on ice for at least 20 min.

   Note: Most of the proteins and polysaccharides are removed as a complex with the insoluble potassium dodecyl sulphate precipitate.
6. Spin the tubes at 16,000 × g with a Beckman JA-20 rotor for 15 min.

7. Transfer the supernatant into a 50-mL sterile centrifuge tube containing an equal volume of cold isopropanol.
8. Mix the tube gently and incubate on ice for a minimum of 30 min.
   Note: A DNA clot appears.
9. Centrifuge at 15,000 × g for 15 min.
10. Pour off the supernatant and wash the DNA pellet with 85% ethanol twice.
11. Follow Section 2.2.3 to remove RNA.

2.2.3 RNase A Digestion

Equipment

- Benchtop centrifuge

Reagents

- Chloroform/isoamyl alcohol (24:1)
- Ethanol, 70%
- Ethanol, 100%
- Phenol/chloroform/isoamyl alcohol (25:24:1)
- RNase A, 10 mg/mL
- Sodium acetate, 3 M
- TE buffer, pH 8.0
  - 1 mM EDTA, pH 8.0
  - 10 mM Tris-HCl, pH 8.0

Procedures

1. Add an appropriate amount of RNase A (10 mg/mL) to the DNA solution such that the final concentration is 0.5 mg/mL and incubate it at 50°C for 1 h.
2. Add an equal volume of phenol/chloroform/isoamyl alcohol and gently emulsify. Separate the phases by centrifugation

at 13,000 × g for 10 min. Transfer the supernatant to a new microcentrifuge tube.

3. Repeat once with chloroform/isoamyl alcohol extraction.
4. Add 0.1-fold volume of 3 M sodium acetate followed by a 2.5-fold volume of 100% ethanol and precipitate at −20°C overnight.
5. Collect the pellet by centrifugation and wash with 70% ethanol twice.
6. Air-dry and redissolve the pellet in an appropriate volume of TE or distilled water.
7. Check DNA purity and concentration.

2.3 Materials and Methods

2.3.1 Sample Information and Storage

Decoction slices of 15 plant-derived CMMs and six animal-derived CMMs collected from Hong Kong were used in this study. They were deposited in the Li Dak Sum Yip Yio Chin R & D Centre of Chinese Medicine. The CMMs were carefully chosen to include CMMs derived from different parts of plants and animals, such as stems, roots, leaves, flowers, fruits, seeds, animal skin, animal nest and shell. Compared with leaves, flowers and whole herbs, samples originated from stems, roots, rhizomes and barks are generally believed to have less DNA quantity and lower DNA integrity because of DNA degradation. There are also some 'difficult' samples containing secondary metabolites that may hinder DNA extraction. For instance, Caryophylli Flos has a high total phenolic content (Guo, Cheng, Chan, & Yu, 2008) and Corni Fructus is rich in iridoids, tannins, flavonoids and polysaccharides (Dong, Feng, Chen, Wang, & Lu, 2018). The plant-derived and animal-derived CMMs selected are listed in Tables 2.1 and 2.2, respectively.

Table 2.1 Plant-Derived CMMs in this Study

Sample code	Chinese name	Latin pharmaceutical name	Species name	Medicinal part
Stems, roots and rhizomes				
T5353	竹茹	Bambusae Caulis in Taenias	*Bambusa tuldoides* Munro, *Sinocalamus beecheyanus* (Munro) McClure var. *pubescens* P.F. Li, or *Phyllostachys nigra* (Lodd.) Munro var. *henonis* (Mitf.) Stapf ex Rendle	Dried centre layer of stem
T5354	黄芪	Astragali Radix	*Astragalus membranaceus* (Fisch.) Bge. var. *mongholicus* (Bge.) Hsiao, or *Astragalus membranaceus* (Fisch.) Bge.	Dried root
T5355	牡丹皮	Moutan Cortex	*Paeonia suffruticosa* Andr.	Dried root bark
T5359	新疆紫草	Arnebiae Radix	*Arnebia euchroma* (Royle) Johnst.	Dried root
Leaves, flowers and whole herbs				
T5356	山銀花	*Lonicerae Flos*	*Lonicera macranthoides* Hand. — Mazz., *Lonicera hypoglauca* Miq., *Lonicera confusa* DC. or *Lonicera fulvotomentosa* Hsu et S. C. Cheng	Dried flower bud or flower that have just opened
T5357	丁香	Caryophylli Flos	*Eugenia caryophyllata* Thunb.	Dried flower bud
T5358	月季花	Rosae Chinensis Flos	*Rosa chinensis* Jacq.	Dried flower
T5360	番瀉葉	Sennae Folium	*Cassia angustifolia* Vahl or *Cassia acutifolia* Delile	Dried small leaf

(*Continued*)

Table 2.1 (*Continued*)

Sample code	Chinese name	Latin pharmaceutical name	Species name	Medicinal part
T5376	麻黄	Ephedrae Herba	*Ephedra sinica* Stapf, *Ephedra equisetina* Bge., *Ephedra intermedia* Schrenk et C. A. Mey.	Dried herbaceous stem
Fruits and seeds				
T5361	核桃仁	Juglandis Semen	*Juglans regia* L.	Dried mature seed
T5362	王不留行	Vaccariae Semen	*Vaccaria segetalis* (Neck.) Garcke.	Dried mature seed
T5363	淡豆豉	Sojae Semen Praeparatum	*Glycine max* (L.) Merr.	Dried, fermented mature seed
T5365	芡實	Euryales Semen	*Euryale ferox* Salisb.	Dried mature kernel
T5366	山茱萸（山萸肉）	Corni Fructus	*Cornus officinalis* Sieb. et Zucc.	Dried mature fruit
Resin				
T5375	乳香	Olibanum	*Boswellia carterii* Birdw., *Boswellia bhaw-dajiana* Birdw. or *Boswellia neglecta* M. Moore	Oily, gummy resin (with residual bark)

All samples in this study are dried decoction slices. We stored them with silica beads in airtight boxes. Each sample has been visually examined to ensure it is free of mould and insect/bug infestation, before being double-bagged and placed in the airtight

Table 2.2 Animal-Derived CMMs in this Study

Sample code	Chinese name	Latin pharmaceutical name	Species name	Medicinal part	Weight
T5367	蛇蜕	Serpentis Periostracum	*Elaphe taeniura* Cope, *Elaphe carinata* (Guenther) or *Zaocys dhumnades* (Cantor)	Dried sloughed outer skin	50 mg
T5369	烏梢蛇	Zaocys	*Zaocys dhumnades* (Cantor)	Dried body	70 mg
T5370	蜂房	Nidus Vespae	*Polistes olivaceous* (DeGeer), *Polistes japonicus* Saussure or *Parapolybia varia* Fabricius	Dried nest	70 mg
T5371	甘草泡地龍	Pheretima	*Pheretima aspergillum* (E. Perrier), *Pheretima vulgaris* Chen, *Pheretima guillelmi* (Michaelsen) or *Pheretima pectinifera* Michaelsen	Dried body	100 mg
T5373	龜甲	Testudinis Carapax et Plastrum	*Chinemys reevesii* (Gray)	Dorsal and ventral shell	100 mg
FBN01	花膠	Fish maw (common name)	Mostly Sciaenidae family	Dried bladder	70 mg

box. In the case of freshly collected samples, fresh plant samples (leaves, flowers, small fruits and seeds) can be placed in paper bags and dried with silica beads. Fresh animal tissues should be snap-frozen with liquid nitrogen or dried ice as soon as possible and further stored at –80°C before DNA extraction.

2.3.2 Methods

2.3.2.1 *DNA Extraction from Plant-Derived CMMs*

Equipment, apparatus and accessories

- Tissue homogeniser from Precellys Evolution, Bertin Instrument
- Hard tissue grinding lysing kit, Precellys MK28, Bertin Instrument
- Heat block or thermomixer
- Ambient temperature microcentrifuge (Maximum RCF higher than or equal to 16,000 ×g)
- Vortex
- Sterilised stainless steel scissors and forceps

Reagents

- Modified CCDB/GCMTI spin column-based DNA extraction protocol for plant-derived medicinal materials
    - Lysis Buffer (LB; Guanidine thiocyanate 700 mM, EDTA pH 8.0 30 mM, Tris-HCl pH 8.0 30 mM, Triton X-100 0.5%, Tween-20 5%)
    - Proteinase K (20 mg/mL)
    - α-amylase (Sigma A4582)
    - RNase A (100 mg/mL)
    - Extraction Binding Buffer EBB (Guanidine thiocyanate 6M, EDTA pH 8.0 20 mM, Tris-HCl pH 6.4, Triton X-100, 4%). *Pre-warm at 60°C if precipitation occurs

  - MB Spin Column, Qiagen
  - 2-mL collection tube
  - Extraction Wash Buffer EWB (Ethanol 60%, Sodium chloride 50 mM, Tris-HCl pH 7.4, EDTA pH 8.0)
  - Molecular Biology Grade Water
- DNeasy Plant Pro Kit, Qiagen
  - Solution CD1
  - Solution PS
  - Solution CD2
  - Buffer APP *Pre-warm at 60°C if precipitation occurs
  - MB Spin Column
  - 2-mL collection tube
  - Buffer AW1 *Ethanol added
  - Buffer AW2 *Ethanol added
  - Buffer EB

2.3.2.1.1 Sample Preparation

- Clean the working area with 75% ethanol and wear a new pair of gloves before handling each sample.

Procedure

1. Clean the surface of the medicinal materials with 75% ethanol and wipe dry with a multi-fold paper towel.
2. Cut and weigh about 100 mg dried plant-derived CMM. Further cut into smaller pieces (about 4 × 4 mm) and put into a Precellys MK28 hard tissue grinding lysing kit.
   Note: Perform cutting in a plastic container or paper bag to prevent contaminating the area.
3. For samples T5357, T5363 and T5366, check to make sure they are in small pieces and place the lysing kits with these three samples into a −80°C to −20°C freezer for a few minutes to freeze the samples before homogenisation.

Note: If homogenised at room temperature, these three samples would form a sticky paste at the top of the lysing kit and cannot be ground thoroughly.

4. Put the lysing kit into a Precellys Evolution tissue homogeniser for grinding with five cycles of 6,800 rpm at 30 s.
5. Briefly centrifuge the lysing kit before opening it to check whether the sample has been completely pulverised. Repeat Steps 3–5 once if necessary. For samples T5357, T5363 and T5366, the samples would not be in dried powder form but would be more like ground paste.
6. IMPORTANT: Check the bottom of the lysing kits to make sure they are all intact without cracks, before proceeding to DNA extraction. Transfer to a new lysing kit with care if necessary.

2.3.2.1.2 Modified CCDB/GCMTI Spin Column-Based DNA Extraction Protocol for Plant-Derived Medicinal Materials

- With a pair of new, clean gloves, take out and label all the 1.5-mL tubes, MB Spin Columns and 2-mL collection tubes before the following steps.
- Freshly prepare Buffer PLB by mixing LB with Proteinase K (20 mg/mL) at a 10:1 ratio. For example, add 2 mL Proteinase K into 20 mL LB and mix.
- An empty extraction blank control should be carried out together with the samples.
- Pre-warm Molecular Biology Grade Water to 40°C (Optional).

Procedure

1. Briefly centrifuge the lysing kit with sample powder. Add 1 mL Buffer PLB, 25 μL α-amylase and 5 μL RNase A into the lysing kit.

2. Vortex at maximum speed or homogenise with tissue homogeniser again with three cycles of 6,000 ×g at 30 s to ensure all powder is mixed with the solution but not stuck to the top or bottom of the tube.
3. Incubate at 56°C for 30 min, followed by incubation at 65°C for 1 h. Vortex intermittent for every 15–20 min.
4. Centrifuge at maximum speed for 5 min at room temperature to pellet the debris.
5. Transfer the supernatant (500–650 μL) to a new 1.5-mL tube. *Note: Sample T5361 would give a thin pale-coloured layer on top of the aqueous layer. Some samples would have small particles floating in the upper part of the supernatant. Carefully avoid them during aspiration of supernatant. Repeat centrifugation if necessary.*
6. Add an equal volume of Buffer EBB to the lysate. Mix thoroughly by pipetting up and down.
7. Transfer 600 μL of the mixture in Step 6 into an MB Spin Column and centrifuge at 6,000 ×g for 2 min.
8. Discard the flow-through and repeat Step 7 until all mixture in Step 6 has passed through the MB Spin Column.
9. Place the MB Spin Column into a clean 2-mL collection tube.
10. Add 600 μL Buffer EWB to the column. Centrifuge at 6,000 ×g for 2 min.
11. Discard the flow-through and place the MB Spin Column back into the same 2-mL collection tube.
12. Add 600 μL Buffer EWB to the column. Centrifuge at 6,000 ×g for 4 min.
13. Discard the flow-through and place the MB Spin Column back into the same 2-mL collection tube.
14. Centrifuge at maximum speed for 3 min. Place the MB Spin Column to a new 1.5-mL tube (pre-labelled).

Note: This step is to remove any residual ethanol in the membrane of the spin column. It is important to take out the spin column from the collection tube and place it into a new tube immediately after the centrifugation is finished.

15. Add 50 μL pre-warmed Molecular Biology Grade Water directly onto the membrane of the MB Spin Column. Incubate at room temperature for 2–3 min.
16. Centrifuge at maximum speed for 2 min to elute the DNA. Discard the MB Spin Column. The eluted DNA solution can be stored at –20°C or a lower temperature.

2.3.2.1.3 Modified DNA Extraction Protocol Using DNeasy Plant Pro Kit

- With a pair of new, clean gloves, take out and label all the 1.5-mL tubes, MB Spin Columns and 2-mL collection tubes before the following steps.
- Pre-warm Buffer EB to 40°C (optional).

Procedures

1. Briefly centrifuge the lysing kit with sample powder. Add 950 μL Solution CD1 and 50 μL Solution PS.
2. Vortex at maximum speed or homogenise with a tissue homogeniser again with three cycles of 6,000 ×g at 30 s to ensure all powder is mixed with the solution but not stuck to the top or bottom of the tube.
3. Incubate at 60°C for 1 h. Vortex intermittent for every 15–20 min.
4. Centrifuge at maximum speed for 5 min at room temperature.
5. Transfer the supernatant (600–750 μL) to a 1.5-mL tube.

   Note: Samples T5361 and T5362 would give a pale-coloured layer on the top of the aqueous layer. Carefully scrape away the upper layer or avoid that layer during aspiration of supernatant.

6. Add 400 μL Solution CD2 and vortex for 5 s.
7. Centrifuge at maximum speed for 5 min at room temperature. Carefully avoid the pellet and transfer the supernatant (700–900 μL) to a 1.5-mL tube.

   Note: It is important to avoid any debris in the pellet in this step. Repeat centrifugation if necessary.
8. Add an equal volume of Buffer APP and vortex for 5 s.
9. Transfer 600 μL of the mixture in Step 8 into an MB Spin Column and centrifuge at 6,000 ×g for 2 min.
10. Discard the flow-through and repeat Step 9 until all mixture in Step 8 has passed through the MB Spin Column.
11. Place the MB Spin Column into a clean 2-mL collection tube.
12. Add 650 μL Buffer AW1 to the MB Spin Column. Centrifuge at 6,000 ×g for 2 min.
13. Discard the flow-through and place the MB Spin Column back into the same 2-mL collection tube.
14. Add 650 μL Buffer AW2 to the MB Spin Column. Centrifuge at 6,000 ×g for 3 min.
15. Discard the flow-through and place the MB Spin Column back into the same 2-mL collection tube.
16. Centrifuge at maximum speed for 3 min. Place the MB Spin Column to a new 1.5-mL tube (pre-labelled).

    Note: This step is to remove any residual ethanol in the membrane of the spin column. It is important to take out the spin column from the collection tube and place it into a new tube immediately after the centrifugation is finished.
17. Add 50 μL Buffer EB to the centre of the white filter membrane of the MB Spin Column. Incubate at room temperature for 2–3 min.

18. Centrifuge at maximum speed for 2 min to elute the DNA. Discard the MB Spin Column. The eluted DNA solution can be stored at –20°C or a lower temperature.

2.3.2.2 *DNA Extraction from Animal-derived CMMs*

Equipment, apparatus and accessories

- Tissue homogeniser from Precellys Evolution, Bertin Instrument
- Hard tissue grinding lysing kit, Precellys MK28, Bertin Instrument
- Heat block or thermomixer
- Ambient temperature microcentrifuge (Maximum RCF ≥ 17,900 × g)
- Vortex
- Sterilised stainless steel scissors and forceps

Reagents

- DNeasy Mericon Food Kit, Qiagen
  - Food Lysis Buffer
  - Proteinase K solution
  - Chloroform
  - Buffer PB
  - QIAquick spin column
  - Buffer AW2 *Ethanol added
  - Buffer EB
- Modified CCDB spin column-based DNA extraction protocol for animal-derived medicinal materials
  - Lysis Buffer LB (Guanidine thiocyanate 700 mM, EDTA pH 8.0 30 mM, Tris-HCl pH 8.0 30 mM, Triton X-100 0.5%, Tween-20 5%)

- Proteinase K (20 mg/mL)
- RNase A (100 mg/mL)
- Extraction Binding Buffer EBB (Guanidine thiocyanate 6M, EDTA pH 8.0 20 mM, Tris-HCl pH 6.4, Triton X-100 4%). *Pre-warm at 60°C if precipitation occurs
- QIAquick spin column, Qiagen
- 2-mL collection tube
- Extraction Wash Buffer EWB (Ethanol 60%, Sodium chloride 50 mM, Tris-HCl pH 7.4, EDTA pH 8.0)
- Molecular Biology Grade Water

2.3.2.2.1 Sample Preparation

- Clean the working area with 75% ethanol and wear a new pair of gloves before handling each sample.

Procedures

1. Clean the surface of the medicinal materials with 75% ethanol and wipe dry with a multi-fold paper towel.
2. Cut and weigh the samples. Weight amount of each sample is shown in Table 2.2. Further cut into smaller pieces (about 4 × 4 mm). For sample FBN01 (fish maw), put the sample pieces into a 1.5-mL microcentrifuge tube. For other samples, put into a Precellys MK28 hard tissue grinding lysing kit with shearing beans.
   Note: For sample T5369, we mainly cut out the muscle for experiment. Sample T5370 contains some sand and dirt at the bottom of the CMM. Care should be given to remove the sand/dirt before cutting and weighing. Sample FBN01 (fish maw) can be completely digested by proteinase K without further homogenisation.

Note: Perform cutting in a plastic container or a paper bag to prevent contaminating the area.

3. Put the lysing kit with sample into a −80°C to −20°C freezer for a few minutes to freeze the sample before homogenisation.
Note: If homogenised at room temperature, some loose samples, such as T5367 and T5370, might pack together at the top of the tube and cannot be ground thoroughly.
4. Put the lysing kit with sample into a Precellys Evolution tissue homogeniser for grinding with three cycles of 6,000 ×g at 30 s.
5. Briefly centrifuge the lysing kit before opening it to check whether the sample has been completely pulverised. Repeat Steps 3–5 once if necessary.
6. IMPORTANT: Check the bottom of the lysing kit to make sure they are all intact without cracks, before proceeding to DNA extraction. Transfer to a new lysing kit with care if necessary.

2.3.2.2.2 Modified CCDB Spin Column-Based DNA Extraction Protocol for Animal-Derived Medicinal Materials

- With a pair of new, clean gloves, take out and label all the 1.5-mL tubes, QIAquick Spin Columns and 2-mL collection tubes before the following steps.
- Freshly prepare Buffer PLB by mixing LB with Proteinase K (20 mg/mL) at a 10:1 ratio. For example, add 2 mL Proteinase K into 20 mL LB and mix.
- An empty extraction blank control should be carried out together with the samples.
- Pre-warm Molecular Biology Grade Water to 40°C (optional).

Procedures

1. Briefly centrifuge the lysing kit with sample powder. Add 1 mL Buffer PLB and 5 μL RNase A into the lysing kit or 1.5-mL microcentrifuge tube (for sample FBN01).
2. Vortex at maximum speed to ensure all powder is mixed with the solution but not stuck to the top or bottom of the tube.
3. Incubate at 56°C for 1 h. Vortex intermittent for every 15–20 min.
4. Centrifuge at maximum speed for 5 min at room temperature to pellet the debris.
5. Transfer the supernatant (500–700 μL) to a new 1.5-mL tube. *Note: Some samples would have small particles floating in the upper part of the supernatant. Carefully avoid them during aspiration of supernatant. Repeat centrifugation if necessary.*
6. Add an equal volume of Buffer EBB to the lysate. Mix thoroughly by pipetting up and down.
7. Transfer 600 μL of the mixture in Step 6 into a QIAquick Spin Column and centrifuge at 6,000 ×g for 2 min.
8. Discard the flow-through and repeat Step 7 until all the mixture in Step 6 has passed through the Spin Column.
9. Place the Spin Column into a clean 2-mL collection tube.
10. Add 600 μL Extraction Wash Buffer (EWB) to the column. Centrifuge at 6,000 ×g for 2 min.
11. Discard the flow-through and place the Spin Column back into the same 2-mL collection tube.
12. Add 600 μL Extraction Wash Buffer (EWB) to the column. Centrifuge at 6,000 ×g for 4 min.
13. Discard the flow-through and place the Spin Column back into the same 2-mL collection tube.

14. Centrifuge at maximum speed for 3 min. Place the Spin Column to a new 1.5-mL tube (pre-labelled).
Note: This step is to remove any residual ethanol in the membrane of the spin column. It is important to take out the spin column from the collection tube and place it into a new tube immediately after the centrifugation is finished.
15. Add 80 μL pre-warmed Molecular Biology Grade Water directly onto the membrane of the Spin Column. Incubate at room temperature for 2–3 min.
16. Centrifuge at maximum speed for 2 min to elute the DNA. Discard the Spin Column. The eluted DNA solution can be stored at −20°C or a lower temperature.

2.3.2.2.3 Modified DNA Extraction Protocol Using DNeasy Mericon Food Kit

- With a pair of new, clean gloves, take out and label all the microcentrifuge tubes, QIAquick Spin Columns and 2-mL collection tubes before the following steps.
- Pre-warm Buffer EB to 40°C (optional).

Procedures

1. Briefly centrifuge the lysing kit with sample powder. Add 1 mL Food LB and 2.5 μL Proteinase K solution into the lysing kit or 1.5-mL microcentrifuge tube (for sample FBN01).
2. Vortex at maximum speed to ensure all powder is mixed with the solution but not stuck to the top or bottom of the tube.
3. Incubate at 60°C for 1 h. Vortex intermittent for every 15–20 min.
4. Cool the sample to room temperature by incubating at −20°C freezer for about 5 min to enhance inhibitor precipitation.

5. Centrifuge at maximum speed for 5 min at room temperature to pellet the debris.
6. Pipet 500 μL chloroform into a 2-mL microcentrifuge tube.
Note: Chloroform easily leaks from pipet tips. Minimise the leakage by repeatedly pipetting the chloroform up and down several times and transfer the solvent quickly.
7. Transfer the clear supernatant in Step 5 (500–700 μL) to the microcentrifuge tube containing the chloroform.
Note: Carefully avoid the inhibitor precipitate at the bottom and the upper phase, if any, of the tube in Step 5. Repeat centrifugation if necessary.
8. Vortex the microcentrifuge tube from Step 7 for 15 s and centrifuge at 16,000 ×g for 15 min.
9. Transfer the clear aqueous supernatant (400–500 μL) to a new 1.5-mL microcentrifuge tube.
10. Add an equal volume of Buffer PB to the aqueous supernatant. Mix thoroughly by pipetting up and down.
11. Transfer 600 μL of the mixture in Step 10 into a QIAquick Spin Column and centrifuge at 6,000 ×g for 2 min.
12. Discard the flow-through and repeat Step 11 until all mixture in Step 10 has passed through the Spin Column.
13. Add 500 μL Buffer AW2 to the Spin Column. Centrifuge at 6,000 ×g for 2 min. Discard the flow-through.
14. Centrifuge the empty Spin Column at maximum speed for 3 min. Place the MB Spin Column to a new 1.5-mL tube (pre-labelled).
Note: This step is to remove any residual ethanol in the membrane of the spin column. It is important to take out the spin column from the collection tube and place it into a new tube immediately after the centrifugation is finished.

16. Add 80 μL pre-warmed Buffer EB directly onto the membrane of the Spin Column. Incubate at room temperature for 2–3 min.
17. Centrifuge at maximum speed for 2 min to elute the DNA. Discard the Spin Column. The eluted DNA solution can be stored at −20°C or lower temperature.

2.3.2.3 *Nucleic Acid Quantification*

NanoDrop Lite spectrophotometer was used to measure the OD 260 and OD 280 of all DNA extracts. The corresponding eluents, Buffer EB are Molecular Biology Grade Water, were used as blank.

2.3.2.4 *PCR Amplification and Agarose Gel Electrophoresis*

To assess whether the DNA extracts are in good PCR quality, i.e., amplifiable by PCR, PCR was performed to amplify two commonly used DNA barcodes using universal primers. For plant-derived CMMs, ribulose bisphosphate carboxylase large subunit (*rbcL*) and internal transcribed spacer 2 (ITS2) were amplified. For animal-derived CMMs, mitochondrial cytochrome c oxidase subunit I gene (*COI*) and mitochondrial 16S rRNA gene were amplified. Primer sequences are listed in Table 2.3. For each 30 μL reaction, there was 1× PCR buffer, 2.5 mM $MgCl_2$, 200 μM dNTPs, 500 nM forward primer, 500 nM reverse primer, 1U GoTaq DNA polymerase and 10–30 ng DNA template (or 5 μL undiluted DNA extracts). PCR was carried out at 95°C for 3 min, 35 cycles of 95°C for 30 s, 47°C for 30 s and 72°C for 1 min, with a final elongation at 72°C for 5 min. A relatively high concentration of magnesium ions in the PCR reaction and a low annealing temperature were selected to give a less stringent PCR condition in order to show the

Table 2.3 Primers Used in This Study

Target region	Primer name	Sequence (5′ to 3′)	Reference
ITS2	ITS-S2F	ATG CGA TAC TTG GTG TGA AT	(Chen *et al.*, 2010)
	ITS-S3R	GAC GCT TCT CCA GAC TAC AAT	(Chen *et al.*, 2010)
	ITS3	GCA TCG ATG AAG AAC GCA GC	(White, Burns, Lee, & Taylor, 1990)
	ITS4	TCC TCC GCT TAT TGA TAT GC	(White *et al.*, 1990)
rbcL	rbcLa_F	ATG TCA CCA CAA ACA GAG ACT AAA GC	(CBOL Plant Working Group, 2009)
	rbcLa_R	GTA AAA TCA AGT CCA CCR CG	(CBOL Plant Working Group, 2009)
COI	FISHCOIHBC	TCA ACY AAT CAY AAA GAT ATY GGC AC	(Handy *et al.*, 2011)
	FISHCOILBC	ACT TCY GGG TGR CCR AAR AAT CA	(Handy *et al.*, 2011)
16S rRNA	16H1	CTG ACC GTG CAA AGG TAG CGT AAT CAC T	(Hedges, 1994)
	16L1	CTC CGG TCT GAA CTC AGA TCA CGT AGG	(Hedges, 1994)

amplifiability of the 'difficult' samples. PCR products were subject to agarose gel electrophoresis in 1.5% agarose gel for visualisation.

2.4 Results

2.4.1 DNA Yield and Purity

Modified CCDB/GCMTI method generally gave a higher DNA yield than the commercial kit counterparts in both plant-derived and animal-derived CMMs (Tables 2.4 and 2.5). A higher DNA concentration was obtained from 13 out of 15 plant-derived CMMs using modified CCDB/GCMTI protocol, except for samples T5357 and T5375. The difference in DNA yield is quite signif-

Table 2.4 DNA Concentration and OD Ratio of DNA Extracts from Plant-Derived CMMs

			Modified CCDB/ GCMTI method		Modified DNeasy Plant Pro Kit	
Sample code	Chinese name	Latin pharmaceutical name	DNA concentration (ng/μL)	A260/ A280	DNA concentration (ng/μL)	A260/ A280
Stems, roots and rhizomes						
T5353	竹茹	Bambusae Caulis in Taenias	9.2	1.63	1.9	3.16
T5354	黃芪	Astragali Radix	157.7	1.72	23.6	1.93
T5355	牡丹皮	Moutan Cortex	145.8	1.58	76.8	1.25
T5359	新疆紫草	Arnebiae Radix	238.1	1.76	21.3	0.96
Leaves, flowers and whole herbs						
T5356	山銀花	Lonicerae Flos	97.7	1.74	12.6	5.67
T5357	丁香	Caryophylli Flos	58.7	1.10	189.6	0.94
T5358	月季花	Rosae Chinensis Flos	193.6	1.61	93.3	1.16
T5360	番瀉葉	Sennae Folium	371.6	1.84	42.4	1.33
T5376	麻黃	Ephedrae Herba	1056.9	1.85	111.8	1.82
Fruits and seeds						
T5361	核桃仁	Juglandis Semen	143.6	1.48	61.6	1.90
T5362	王不留行	Vaccariae Semen	350.9	1.84	9.9	2.15
T5363	淡豆豉	Sojae Semen Praeparatum	42.6	1.68	4.0	2.56
T5365	芡實	Euryales Semen	312.4	1.88	13.0	1.88
T5366	山萸肉	Corni Fructus	2.0	0.88	3.4	1.70
Resin						
T5375	乳香	Olibanum	3.5	1.12	3.9	1.35

Table 2.5 DNA Concentration and OD Ratio of DNA Extracts from Animal-Derived CMMs

			Modified CCDB/ GCMTI method		Modified DNeasy Mericon Food Kit	
Sample code	**Chinese name**	**Latin pharmaceutical name**	**DNA concentration (ng/μL)**	**A260/ A280**	**DNA concentration (ng/μL)**	**A260/ A280**
T5367	蛇蛻	Serpentis Periostracum	381.0	1.84	232.3	1.84
T5369	烏梢蛇	Zaocys	91.4	1.88	161.0	1.92
T5370	蜂房	Nidus Vespae	53.2	1.72	33.3	1.82
T5371	甘草泡地龍	Pheretima	162.5	1.86	142.2	1.86
T5373	龜甲	Testudinis Carapax et Plastrum	30.0	1.68	−0.8	2.48
FBN01	花膠	Fish maw (common name)	13.9	1.62	12.0	1.75

icant among those 13 samples, with DNA concentration 1.9–35.3 times of that obtained from the modified DNeasy Plant Pro Kit. Modified CCDB/GCMTI method also gave better DNA purity in terms of an A260/A280 ratio, with 7 out of 15 samples having an A260/A280 ratio within the range of 1.70–1.90, whereas the modified DNeasy Plant Pro Kit only had two samples within the range. For animal-derived CMMs, the difference in DNA yield between the two methods is less drastic. Modified CCDB/GCMTI method gave a higher DNA concentration in four out of six animal-derived samples, which are 1.1–1.6 times of that DNA concentration obtained from the modified DNeasy Mericon Food Kit.

2.4.2 PCR Success Rate

To test the amplifiability of the DNA extracts, two DNA barcode regions were amplified from each DNA extract. PCR results of

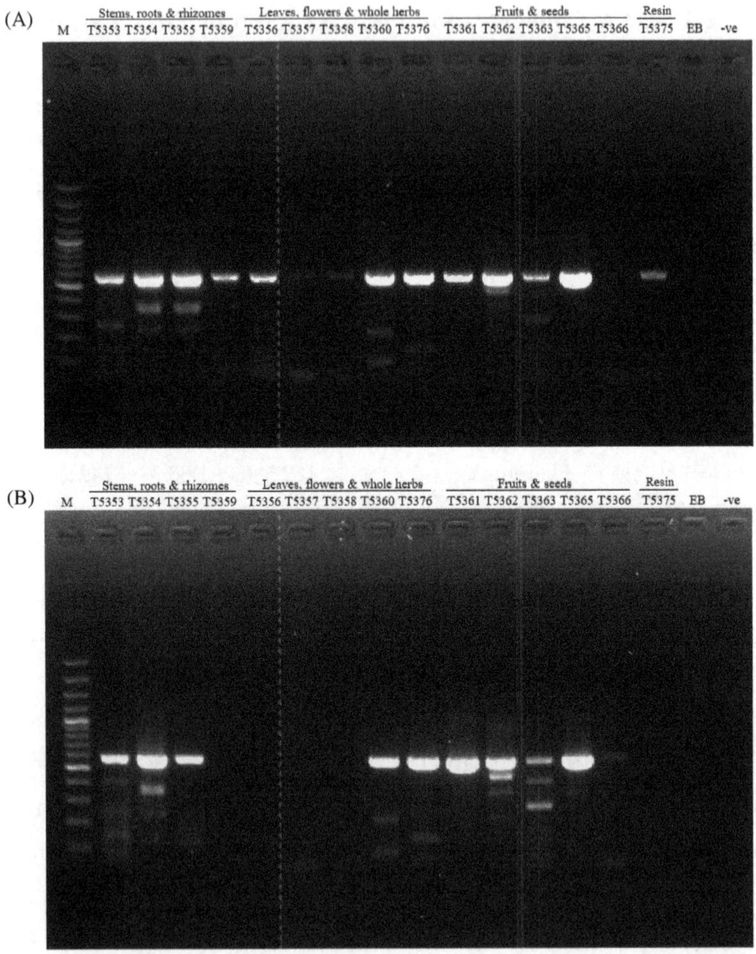

Fig. 2.1 PCR amplification of *rbcL* from DNA extracts of plant-derived CMMs isolated using (A) modified CCDB/GCMTI method and (B) modified DNeasy Plant Pro kit. EB: Extraction blank control; M: 100 bp DNA size marker; –ve: PCR negative control (without template DNA).

plant-derived CMMs are shown in Figure 2.1–2.2 and summarised in Table 2.6. In general, modified CCDB/GCMIT method outperformed the modified DNeasy Plant Pro Kit. Both the *rbcL* gene and ITS2 region were successfully amplified from 11 out of 15 plant-derived CMMs extracted by the modified CCDB/GCMTI method. Three samples, T5357, T5358 and T5375, gave weak

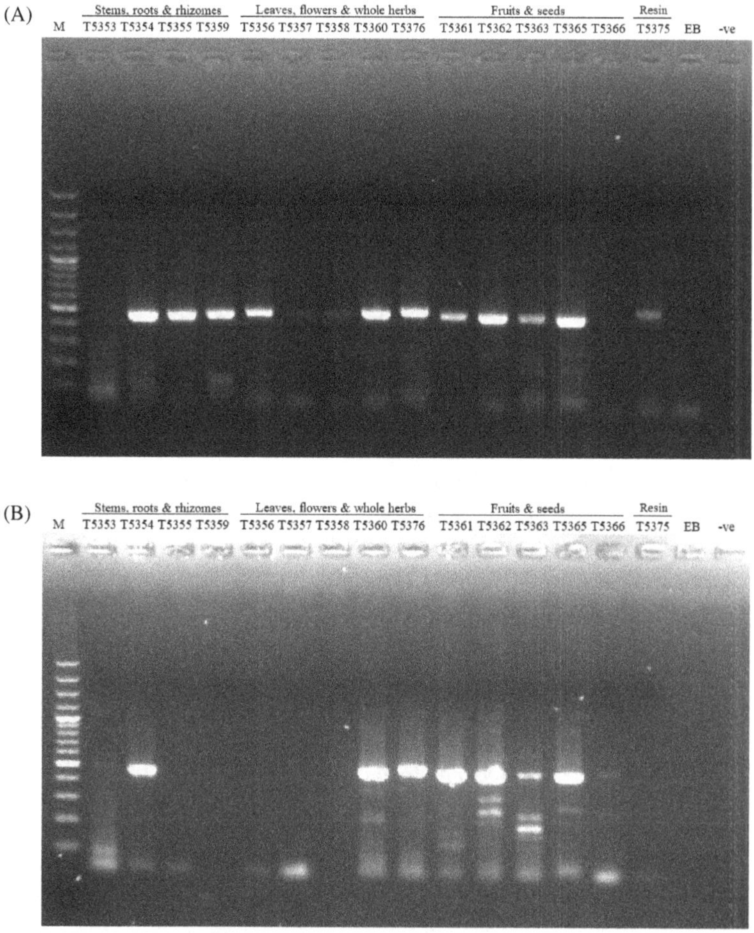

Fig. 2.2 PCR amplification of ITS2 from DNA extracts of plant-derived CMMs isolated using (A) modified CCDB/GCMTI method and (B) modified DNeasy Plant Pro kit. EB: Extraction blank control; M: 100 bp DNA size marker; –ve: PCR negative control (without template DNA).

bands in both regions. Only one sample, T5366, failed to be amplified. For animal-derived CMMs, both extraction methods had good PCR success rates. PCR results of animal-derived CMMs are shown in Figure 2.3 and summarised in Table 2.7. *COI* gene could be amplified from all animal-derived samples, albeit with two weak bands. Even a sample without detectable DNA, T5373, extracted by the modified DNeasy Mericon Food Kit, could

Table 2.6 Amplifiability of DNA Extracts of Various Plant-Derived CMMs

Sample code	Chinese name	Latin pharmaceutical name	Modified CCDB/GCMTI method		Modified DNeasy Plant Pro Kit	
			rbcL	ITS2	*rbcL*	ITS2
Stems, roots and rhizomes						
T5353	竹茹	Bambusae Caulis in Taenias	+	–/+*	+	+wk/+*
T5354	黃芪	Astragali Radix	+	+	+	+
T5355	牡丹皮	Moutan Cortex	+	+	+	–
T5359	新疆紫草	Arnebiae Radix	+	+	–	–
Leaves, flowers and whole herbs						
T5356	山銀花	Lonicerae Flos	+	+	–	–
T5357	丁香	Caryophylli Flos	+wk	+wk	–	–
T5358	月季花	Rosae Chinensis Flos	+wk	+wk	–	–
T5360	番瀉葉	Sennae Folium	+	+	+	+
T5376	麻黃	Ephedrae Herba	+	+	+	+
Fruits and seeds						
T5361	核桃仁	Juglandis Semen	+	+	+	+
T5362	王不留行	Vaccariae Semen	+	+	+	+
T5363	淡豆豉	Sojae Semen Praeparatum	+	+	+wk	+
T5365	芡實	Euryales Semen	+	+	+	+
T5366	山萸肉	Corni Fructus	–	–	+wk	+wk
Others						
T5375	乳香	Olibanum	+wk	+wk	–	–

+: clear band at expected size; +wk: weak band at expected size; –: no band at expected size.

*Clear band obtained when primers ITS3 and ITS4 were used. Gel photo not shown.

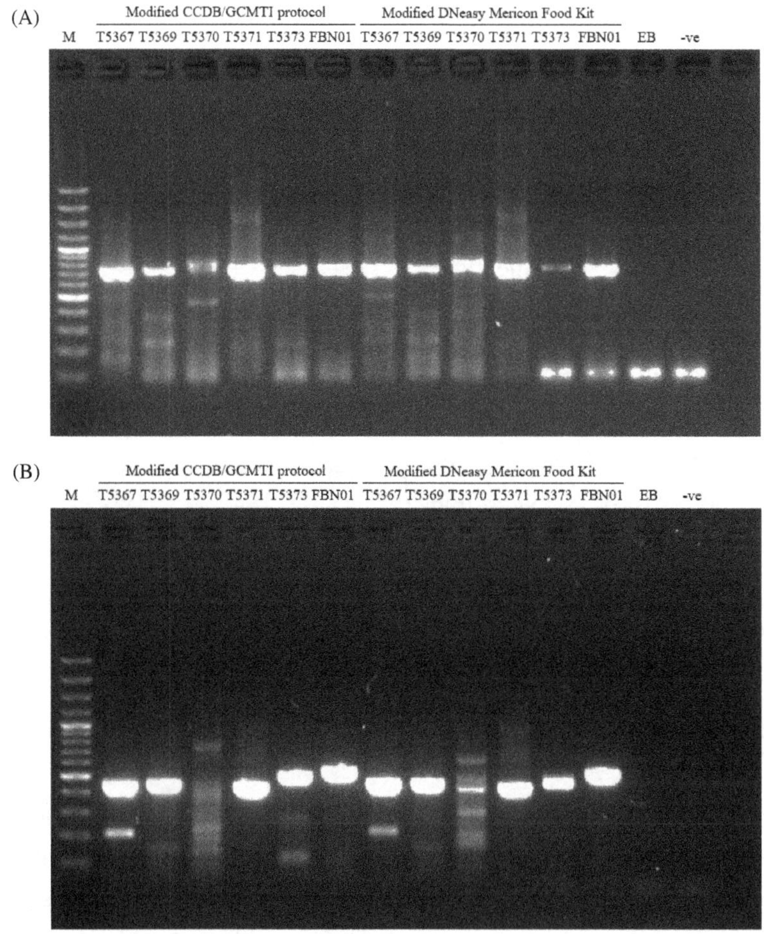

Fig. 2.3 PCR amplification of (A) *COI* and (B) 16S rRNA region from DNA extracts of animal-derived CMMs isolated using modified CCDB/GCMTI method and modified DNeasy Mericon Food Kit. EB: Extraction blank control; M: 100 bp DNA size marker; –ve: PCR negative control (without template DNA).

produce a weak but distinct band at the right size. The 16S rRNA gene could not be amplified from sample T5370, irrespective of the DNA extraction method. This might be due to primer mismatch, as *COI* could still be amplified from this sample.

Table 2.7 Amplifiability of DNA Extracts of Various Animal-Derived CMMs

Sample code	Chinese name	Latin pharmaceutical name	Modified CCDB/GCMTI method		Modified DNeasy Mericon Food Kit	
			COI	16S rRNA	*COI*	16S rRNA
T5367	蛇蛻	Serpentis Periostracum	+	+	+	+
T5369	烏梢蛇	Zaocys	+	+	+	+
T5370	蜂房	Nidus Vespae	+wk	–	+	–
T5371	甘草泡地龍	Pheretima	+	+	+	+
T5373	龜甲	Testudinis Carapax et Plastrum	+	+	+wk	+
FBN01	花膠	Fish maw (common name)	+	+	+	+

+: clear band at expected size; +wk: weak band at expected size; –: no band at expected size

2.5 Discussion

The traditional CTAB extraction method relies on the selective precipitation of nucleic acid by CTAB. The CTAB extraction buffer has a high salt concentration (0.7 M), at which DNA is soluble but many polysaccharides are not (Murray & Thompson, 1980). Repeated extraction with CTAB at high salt concentration followed by chloroform/isoamyl alcohol, firstly with a CTAB extraction buffer, and secondly with 10% CTAB, allows the removal of polysaccharides and protein. Addition of the CTAB precipitation buffer at equal volume with no salt would reduce the salt concentration from 0.7 M to 0.35 M, at which CTAB would selectively precipitate with nucleic acids. The precipitated CTAB-nucleic acid is then redissolved in 1 M NaCl and precipitated with ethanol to remove CTAB. This method is a classical method for DNA extraction from a plant sample, but it is laborious with two precipitations.

Potassium acetate/SDS precipitation removes proteins and polysaccharides, followed by DNA precipitation with isopropanol. The volume of isopropanol required for DNA precipitation is usually 0.6–0.7 volume of the lysate, much less than that of ethanol (usually 2–3 volumes). However, salts are less soluble in 35% isopropanol than in 60%–70% ethanol, leading to a higher chance of co-precipitation of salt in the DNA pellet.

In this chapter, we have shown that the modified CCDB/GCMTI method has outperformed popular commercial kits in both plant-derived and animal-derived CMM samples. This method gave more amplifiable DNA of PCR-quality with higher yield, compared with the commercial kit methods. When this method was first published, it showed that the combination of LB with guanidine thiocyanate, Triton X-100 and Tween-20 and binding buffer with 6M guanidine thiocyanate but no ethanol gave a consistently higher or comparable PCR success rate in fresh or dried plant materials, when compared with LB with CTAB or sodium dodecyl sulphate and binding buffer with ethanol. GCMTI of Department of Health in Hong Kong further improved this method by adding α-amylase in the LB for plant-based materials. Here, we show that this is a useful method that could isolate PCR-quality DNA from CMMs collected from different parts of plants and animals. It could be adapted as a standard/basic DNA extraction method in molecular testing laboratory for food and CMM samples. In our laboratory, we have adapted the method based on our existing bead-beating homogeniser with minor optimisations and written it into an in-house extraction method, which was basically shared previously, with points-to-note that we think would be important in carrying out the experiment.

Further optimisation of the protocol may be required for some challenging samples that are not uncommon among Chinese medicinal materials, as they could be from a variety of plants and be heavily processed. Here are some optimisation approaches we would suggest considering:

i. Adjusting the starting material: LB ratio and the scale of extraction — For samples rich in PCR inhibitors, lower the starting material: LB ratio by reducing the amount of starting material from 100 mg to 20–50 mg per millilitre of LB. To avoid a decrease in DNA yield, make several replicates of the same sample, i.e., scale up the reaction, and pool them together to the same silica spin column.
ii. Addition of PVP or PVPP — For samples rich in phenolic compounds, 2% (final concentration) polyvinylpyrrolidone (PVP) can be added to the LB. Or, add ~50 mg polyvinylpolypyrrolidone (PVPP) directly into the lysing kit to grind/homogenise together with the dried sample. Addition of 2-Mercaptoethanol alongside PVP is quite common in other plant DNA extraction protocols. However, it has been reported that the presence of 2-Mercaptoethanol in LB was detrimental for isolation of high molecular weight DNA from freshwater microalgae (Yee, Kumar, & Muthusamy, 2018). Whether 2-Mercaptoethanol would affect DNA isolation from algae-derived CMMs remains to be investigated.
iii. Prolonging incubation time with shaking — Samples can be incubated in LB at 55°C–60°C for a longer period, or overnight, with constant or occasional shaking to enhance the release of DNA.
iv. Dilution of DNA solution in subsequent PCR — Perform 1:50 to 1:5 dilution of DNA solution with Molecular Biology

Grade Water for downstream PCR so as to reduce the amount of PCR inhibitors in the reaction.

In our experience, samples that give weak but specific band after PCR, as in samples T5357, T5358 and T5375 extracted by the modified GCMTI/CCDB method (Figure 2.1A and 2.2A), could be improved after adapting these optimisations. For example, as samples T5357 and T5358 gave decent amount of DNA (58.75 ng/μL and 193.45 ng/μL) in the first extraction, one may consider reducing the amount of starting material to 30 mg and add PVPP into the lysing kit before grinding. This protocol was originally developed by Ivanova and collaborators in 2006 to make it automation-friendly and suitable for most fresh and dried plant materials. However, the nature of CMMs is much more complex and diverse than the general plant, from parts of plants/animals to a degree of processing to storage conditions and duration. There may not be a one-size-fits-all method to all CMMs. The target DNA yield and DNA purity depend on the requirement of the subsequent experiments. The DNA quantity required for a few PCR is, expectedly, much lower than that for high-throughput sequencing. This would, in turn, affect the amount of starting material and scale of the extraction needed.

2.6 Conclusion

The applicability of the modified CCDB/GCMTI method to different kinds of plant-derived and animal-derived CMMs have been shown. Equipment, apparatus and procedures are listed in detail to demonstrate how the method can be easily adopted with an existing setup of a molecular biology laboratory. Further optimisations would be needed for some difficult samples, but this protocol can serve as a good starting point for experimentation.

References

Bahnweg, G., Schulze, S., Moller, E. M., Rosenbrock, H., Langebartels, C., & Sandermann, H., Jr. (1998). DNA isolation from recalcitrant materials such as tree roots, bark, and forest soil for the detection of fungal pathogens by polymerase chain reaction. *Anal Bioche, 262*(1), 79–82. doi:10.1006/abio.1998.2769

CBOL Plant Working Group. (2009). A DNA barcode for land plants. *Proc Nat Acad Sci USA, 106*(31), 12794–12797. doi:10.1073/pnas.0905845106

Chen, S., Yao, H., Han, J., Liu, C., Song, J., Shi, L., Zhu, Y., Ma, X., Gao, T., Pang, X., Luo, K., Li, Y., Li, X., Jia, X., Lin, Y., & Leon, C. (2010). Validation of the ITS2 region as a novel DNA barcode for identifying medicinal plant species. *PLoS One, 5*(1), e8613. doi:10.1371/journal.pone.0008613

Dellaporta, S. L., Wood, J., & Hicks, J. B. (1983). A plant DNA minipreparation: Version II. *Plant Mol Biol Rep, 1*(4), 19–21. doi:10.1007/BF02712670

Dong, Y., Feng, Z. L., Chen, H. B., Wang, F. S., & Lu, J. H. (2018). Corni Fructus: A review of chemical constituents and pharmacological activities. *Chin Med, 13*, 34. doi:10.1186/s13020-018-0191-z

Draper, J., & Scott, R. (1988). The isolation of plant nucleic acids. In J. Draper, R. Scott, P. Armitage & R. Walden (Eds.), *Plant Genetic Transformation and Gene Expression. A Laboratory Manual* (pp. 199–236). London: Blackwell.

Grazina, L., Amaral, J. S., & Mafra, I. (2020). Botanical origin authentication of dietary supplements by DNA-based approaches. *Compr Rev Food Sci Food Saf, 19*(3), 1080–1109. doi:10.1111/1541-4337.12551

Guo, D. J., Cheng, H. L., Chan, S. W., & Yu, P. H. (2008). Antioxidative activities and the total phenolic contents of tonic Chinese medicinal herbs. *Inflammopharmacology, 16*(5), 201–207. doi:10.1007/s10787-008-8016-9

Handy, S. M., Deeds, J. R., Ivanova, N. V., Hebert, P. D., Hanner, R. H., Ormos, A., Weigt, L. A., Moore, M. M., & Yancy, H. F. (2011). A single-laboratory validated method for the generation of DNA barcodes for the identification of fish for regulatory compliance. *J AOAC Int, 94*(1), 201–210.

Hedges, S. B. (1994). Molecular evidence for the origin of birds. *Proc Nat Acad Sci USA, 91*(7), 2621–2624. doi:10.1073/pnas.91.7.2621

Ivanova, N. V., Dewaard, J. R., & Hebert, P. D. N. (2006). An inexpensive, automation-friendly protocol for recovering high-quality DNA. *Mol Ecol Notes,* 6(4), 998–1002. doi:10.1111/j.1471-8286.2006.01428.x

Murray, M. G., & Thompson, W. F. (1980). Rapid isolation of high molecular weight plant DNA. *Nucl Acids Res,* 8(19), 4321–4325. doi:10.1093/nar/8.19.4321

Porebski, S., Bailey, L. G., & Baum, B. R. (1997). Modification of a CTAB DNA extraction protocol for plants containing high polysaccharide and polyphenol components. *Plant Mol Biol Rep, 15*(1), 8–15. doi:10.1007/BF02772108

White, T. J., Burns, T., Lee, S., & Taylor, J. (1990). *PCR Protocols: A Guide to Methods and Applications*. San Diego: Academic Press.

Yee, W., Kumar, J. N., & Muthusamy, P. D. (2018). Inclusion of 2-Mercaptoethanol in lysis buffer could interfere with isolation of high molecular weight DNA from freshwater microalgae. *Ind J Microbiol,* 58(1), 109–113. doi:10.1007/s12088-017-0698-5

Chapter 3

General Methodology

Mavis Hong-Yu Yik

3.1 Introduction

Traditional ways to authenticate medicinal materials include morphological characterisation, microscopic identification and chemical markers/fingerprints. With the advancement of DNA technology, molecular authentication has provided an independent and reliable approach. According to the Pharmacopoeia of the People's Republic of China (2020), *Fritillaria cirrhosa*, *Zaocys dhumnades*, *Agkistrodon acutus*, *Bungarus multicinctus* and *Dendrobium huoshanense* already have their own DNA-based molecular authentication assays. The application of molecular techniques for authentication is prevailing worldwide. In this chapter, we are going to describe the general molecular techniques that have been commonly adopted for molecular authentication. This chapter is divided into five sections: (1) DNA concentration and purity measurement, (2) polymerase chain reaction (PCR), (3) DNA gel electrophoresis, (4) PCR product purification and (5) molecular cloning.

Obtaining high-quantity and purified DNA is of paramount importance for performing subsequent molecular analysis. Measurement of the amount and purity of extracted DNA is a prerequisite for downstream procedures. DNA concentration and purity can be measured by spectrophotometry, for example, ultraviolet (UV) spectrometer, NanoDrop™ micro-UV/Vis spectrophotometer and Qubit® fluorometer (Section 3.2). PCR is an enzymatic amplification of a specific DNA region, which is flanked by two specific primers. The amplification involves repeated cycles of three critical steps: (1) heat denaturation of the DNA templates, (2) annealing of primers to complementary sequences and (3) extension of annealed primers by DNA polymerase (Section 3.3). This allows the target DNA to be exponentially amplified millions of times in a short period of time. Primer design and factors affecting PCR are described in Section 3.3.2–3.3.3.

Agarose gel electrophoresis is a common lab technique used for resolving the amplified DNA from PCR. PCR products are loaded into wells of an agarose gel and subjected to an electric field. The negatively charged DNA fragments move toward the positive electrode (Section 3.4.1). Denaturing polyacrylamide gel electrophoresis (PAGE) and autoradiography are discussed in Section 3.4.2. Factors affecting electrophoresis are discussed in Section 3.4.3. The use of a gel extraction kit to purify PCR products from agarose gel is also illustrated in Section 3.5.

The final section introduces the preparation, ligation and transformation of *Escherichia coli*, which are required for DNA to be cloned into a plasmid. Blue-white screening is also described for selecting successful recombinant clones (Section 3.6).

3.2 DNA Concentration and Purity Measurement

3.2.1 UV Spectrophotometer

Equipment

- UV Spectrophotometer

Procedures

The concentration of the sample can be determined by measuring the absorbance at 260 nm and 280 nm using UV spectrophotometer and calculating through the following formula:

$$[DNA] = A260 \times Dilution\ factor \times 50\ \mu g/mL$$

Remark

1. *The amount of UV absorbed is directly proportional to the amount of DNA in the sample.*
2. *One A260 unit corresponds to 50 μg of double-stranded DNA per millilitre.*
3. For purity, the A260/A280 purity ratio is the ratio of corrected absorbance at 260 nm to corrected absorbance at 280 nm. The ratio reached ~1.8 is generally considered as 'pure' DNA.

3.2.2 NanoDrop™ Spectrophotometer

Equipment

- NanoDrop™ Micro-UV/Vis Spectrophotometer

Reagent

- Double-distilled water

Procedures

1. Select the 'Nucleic Acids' and 'dsDNA' at the Home screen.
2. Clean both pedestals with a laboratory wipe.
3. Pipette 1–2 μL double-distilled water onto the lower pedestal and lower the arm.
4. Tap 'Blank' and wait for the measurement to complete.
   Remark: If Auto-Blank is 'On', the blank measurement starts automatically after the arm is lowered.
5. Lift the arm and clean both pedestals with a new laboratory wipe.
6. Pipette 1–2 μL sample solution onto the pedestal and lower the arm.
7. Tap 'Measure' and wait for the sample measurement.
   Remark: If Auto-Measure is 'On', the sample measurement starts automatically after the arm is lowered.
8. The spectrum and reported values, including nucleic acid concentration, A260/A280 and A260/A230 purity ratio, are displayed when the sample measurement is completed.
   Remark: A260/A230 purity ratio between 1.8 and 2.2 is generally considered as 'pure' DNA.

Source

Product guide of NanoDrop™ Micro-UV/Vis Spectrophotometer (Thermo Fisher Scientific, Waltham, MA)

3.2.3 Qubit® Fluorometer

Equipment

- Qubit® fluorometer (Thermo Fisher Scientific, Waltham, MA)

Reagent

- Qubit® assay kit (Thermo Fisher Scientific, Waltham, MA)

Procedures

1. Set up two assay tubes for the standards (S1 and S2) and one assay tube for each sample.
2. Use Qubit® buffer to dilute the Qubit® reagent into Qubit® working solution in 1:200.
3. Prepare 200 μL of working solution for each standard and sample.
4. Prepare the assay tubes according to the following table:

	Standard assay tube	Sample assay tube
Volume of Qubit® Working Solution	190 μL	180–199 μL
Volume of Standard (from Qubit® assay kit)	10 μL	/
Volume of Sample	/	1–20 μL
Total Volume	200 μL	200 μL

5. Vortex all tubes for 2–3 s.
6. Incubate the tubes for 2 min at room temperature.
7. Insert the tubes in the Qubit® fluorometer.
8. Select the 'dsDNA' quantitation assays.
9. Tap 'Read standards' for calibration.
10. Insert Standard #1 into the sample chamber and tap 'Read standard'.
11. Insert Standard #2 into the sample chamber and tap 'Read standard'. The calibration is then completed.
    Remark: For successful calibration, a Fluorescence versus Concentration graph with a straight line connecting the two standard data points will be shown.
12. Insert the sample tube into the sample chamber. Tap 'Run samples' and select the sample volume and units.

13. Tap 'Read tube' and take the reading.

Source

Product guide of Qubit® fluorometer (Thermo Fisher Scientific, Waltham, MA)

3.3 Polymerase Chain Reaction

3.3.1 Workflow of PCR

Equipment

- Benchtop centrifuge
- Thermal cycler

Reagents

- GoTaq® G2 Flexi DNA Polymerase kit (Promega, Madison, WI)

Procedures

1. Prepare the reaction mixture by combing the following components:

	Component	Volume
1.	5× Green or Colorless GoTaq® Flexi buffer#	5 μL
2.	$MgCl_2$ solution, 25 mM#	4 μL
3.	PCR Nucleotide Mix, 10 mM each#	0.5 μL
4.	Forward primer (10 μM)	2.5 μL
5.	Reverse primer (10 μM)	2.5 μL
6.	GoTaq® G2 Flexi DNA Polymerase (5 u/μL)#	0.25 μL
7.	DNA template	1 μL
8.	Double-distilled water	9.25 μL
	Total volume	**25 μL**

#*From the GoTaq® G2 Flexi DNA Polymerase kit.*

2. Prepare the positive control by combining the earlier reaction components with known PCR-amplifiable DNA as the DNA template.
3. Prepare the negative control by combining the earlier reaction components with double-distilled water as the DNA template.
4. Put the prepared samples, positive control and negative control into a thermal cycler with the following setting:

Temperature	**Duration**	**Cycle**
94°C	3 min	1×
94°C	30 s	
55°C–60°C*	20 s	35×
72°C	30 s	
72°C	5 min	1×

**Please refer to Section 3.3.3.2 for a discussion on annealing temperature.*

Demonstration video on PCR

Cantonese Version with English Subtitles

Putonghua Version with English Subtitles

Source

Product guide of GoTaq® G2 Flexi DNA Polymerase kit (Promega, Madison, WI)

3.3.2 Primer Design

Computer software

- Biological Sequence Alignment Editor (BioEdit, Ibis Biosciences)

Procedures

1. Download the sequences at particular DNA loci of concerned species from the GenBank of National Center for Biotechnology Information (NCBI).
2. Align the sequences by BioEdit.
3. Find out the conserved sequences that flank the region of interest in the template DNA.
4. Design primers at the conserved sequences with consideration of the following factors (Table 3.1):

Table 3.1 Factors Need to be Considered in Primer Design

Factor	Recommendation	Remark
1. Length	18–30 nucleotides	This length is good for the primers to bind DNA template effectively with high specificity
2. Melting temperatures (T_m)	55°C–70°C	The difference of melting temperatures of the two primers should be less than 5°C. The primer melting temperature helps in determining the annealing temperature (Section 3.3.3.2)
3. GC content	40%–60%	Uniform distribution of C and G bases can avoid mis-priming

Table 3.1 (*Continued*)

Factor	Recommendation	Remark
4. Primers' ends	One C or G at 3' end	C or G base at the 3' end of the primer can facilitate primer anchoring and extension. To minimise non-specific priming, the number of C or G bases at 3' end should be less than three
5. Homo-dimer	No complementary sequences within the primer	The formation of secondary structures reduces the availability of primers and affects primer-template annealing
6. Hetero-dimer	No complementary sequences between the forward and reverse primers	The formation of primer dimers reduces the availability of primers and affects primer-template annealing

3.3.3 Factors Affecting PCR

3.3.3.1 *PCR Reaction Components*

There are six basic components playing critical roles in PCR. Their function, recommended concentration and key considerations in setting up the reactions are described in Table 3.2.

Apart from PCR buffer, each component has its own recommended range of concentration. In general, the higher the concentration of each ingredient, the more the PCR products will be. But the accuracy and specificity of the reaction will be lowered. Conversely, the lower the concentration of each ingredient, the fewer the PCR products can be obtained. But in that case, the accuracy and specificity of the reaction will be higher.

Table 3.2 Components and Recommended Concentration/Amount for PCR

Component	Recommended final concentration/amount	Function	Remark
1. PCR Buffer	1×	To provide a suitable chemical environment for DNA polymerase	The buffer pH is usually between 8.0 and 9.5 and is often stabilised by Tris-HCl
2. Magnesium chloride ($MgCl_2$)	1–4 mM	Mg^{2+} acts as a cofactor for the activity of DNA polymerase by enabling incorporation of dNTPs during polymerisation	High [Mg^{2+}] produces non-specific PCR products, whereas low [Mg^{2+}] gives little or no PCR product
3. Deoxynucleotide triphosphates (dNTPs)	0.2 mM of each dNTP	The four basic nucleotides (dATP, dCTP, dGTP and dTTP) act as building blocks of new DNA strands	Inhibition of PCR may occur when dNTPs exceed optimal concentration
4. Primers (forward and reverse)	0.1–1 μM	To bind complementary sequences that flank the region of interest in the template DNA	High amount of primers increases the chance of primer dimer formation. Low amount of primers reduces the yield of the PCR product
5. DNA Taq Polymerase	1–2 units	To catalyse 5′ to 3′ synthesis of DNA	Increasing the amount of DNA polymerase may improve PCR yields when inhibitors are present in the DNA sample. However, this may increase non-specific PCR products
6. DNA Template	0.1–1 ng/μL	To provide a template for DNA synthesis	High amount of DNA template increases the risk of non-specific amplification, whereas low amount reduces the yields

3.3.3.2 *Annealing Temperature*

PCR specificity is highly dependent on the annealing temperature (T_A). If the T_A is too high, it may result in low PCR product yield as there is insufficient primer-template hybridisation. If the T_A is too low, non-specific products may result because of the increase of base pair mismatches. T_A is set based on the melting temperature of forward and reverse primers. In general,

$$\text{Annealing Temperature} = \frac{\text{Forward primer } T_m + \text{Reverse primer } T_m}{2} - 5$$

Source

PCR Setup — Six Critical Components to Consider (Thermo Fisher Scientific, Waltham, MA)

3.4 Electrophoresis

3.4.1 Agarose Gel Electrophoresis

Equipment

- Microwave oven
- Gel electrophoresis apparatus and tank
- Power pack
- Gel documentation system

Reagents

- Agarose
- 1× Tris-acetate-EDTA (TAE) buffer
  - 40 mM Tris
  - 20 mM Acetate
  - 1 mM EDTA
- SYBR® Safe DNA gel stain
- 6× DNA gel loading dye

Procedures

1. Depending on the fragment size for analysis, prepare agarose gel accordingly.* For example, to prepare a 1.5% agarose gel, weigh 0.6 g agarose powder and add to a conical flask.
   **Please refer to Section 3.4.3.2 for a discussion on the concentration of agarose gel.*
2. Add 40 mL of 1× TAE buffer.
   Remark: The TAE buffer added should be lower than 50% of the conical flask volume.
3. Cover the conical flask with microwave-safe cling wrap and poke a few holes.
4. Heat to dissolve using microwave oven. Swirl gently to avoid bubbles.
5. Add 4 μL of 10,000× SYBR® Safe DNA gel stain when the solution cools down to about 56°C.
6. Swirl gently and pour into the gel tray.
7. Remove bubbles and let the gel harden for about 30 min or until it becomes opaque.
8. Remove the comb and place the gel set into the electrophoresis tank filled with 1× TAE buffer.
9. Mix the DNA samples with the appropriate amount of 6× DNA gel loading dye.
10. Load the sample and DNA ladder into the slots of the gel.
11. Run at 5–10 V/cm until the dye front migrates to around two-third of the gel.
12. Examine the gel using the gel documentation system.

Demonstration video on gel electrophoresis

Cantonese Version with English Subtitles

Putonghua Version with English Subtitles

3.4.2 Denaturing PAGE

Equipment

- Gel dryer
- Heat block
- Kodax X-OMAT AR diagnostic film or Fuji RX Medical X-ray Film
- Kodax X-Omatic cassette
- Power supply system with high-voltage supply (e.g., BioRad PowerPac 3000)
- Radioisotope protection shield
- Saran wrap
- Sequencing apparatus (e.g., BioRad Sequi-Gen® nucleic acid sequencing cell)
- Whatman 3MM filter paper

Reagents

- Acetone
- Acrylamide solution, 40%

  - 38% (w/v) Acrylamide
  - 2% (w/v) N, N'-methylene-bisacrylamide
- Ammonium persulphate (APS), 10%
  - 10% (w/v) APS in distilled water
- Dimethyldichlorosilane solution (DMDCS), 2%
  - 2% (w/v) DMDCS in 1,1,1-trichloroethane
- Ethanol, 70%
- 1× TBE (Tris-borate-EDTA) buffer
  - 90 mM Tris-borate
  - 2 mM Na_2EDTA
- Tetramethylethylenediamine (TEMED)
- Urea

Procedures

Preparation of 6% polyacrylamide gel solution

1. Add 11.7 g urea, 7.5 mL 40% acrylamide and 5 mL 10× TBE.
2. Make up to 50 mL with distilled water.

Gel casting

1. Clean the glass surface with distilled water, 70% ethanol and acetone before use.
2. Wipe one side of the glass with DMDCS.
3. Assemble the gel sandwich.
4. Mix 5 mL 6% acrylamide gel solution, 8 μL 10% APS and 7 μL TEMED to seal the bottom of the sandwich.
5. Place the cell horizontally and inject the gel solution into the base of the glass plates.
6. Seal with tape and lay it vertically for 3 min.
7. After the bottom of the cell is sealed, place in an inclined position at about 20 degrees.
8. Add 250 μL 10% APS and 40 μL TEMED to the remaining acrylamide gel solution.

9. Pour immediately into the gap between the glass plates.
10. Insert a 0.4-mm thick shark-tooth comb between the glass plates with its flat side facing inward.
11. Allow the gel to set for 1 h.

Electrophoresis of sequencing gel

1. Remove the comb and insert with its toothed side pointing inward.
2. Remove the tape and insert sandwich assembly into the gel tank.
3. Fill reservoirs with 1× TBE and pre-run the gel at a constant power of 50 W for 30 min.
4. Denature the sample for 3 min.
5. Flush the wells with running buffer to remove urea.
6. Load a 3 μL sample into the well and run at a constant power of 50 W until the dyes reach the desired position.
   Remark: Higher power is sometimes required to maintain the optimal sequencing temperature at 55°C.
7. Dissemble the casting unit and transfer the gel to a 3MM Whatman filter paper.
8. Cover it with Saran wrap and dry it in a gel dryer for 1.5 h.
   Remark: Excessive boiling of the sample in formamide or dye may cause DNA chain breakage, resulting in smeared bands. If repeated loading is necessary, remove required amount of the sample for denaturing prior to loading.

Autoradiography

1. Place an X-ray film onto the gel in a darkroom and expose in a Kodak X-Omatic cassette at room temperature (for ^{35}S or ^{33}P isotopes) or −70°C (for ^{32}P isotope).
   Remark: The exposure time depends on the gel signal. It may take from a few hours to several days.

2. Develop the film with an automatic developer (e.g., X-ray film processor Kodak M35).

3.4.3 Factors Affecting Agarose Gel Electrophoresis

3.4.3.1 *Voltage of Electric Field*

- Low voltage decreases resolution of small fragments.
- High voltage decreases the separation of large fragments.
- Too high a voltage may melt the gel or cause smearing or distortion of DNA bands.

3.4.3.2 *Concentration and Thickness of Agarose Gel*

3.4.3.2.1 Concentration

- Optimal concentration for high resolution varies inversely with the size of DNA (Table 3.3).

Table 3.3 The Optimum Resolution of DNA Molecular Size with Different Agarose Gel Concentrations

% Gel	Optimum resolution for linear DNA molecule (kb)
0.5	1.0–30
0.7	0.8–12
1.0	0.5–10
1.2	0.4–7
1.5	0.2–3

3.4.3.2.2 Thickness

- Thin gels are preferred for high resolution; however, overloading of samples may occur.

3.4.3.3 *Temperature of Electrophoresis*

- Migration of DNA molecules are slower at lower temperature.

Source

Factors affecting Electrophoresis (Broad Learnings Enterprises LLC).

3.5 PCR Product Purification

Equipment

- Benchtop centrifuge
- Razor blade
- UV transilluminator

Reagent

- DNA gel extraction kit (Biomed, China)

Procedures

1. Cut the band of interest using a sterile razor blade and put into a 1.5-mL microcentrifuge tube.
2. Weigh out the gel slices and add 3 volumes of gel dissolving buffer for <2% TAE gel.
   Remark: If 2% or more TAE gel is used, 6 volumes of gel dissolving buffer should be added.
3. Incubate the mixture at 55°C–60°C until the gel is completely dissolved.
4. Place a spin column in a 2-mL collection tube.
5. Apply the mixture to the spin column and centrifuge for 1 min at 12,100 ×g.
6. Add 500 μL washing buffer and centrifuge for 1 min at 12,100 ×g. Discard the flow-through and repeat once.

7. Discard the flow-through and place the spin column back to the same collection tube.
8. Centrifuge the empty spin column for 2 min at 12,100 ×g to remove any residual ethanol.
9. Place the spin column back in a new 1.5-mL microcentrifuge tube.
10. Add 50 μL elution buffer to the centre of the spin column membrane. Let the column stand for 1 min and then centrifuge for 1 min at 12,100 ×g to obtain the purified PCR products.
    Remark: To increase DNA concentration collected, add back the eluted solution to the centre of the spin column membrane. Let the column stand for 1 min and then centrifuge for 1 min at 12,100 ×g.

Source

Product guide of DNA gel extraction kit (Biomed, China)

3.6 Cloning

3.6.1 *Preparation of E. coli*

Equipment

Rotary shaking incubator

Reagents

- Luria-Bertani (LB) medium
    - 10 g/L NaCl
    - 10 g/L Tryptone
    - 5 g/L Yeast extract
- RF1 medium (pH 5.8)
    - 30mM KAc
    - 100mM $RbCl_2$
    - 10mM $CaCl_2$

- $50mM\ MnCl_2$
- 15% glycerol

Remark: Store at 4°C

- RF2 medium (pH 6.5)
  - 10mM MOPS (pH 6.5)
  - $10mM\ RbCl_2$
  - $75mM\ CaCl_2$
  - 15% glycerol

Remark: Store at 4°C

Procedures

Day 1

1. Streak the competent cell stock on an LB plate.

Day 2

1. Pick a single colony from the plate and inoculate it into a 5 mL LB medium.
2. Shake the cultures overnight at 37°C.

Day 3

1. Add 0.5 mL overnight culture into a 100 mL LB medium.
2. Shake the culture at 37°C for around 2–3 h until the absorbance of the culture reaches 0.45 at OD_{600}.
3. Chill the culture on ice for 5 min.
4. Transfer the culture into 50-mL centrifuge tubes.
5. Centrifuge the centrifuge tubes for 10 min at 1,700 ×g at 4°C.
6. Harvest and resuspend the cells in 40 mL RF1 medium.
   Remark: Swirl gently to resuspend and do not vortex!
7. Chill the culture on ice for 5 min.
8. Centrifuge the cells for 10 min at 1,700 ×g at 4°C.

9. Harvest and re-suspend the cells in 4 mL RF2 medium.
   Remark: Do not vortex!
10. Leave the cells into 70 μL aliquots and freeze in liquid nitrogen.
11. Store the cells at –80°C.

    Remark: Work should be carried out under sterile condition to avoid contamination.

3.6.2 *Ligation and Transformation of E. coli*

Equipment

Rotary shaking incubator

Reagents

- pGEM®-T Easy Vector System (Promega): Vector, control insert DNA, T4 DNA ligase and ligation buffer are included
- 5-Bromo-4-chloro-3-indolyl β-D-galactopyranoside (X-gal), 20 mg/mL
- *E. coli* competent cells
- Isopropyl β-d-1-thiogalactopyranoside (IPTG), 0.1M
- LB medium
  - 10 g/L NaCl
  - 10 g/L Tryptone
  - 5 g/L Yeast extract

Procedures

1. Add ligation buffer, T4 DNA ligase from the kits to the reaction mixture together with the insert and vector in an appropriate ratio.
   Remark: The recommended Vector:Insert molar ratio is between 1:1 and 1:10.
2. Incubate the mixture at 4°C overnight.

3. Add 5 μL ligation mixture (with around 10 ng plasmid DNA) into 100 μL just-thawed *E. coli* competent cells and mix well.
4. Keep the tube on ice for 30 min and then heat-shock it at 42°C for 2 min.
5. Put on ice immediately for 5 min.
6. Add 400 μL 37°C LB medium and incubate at 37°C for 1 h in a rotary shaking incubator for recovery.
7. Spread 50 μL of the culture, 50 μL X-gal and 20 μL IPTG onto an LB plate containing appropriate antibiotics.
8. Invert and incubate at 37°C overnight.
9. Select clones with recombinant DNA on the next day.

Remark

- *Blue-white screening depends on the expression of the β-galactosidase gene in the plasmid and is a well-known technique for the identification of recombinant bacteria for colony selection.*
- *White clones: recombinant cells (with target inserts).*
- *Blue clones: non-recombinant cells (without target inserts).*
- *Should be carried out under sterile conditions to avoid contamination.*

Source

Product guide of pGEM®-T Easy Vector Systems (Promega, Madison, WI)
Blue-white screening & protocols for colony selection (Merck, Darmstadt, Germany)

3.7 Conclusion

Molecular authentication is widely adopted for species identification and authentication. In this chapter, we have introduced five general techniques for molecular authentication, including (1)

DNA concentration and purity measurement, (2) PCR, (3) DNA gel electrophoresis, (4) PCR product purification and (5) molecular cloning. Experimental protocols of each DNA technique are step by step described for general laboratory use. Factors affecting experiments and recommended parameters are discussed for optimising experimental results.

References

Addgene. How to design a primer. Primer design for PCR. Retrieved from https://www.addgene.org/protocols/primer-design/

Biomed. Protocol of gel extraction kit. Retrieved from http://www.biomed168.com/public/uploads/DH101%2020191220.pdf

Broad Learnings. Factors affecting electrophoresis. Retrieved from https://www.broadlearnings.com/lessons/factors-affecting-electrophoresis/

Invitrogen. Qubit® 2.0 fluorometer. User manual. Retrieved from https://www.garvan.org.au/research/capabilities/molecular-genetics/documents/qubit-2-fluorometer-user-manual.pdf

Merck. Blue-white screening & protocols for colony selection. Retrieved from https://www.sigmaaldrich.com/technical-documents/articles/biology/blue-white-screening.html

Promega. Certificate of analysis. Retrieved from https://worldwide.promega.com/-/media/files/resources/protocols/product-information-sheets/g/gotaq-g2-flexi-dna-polymerase-protocol.pdf?la=en

Promega. pGEM®-T Easy Vector Systems. Retrieved from https://worldwide.promega.com/products/pcr/pcr-cloning/pgem-t-easy-vector-systems/?catNum=A1360

Thermo Fisher Scientific. PCR setup — Six critical components to consider. Retrieved from https://www.thermofisher.com/hk/en/home/life-science/cloning/cloning-learning-center/invitrogen-school-of-molecular-biology/pcr-education/pcr-reagents-enzymes/pcr-component-considerations.html

Thermo Fisher Scientific. Nucleic acid: Thermo scientific nanodrop spectrophotometers. Retrieved from https://www.thermofisher.com/document-connect/document-connect.html?url=https%3A%2F%2Fassets.thermofisher.com%2FTFS-Assets%2FCAD%2Fmanuals%2Fts-nanodrop-nucleicacid-olv-r2.pdf

Chapter 4

Bioinformatics for DNA Sequencing Data Analysis

Yat-Tung Lo

4.1 Introduction

Bioinformatics is an interdisciplinary science that utilises mathematics, statistics and computer technologies to analyse, organise and identify biological data, especially for nucleotide sequences generated by DNA sequencing (Luscombe, Greenbaum, & Gerstein, 2001). When compared with DNA fingerprinting-based techniques in Part III, sequencing-based identification is much more informative and reliable than judgement on DNA fingerprint pattern. In addition, DNA barcodes (Chapter 11) are considered as convenient and effective tools due to the quick and accurate sequencing. Bioinformatics assists in DNA sequencing by (1) storing, sorting and retrieving DNA sequences in DNA databases; (2) aiding the design of primers and conducting taxonomic classification and (3) identifying an unknown sample by computational matching with the reference sequences. The general workflow and roles that bioinformatics plays in molecular authentication is illustrated in Figure 4.1.

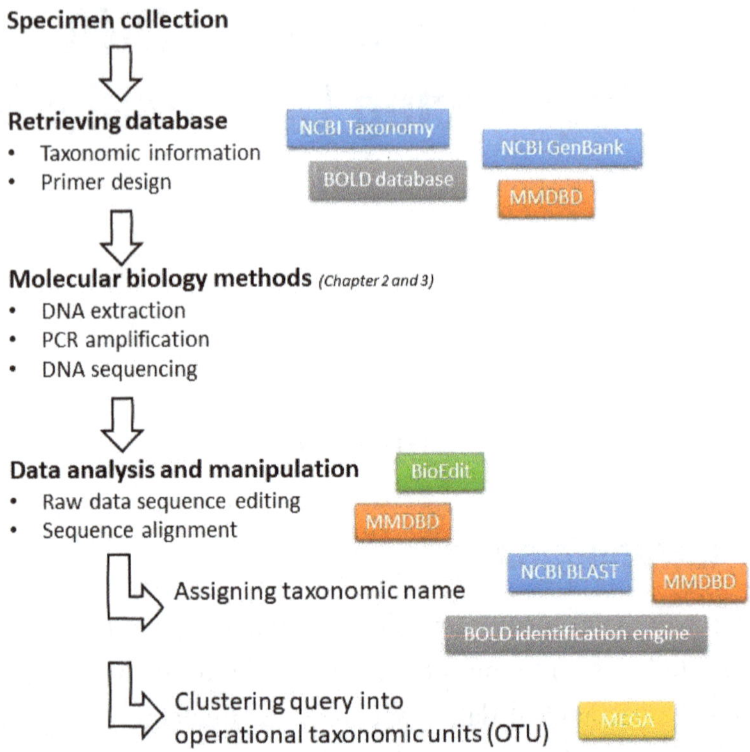

Fig. 4.1 General workflow of molecular authentication and bioinformatics tools involved.

4.2 Databases for Bioinformatics Analysis

To achieve accurate and precise identification, the use of a reliable database as reference for sequence comparison is of paramount importance. There are several commonly available databases for medicinal materials authentication, covering monographs, taxonomies and DNA sequence barcode information.

4.2.1 Useful Resources of Medicinal Materials

The Chinese Pharmacopoeia (ChP) is an official compendium of drugs, covering materials used in traditional Chinese medicine. For medicinal materials, information including the medicinal name in Chinese with Pinyin, scientific binomial name, morphological appearance, description, therapeutic effect, precaution, storage guideline, as well as authoritative authentication methods, are included. Flora of China (http://flora.huh.harvard.edu/china/) is an authoritative document in Chinese plant taxonomy. It describes the botanical nomenclatures, morphologies, literatures, geographical distribution and economic values of more than 30,000 kinds of plants, including brief descriptions, identification keys, essential synonymy, phenology and provincial distribution within or outside China. Medicinal Plant Names Services (MPNS, http://mpns.kew.org/mpns-portal) provides searching of various synonyms such as pharmaceutical, trade and common names besides taxonomy, and provides scientific nomenclature of medicinal plants. In addition, the International Plant Names Index (IPNI, http://www.ipni.org), Tropicos (http://www.tropicos.org) and Index Nominum Genericorum (ING, http://botany.si.edu/ing/) are online databases for the names and associated basic bibliographical details of plant worldwide.

4.2.2 Taxonomy and DNA Sequence Databases

4.2.2.1 *Barcode of Life Data System*

Barcode of Life Data System (BOLD) is an online public database and workbench that supports the assembly and use of DNA barcode data, including acquisition, storage, analysis and publication of DNA barcode records. It is developed by the Centre for Biodiversity Genomics in Canada — more than 9 million DNA barcode records and more than 12 million specimen records are currently included. One of the main features of BOLD is the data trueness and accuracy; for instance, it is connected to other databases of museums, herbaria and other specimen repositories for voucher specimens and taxonomic names. For each record, the voucher specimen with scientific name is required, and the gene sequence must be from a designated gene region. It must meet quality standard and derive from a specimen of which taxonomic assignment can be reviewed; for example, through linkage to a specimen that is held in a major collection (Ratnasingham & Hebert, 2007). Workbench in BOLD is a platform for registered users to access, manage and contribute to DNA barcode projects, as well as the BOLD data analysis tools. It allows users to manage, archive, mine, analyse, publish and share DNA barcoding data. Thus, researchers can assemble, test and analyse their data records in BOLD before uploading them to other databases such as the National Centre for Biotechnology Information (NCBI) GenBank.

Each specimen record involves the following information:

- Identifiers (Sample ID, Museum ID, etc.)
- Taxonomy (Complete taxonomic assignment, BIN ID, etc.)
- Specimen details (Voucher status, detail description of specimen, etc.)
- Collection details (Collector, collection date and location with GPS coordinates)
- Publications
- Sequence (*matK* & *rbcL* for plant, *COI* for animal and ITS for fungi)
- Polymerase chain reaction (PCR) primers used to generate the amplicon
- Electropherogram trace files
- Specimen images

Taxonomy browser in BOLD shows the following information for each taxon:

- Species image
- Taxon description

- Statistics in BOLD database
- Specimen depositories
- Sequencing organisation
- Collection site with distribution maps
- Subspecies involved

4.2.2.2 *Medicinal Materials DNA Barcode Database*

In 2010, our team has created the world's first DNA barcode interactive database for documenting DNA barcode sequences of medicinal materials, namely Medicinal Materials DNA Barcode Database (MMDBD) version 1.0 (Lou *et al.*, 2010). DNA regions commonly used for molecular authentication such as ITS2, *rbcL*, *matK*, *psbA-trnH*, ribosome DNA and other plastid DNA regions are included for medicinal materials listed in the ChP, Dietary Supplements Compendium and Herbal Medicine Compendium of the US Pharmacopoeia, and their selected adulterants. In addition, information including material names, medicinal parts, resources, pharmacopeia information, photographs, biological classification in rank of family, adulterant information, primers used for obtaining the barcodes, references literatures and status on the Convention on International Trade in Endangered Species of Wild Fauna and Flora and the International Union for Conservation of Nature's Red List of Threatened Species, if any, are recorded in MMDBD. In 2018, it has been upgraded into v1.5 with (1) enhancement of the central processing unit (CPU) power and system software integration, (2) expansion of the database to cover the sequences of more medicinal materials and adulterants and (3) optimisation of sequence alignment and primer design accuracy by reducing the copying times when transferring the sequence between different platforms (Wong *et al.*, 2018).

In addition, it allows sequence access, sequence similarity search, multiple sequence alignment and primer design, and to work out these procedures in one platform (Section 4.3.6). MMDBD now has more than 60,000 DNA sequence specimens and more than 2,000 medicinal species, and is a useful resource for researchers in conservation, systematic and forensic study. It can be accessed via: https://rdccm.cuhk.edu.hk/mherbsdb/.

4.2.2.3 *National Centre for Biotechnology Information*

NCBI is part of the United States National Library of Medicine (NLM), a branch of the National Institutes of Health (NIH). It provides biomedical and genomic databases. In molecular authentication, it is essential to understand organism classification and nomenclature in order to define the scope and range of the species to be studied. NCBI Taxonomy database gives the lineage and ranks (order, family, genus, etc.) of the species. In addition, it is interconnected with the NCBI GenBank database to retrieve relevant nucleotide data of a taxon. NCBI GenBank database is a huge and ever-growing public genetic sequence database. It contains all publicly available genomic information, including the species name, DNA sequence and related literatures, etc. DNA sequences of more than 500 species of medicinal materials in ChP have been recorded. In addition, it is part of the International Nucleotide Sequence Database Collaboration, collecting all publicly available sequences such as the DNA Data Bank of Japan (DDBJ) and the European Nucleotide Archive under European Molecular Biology Laboratory (EMBL-DNA). However, the quality and accuracy of the record are the responsibility of the submitting author and not the database, as GenBank does not verify the data and accepts sequences from any kind of materials/specimens by almost anyone, with or without expert taxonomic authentication. For instance, a study on medicinal *Dendrobium* species downloaded from GenBank showed that only 53.06% of the 2,041 accessions downloaded contain reference voucher specimens. Annotations of most accessions are incomplete — only 31.60% and 4.8% of the entries are annotated with the country of origin and collector or assessor, respectively (Wu, Chan, But, & Shaw, 2021). Presence of misidentified or insufficiently annotated sequences in a public database would hamper the reliability of taxonomic identification inferred from such sequences, especially for species with sequences deposited by only one or few research groups. As a result, sequences of GenBank should be used with caution for species-level identification. To alleviate this problem, a user may collect an authenticated specimen with sequencing to compare the similarity, generate reliable DNA sequences directly from curated reference materials deposited in museums or herbaria, compare the sequences deposited in the public database to those reference sequences obtained (Meiklejohn, Damaso, & Robertson, 2019) and assess the percentage of sequence similarity, either by searching against a database with Basic Local Alignment Search Tool (BLAST) or by comparing the downloaded sequences against each other with clustering (Leray, Knowlton, Ho, Nguyen, & Machida, 2019).

4.3 Bioinformatics Tools for Species Identification

4.3.1 Principle of Species Identification

In principle, genome sequence of a species is unique and therefore can be used for identification purpose. Various studies have utilised genetic parameters such as GC% content (Chattopadhyay,

Banerjee, & Banerjee, 2017; Wu *et al.*, 2013), genetic distance (Ginibun *et al.*, 2010; Singh, Parveen, Raghuvanshi, & Babbar, 2012; Tanee, Chadmuk, Sudmoon, Chaveerach, & Noikotr, 2012; Yao *et al.*, 2009), variable sites (Givnish *et al.*, 2015; Tanee *et al.*, 2012), indel appearances (Santos & Pereira, 2018) and monophyletic clusters (Asahina, Shinozaki, Masuda, Morimitsu, & Satake, 2010; Duong *et al.*, 2018; Tang, Yukawa, Bateman, Jiang, & Peng, 2015) for comparison between query and reference sequences. The query sequences are pairwise aligned against the available sequences in certain databases (similarity search) (Parveen, Singh, Malik, Raghuvanshi, & Babbar, 2017; Rajaram, Yong, Azlan, & Go, 2019) or against each other with a selected set of DNA sequences (many-against-each other search) (Chattopadhyay *et al.*, 2017; Feng *et al.*, 2015; Kim, Oh, Bhandari, Kim, & Park, 2014). Even if the reference sequence is not available, one is often able to find a related sequence and obtain the identity at a higher taxonomic rank. Phylogenetic tree (Section 4.4) can also be constructed to understand the evolutionary relationship between related species. Table 4.1 shows the commonly available methods for species identification.

To obtain correct identification results, in which the best hit is the sequence with the species name as expected, and to avoid ambiguous identification in which the best hits are some sequences belonging to different species including the expected species, it is necessary to ensure that the gene regions chosen and sequencing length are sufficient with less intraspecific (within species) variation than interspecific (between species) variation, which is known as the 'Barcoding Gap' (Meyer & Paulay, 2005) (Figure 4.2). In addition, increasing the sequence length for analysis may increase the resolution of species identification at a lower taxonomic rank, with >150 bp in sequence length generally (Meusnier *et al.*, 2008) (Figure 4.3).

Table 4.1 Commonly Available Bioinformatics Methods for Species Identification

Identification method	Alignment method	Identification criteria
BLAST	Similarity search	Correct identification Ambiguous identification Incorrect identification
Genetic distance-based (Nearest distance)	Many-against-each other search	Correct identification Ambiguous identification Incorrect identification
Genetic distance-based (Best match)	Many-against-each other search	Correct (match) Ambiguous Incorrect (mismatch)
Genetic distance-based (Best close match)	Many-against-each other search	Correct (match) Ambiguous Incorrect (mismatch) No-match (under threshold %)
Genetic distance-based (Barcoding gap)	Many-against-each other search	Intra-specific genetic distance Inter-specific genetic distance Barcoding gap
Character-based (Nucleotide polymorphism)	Many-against-each other search	Variable sites Indels Sequence length GC% contents
Tree-based	Many-against-each other search	Monophylectic Paraphylectic Polyphylectic

4.3.2 Raw Data Sequence Pre-editing

In Sanger sequencing, trace files (also known as electropherograms) are produced as digital representation of DNA sequences. The first step of bioinformatics analysis is to 'edit' the sequences in which the 'messy' parts are removed, and only 'reliable' parts are retained.

1. For each sequencing sample, four files are provided, including two sets of files for each forward and reverse sequences with the extensions '.ab1' and '.txt'.

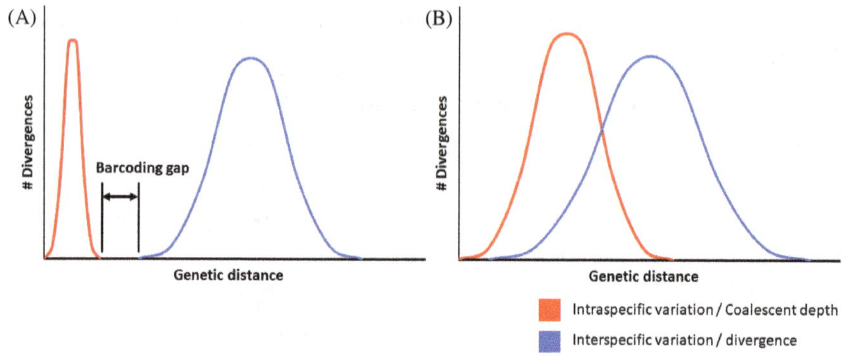

Fig. 4.2 Diagrammatic hypothetical frequency distributions of genetic distances within and between species for two cases: (A) clear 'barcoding gap' formed by the discrete distributions of intraspecific variation and interspecific variation, and (B) overlapping distributions between intra- and interspecific variation and no barcode gap to give ambiguous results.

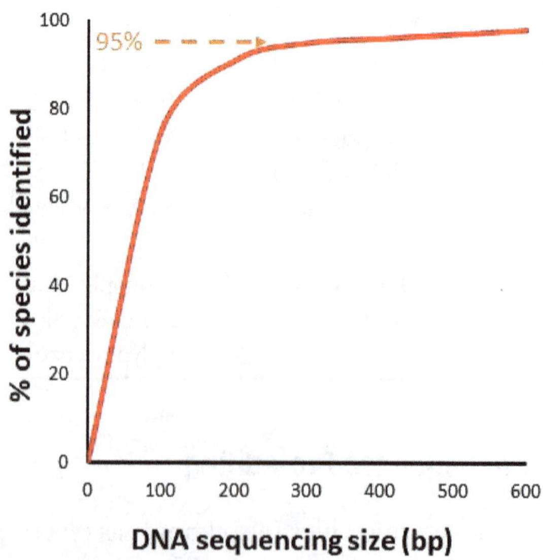

Fig. 4.3 Schematic diagram between the resolution of identification results with a length of DNA sequences for analysis.

2. Open BioEdit program, select *File > New Alignment (Ctrl + N)*.
3. Import both forward and reverse sequences in either '.ab1' or '.txt' by *File >Import > Sequence alignment file*.
4. Reverse complement for the reverse sequence by *Sequence > Nucleic Acid > Reverse complement (Shift + Ctrl + R)*.
5. Align both forward and reverse sequences by *Accessory Application > ClustalW Multiple alignment > Run ClustalW.*
6. Ensure to select mode from 'Select/Slide' to 'Edit' using the dropdown menu (Figure 4.4).
7. Find both forward and reverse primer locations by *Edit > Search > Find (Ctrl + F)* and delete the primer site plus upstream/downstream for forward/reverse primers, respectively (Note: The reverse primer should be reverse complemented in advance for successful searching).

   Remark: For those ambiguous nucleotide (i.e., different nucleotide at same position, or gaps '-'), open the sequencing electropherogram (trace) file (i.e., the '.ab1' file) in SnapGene Viewer program, select 'Show Quality Value' to analyse the Phred quality Scores (Q value) of the corresponding bases (Figure 4.5A). Q value is a measure of the quality of base calling in sequencing — it is logarithmically linked to the base-calling error probabilities. The higher the Q value, the higher the probability that the base

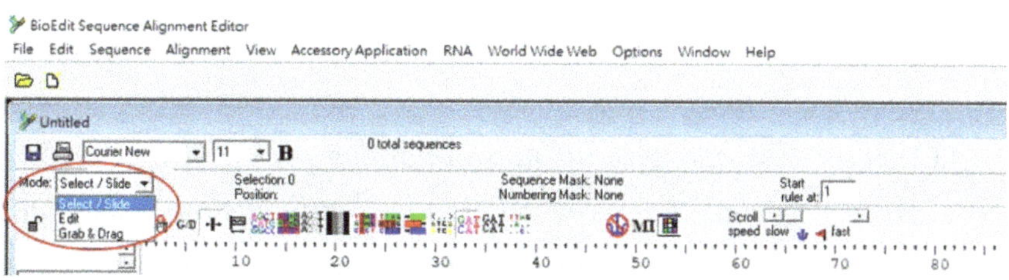

Fig. 4.4 Mode selection in BioEdit program.

(A)

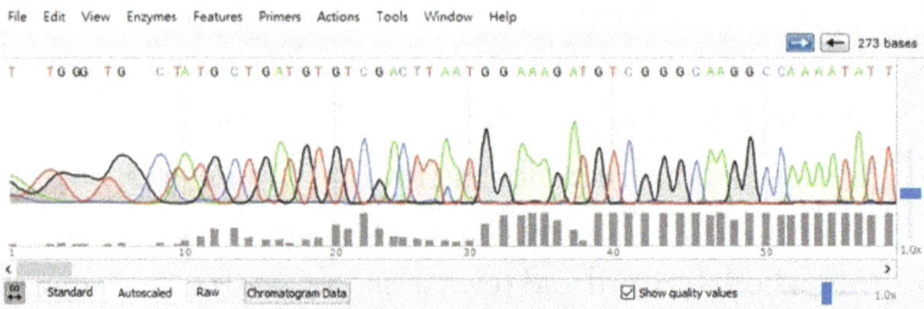

(B)

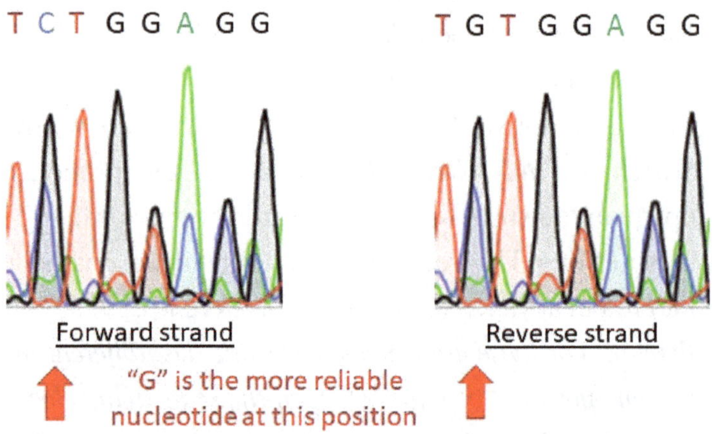

Fig. 4.5 (A) Electropherogram and Q value of raw data showing in SnapGene Viewer program and (B) schematic diagram on ambiguous nucleotide in electropherogram file.

calling is correct, and vice versa. Generally, scores above Q20 (represents 1% error rate) or Q30 (represents 0.1% error rate) are regarded as acceptable. For those traces conflict (i.e., different coloured peaks appear in the same location on the forward and reverse electropherograms), the user can generally decide which one is more reliable based on sequence quality (e.g., higher Q value, less background noise or taller peaks) (Figure 4.5B). User can replace the more reliable nucleotide using 'Edit' mode in BioEdit program to modify the consensus sequences manually.

8. Create a consensus sequence by *Alignment > Create Consensus Sequence*, the conserved sequence sites will show as '·'.

9. In 'Edit' mode, replace the more reliable nucleotide to obtain consensus sequences manually.
10. Export the consensus sequences in Fast Alignment and Search Tool-All (FASTA) format by *Edit > Copy sequence to clipboard (FASTA format)*.

4.3.3 Global Alignment

Sequence alignment is a way to arrange DNA, RNA or protein sequences according to their similarity, and to identify the homologous region, which reflects functional, structural, or evolutionary relationships between the sequences. Since it is assumed that two sequences in an alignment share a common ancestor, mismatches can be interpreted as point mutations and gaps as insertion or deletion mutations (indels in short) introduced in one or both lineages in the time they diverged. In global alignment, the entire length of all query sequences is 'forced' to align and represent as rows within a matrix. Gaps are inserted between the residues so that identical or similar characters are aligned in successive columns. Software such as BioEdit with ClustalW function is the most useful and fully automatic program for small-scale sequence alignment.

1. Open BioEdit program, select *File > New Alignment (Ctrl + N)*.
2. Import all query sequences in '.fasta' format by *File > Import > Sequence alignment file*.
3. Ensure all query sequences are in similar length.
4. For those sequence with wrong orientation, create reverse complement sequence by *Sequence > Nucleic Acid > Reverse Complement (Shift + Ctrl + R)*.
5. Conduct global alignment by *Accessory Application > ClustalW Multiple alignment*, select 'Run ClustalW'.

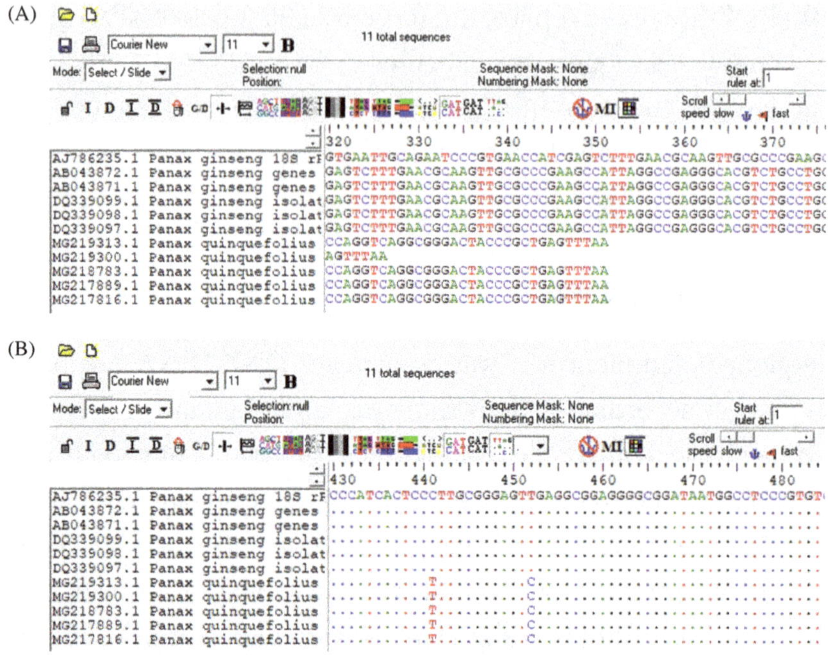

Fig. 4.6 DNA sequences (A) before alignment and (B) after ClustalW global alignment (in Conservation plot view) using BioEdit program.

6. User can simplify the view by *View > Conservation plot*, conserve position will show as '·' while a gap will show as '-', in reference to the first query sequence (Figure 4.6).

However, global alignment is suitable only if all query sequences share global homology with roughly an equal size. If the intergenic spacers are too varied or the two conserved regions are too far apart, global alignment may lead to a missing search and not be able to recognise the conserved ends, then local alignment should be used instead (Section 4.3.4).

4.3.4 Local Alignment

Local alignment analyses the whole sequence in a fragmented way and identify local regions of similarity within long sequences that are often widely divergent overall. It is more useful for dissimilar sequences that are suspected to contain regions of similarity or similar sequence motifs within their larger sequence context. In comparison with global alignment, these sequences may be excluded from the search, since only small portions of sequences are similar to the target with great dissimilarity overall. NCBI BLAST is a widely used local alignment program for the quick authentication of sequence identity by searching the best homologous sequences (i.e., best hits) from the NCBI GenBank database. However, it must be stressed that the identification of local alignment may not be correct when the query coverage is low, even though the sequence similarity is shown as 100%. In a local alignment program, the region of sequences that has no significant similarity will be excluded from the calculation. As an extreme example, suppose sequence A and sequence B are the two candidates with 200 bp for local alignment with a reference sequence. The entire sequence of sequence A is 100% matched with the reference. On the other hand, only the first 100 bp of sequence B is 100% matched with the reference while the rest has no shared similarity to the reference. In spite of this, BLAST will show that the similarities of the two sequences are 100%. In fact, we should conclude that the query sequence is identical to species A but not species B, even if the first 100 nucleotides of species B is identical to the query. In addition, when using the BLAST program, it should be stressed that the success of identification depends on the availability of sequences deposited in databases and the query species must be already exist in the database, otherwise failure of identification will occur (Kim, Kim, Son, & Kim, 2015).

1. Access https://blast.ncbi.nlm.nih.gov/Blast.cgi/, select 'Nucleotide BLAST (BLASTn)'.
2. Paste the query sequence in FASTA format into the box 'Enter accession number(s), gi(s), or FASTA sequence(s)'.

3. Make sure to select database as 'Standard databases (nr etc.)' and optimize the program for 'Highly similar sequences (megablast)' (Figure 4.7 and circled in red).

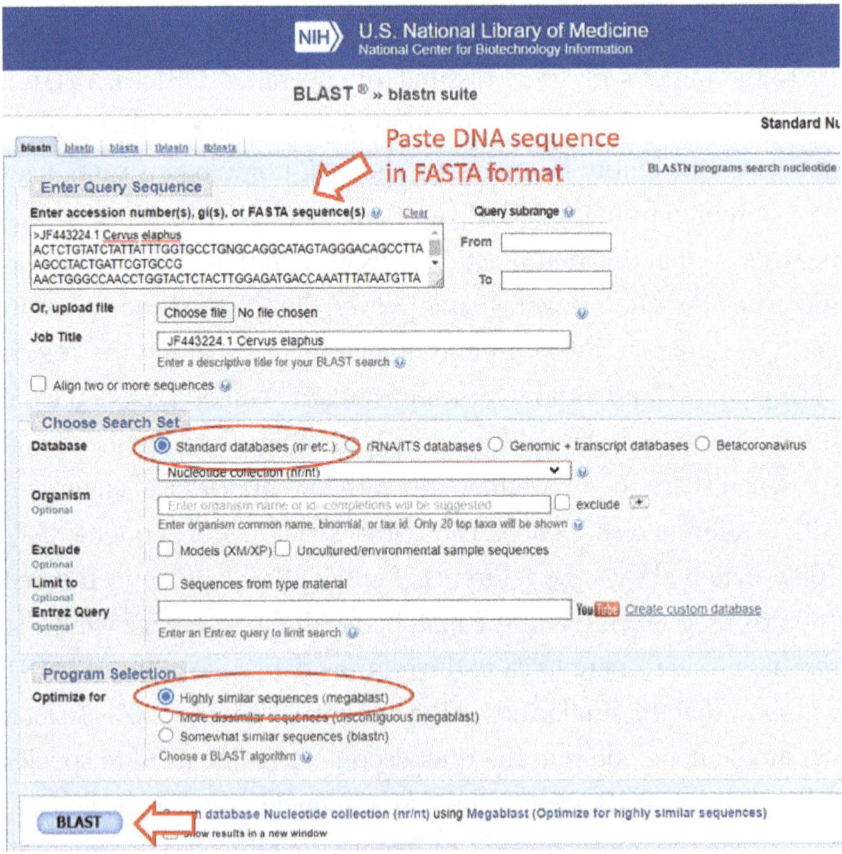

Fig. 4.7 Nucleotide BLAST platform for query sequence input.

BLAST will display the information of the query sequence and BLAST search criteria specified by the user, with search results in four parts:

- Descriptions: Table lists out the sequence accession number, species description and the scores of matched database sequences. Results are arranged according to the closest matched library sequence (i.e., the highest % identity) at the top. Major statistical data are displayed: (1) 'Max Score', which indicates the highest alignment score (bit-score) between the query DNA barcode and the library sequence segment (higher the better — 1,000 is very good), and (2) 'E-value', which indicates the number of alignments expected by chance (closer to zero is better) (Figure 4.8).

- Graphic summary: Showing the alignments between query and database sequences in a graphical way. Five colour keys (black, blue, green, pink and red) denote the score ranges of alignment:

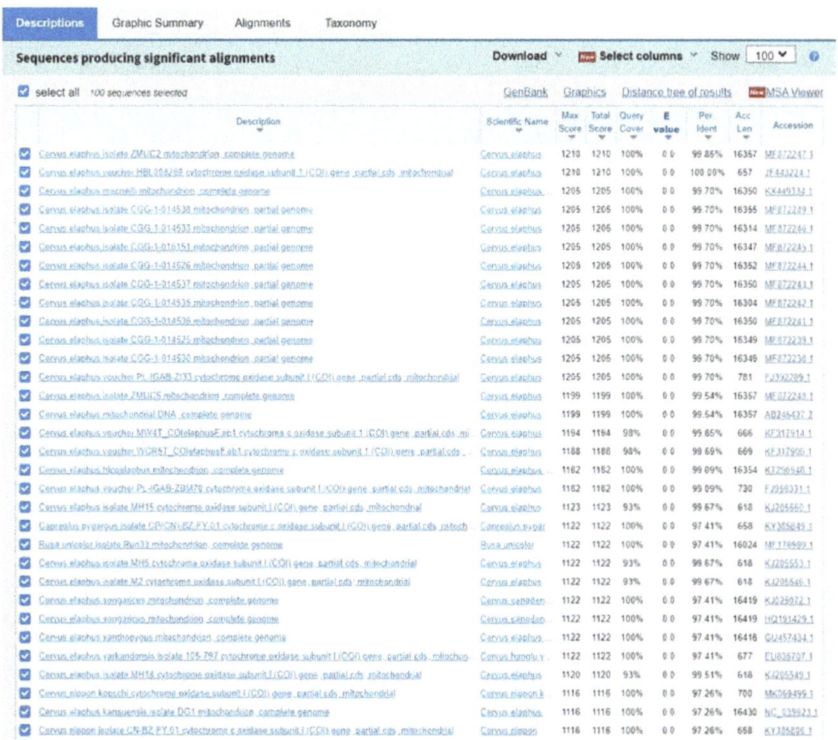

Fig. 4.8 Nucleotide BLAST result — descriptions.

the black key is the lowest while the red key is the highest. Below these keys, the query sequence is represented as a blue-green bar labelled with 'Query'. The numbers underneath the blue-green bar indicate the nucleotide positions. The closest matching library sequence is shown immediately following the query sequence (Figure 4.9).

- Alignments: Showing the local alignment results between the query and database sequence with corresponding BLAST scores (Figure 4.10).
- Taxonomy: Showing the taxonomy of matched database sequences with the query sequence (Figure 4.11).

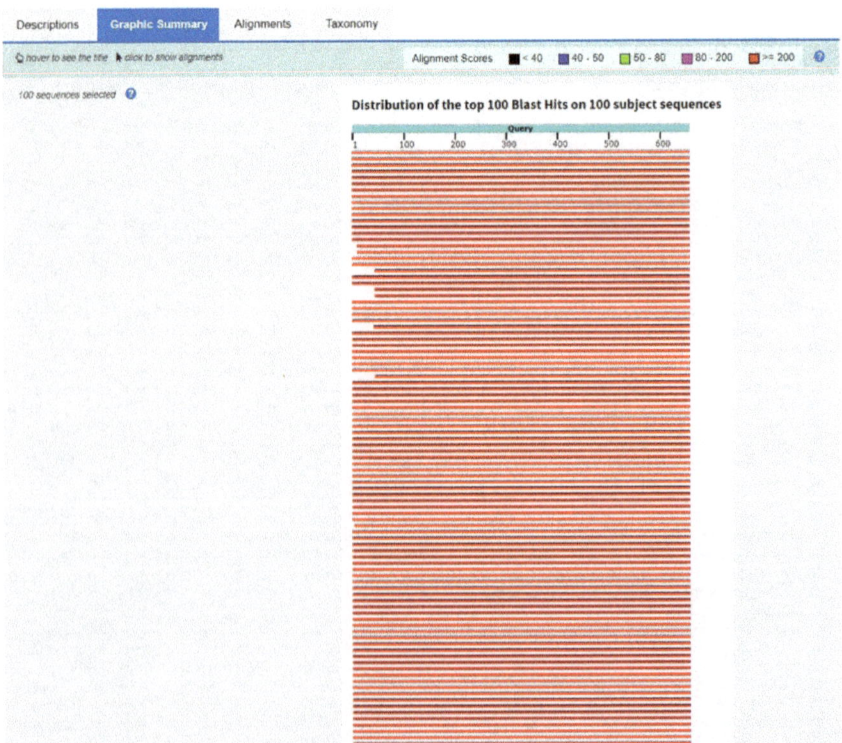

Fig. 4.9 Nucleotide BLAST result — graphic Summary.

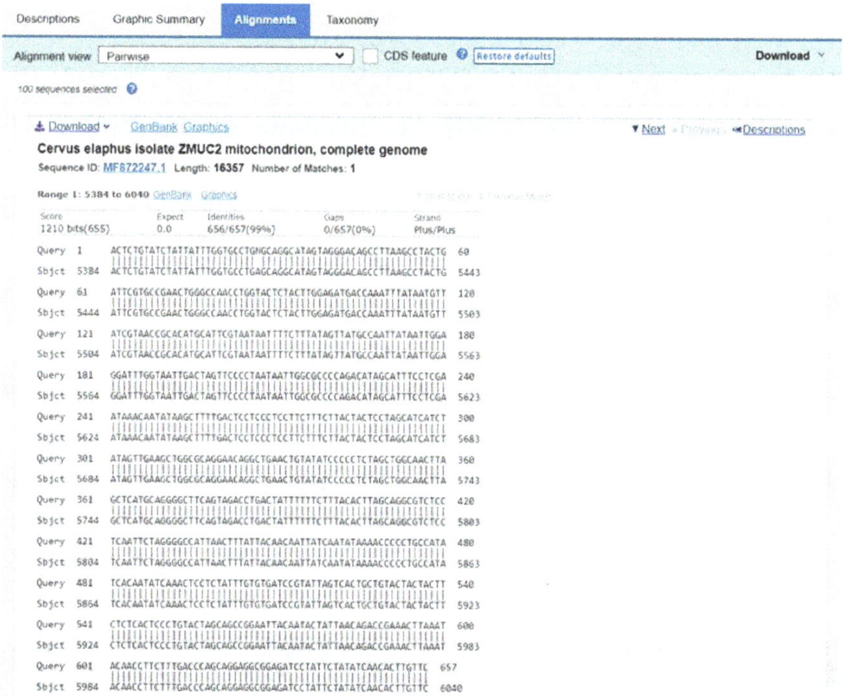

Fig. 4.10 Nucleotide BLAST result — alignments.

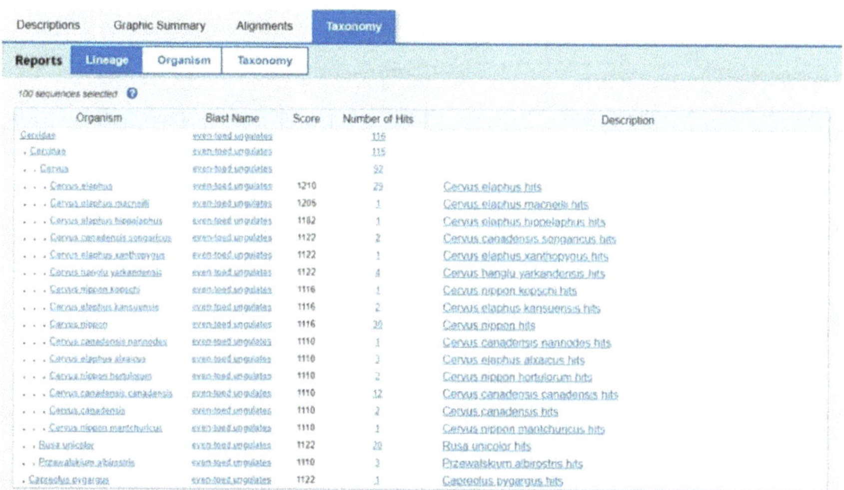

Fig. 4.11 Nucleotide BLAST result — taxonomy.

4.3.5 BOLD Identification Engine

Besides the taxonomy and DNA database, BOLD also provides an identification service in which the user can submit a query sequence for comparison against the BOLD DNA barcode database.

1. Access https://www.boldsystems.org/, select 'Identification'.
2. Select the concerned gene region (circle in red) and database for identification (Figure 4.12).
3. Paste the query DNA sequence in FASTA format into the box and select 'Submit'.
4. In 'Identification engine: Results' page, a list of DNA barcode library records and their similarity to the query

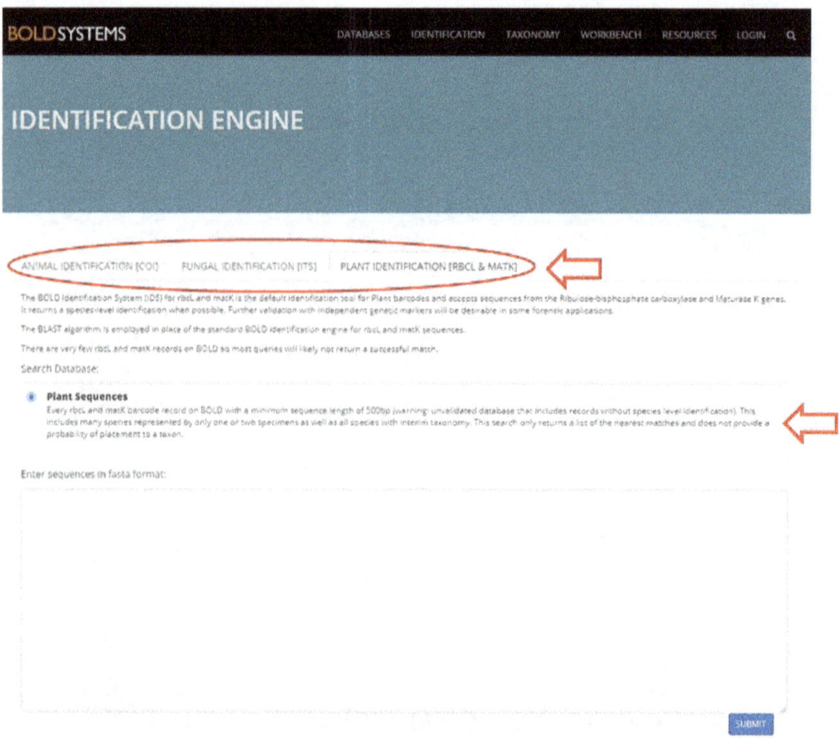

Fig. 4.12 BOLD identification engine.

unknown specimen will be displayed. Taxonomic assignment and sequence similarity between unknown and reference sequences are also available for analysis. User can acquire more information such as a taxonomy record and phylogenetic tree showing the nearest taxa via a hyperlink (Figure 4.13).

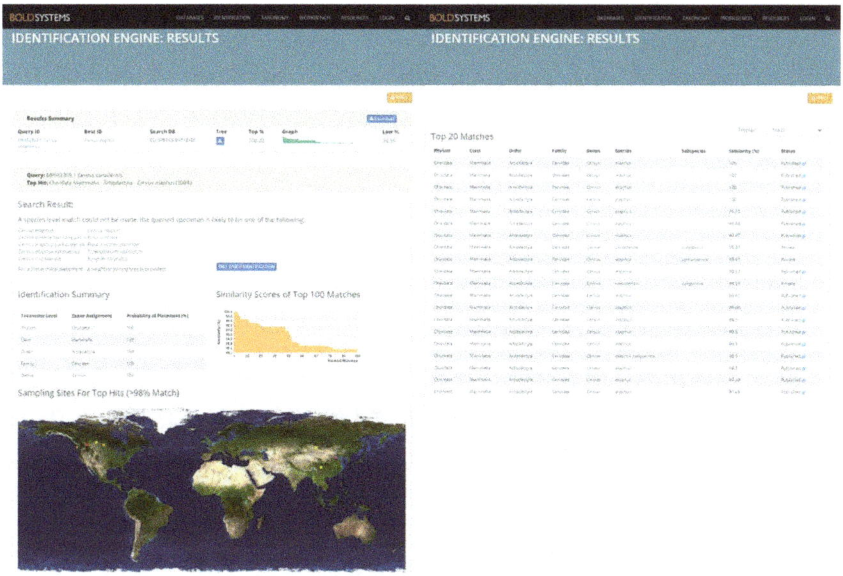

Fig. 4.13 BOLD identification result.

4.3.6 MMDBD, a One-stop Solution

With the upgrade of MMDBD into v1.5, which is a 'One-stop, three steps approach' platform, bioinformatics tools including 'BLAST', 'Clustal Omerga' and 'Primer3' are integrated, which allow users to get the three major identification and primer-designing tools in one platform (Figure 4.14) and avoid the possible errors from repeatedly copying and pasting the sequence across various platforms.

- Step 1: Sample sequence is searched in a built-in BLAST system against all sequences in an MMDBD database.

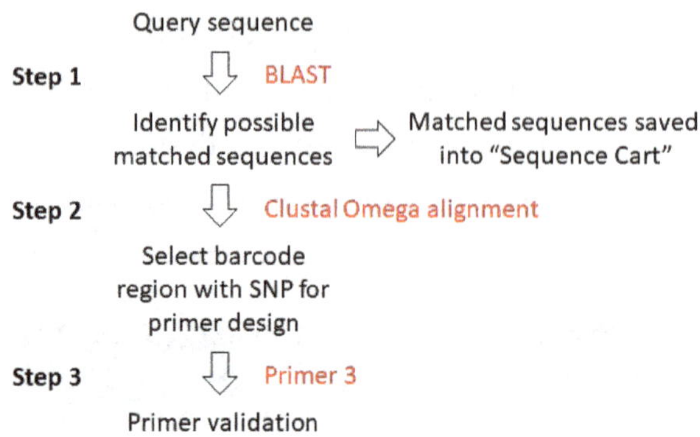

Fig. 4.14 General workflow of 'one-stop, three steps approach' for BLAST, Clustal Omega alignment and primer design.

- Step 2: The best match sequence can be saved into an intermediate sequence storage named 'Sequence Cart', which is generated by the web server automatically for each visitor. Then, on the Alignment & Primer Design page, users can recall the sequences in 'Sequence Cart' and import them for 'Clustal Omega' global alignment.
- Step 3: Users can pick their own primer for amplification based on the alignment results with the built-in 'Primer3' or receive suggested primers from the program.

Workflow of Analysis Using MMDBD

1. Access https://rdccm.cuhk.edu.hk/mherbsdb/, select 'BLAST'.
2. Paste the query sequence in FASTA format into the box, select 'BLAST' to run.
3. Highly similar sequences are shown in red. User can click on each result entry to view the sequence information and add the sequences into the 'Sequence Cart' by clicking 'Place into the cart' (circle in red) (Figure 4.15).
4. The Sequence Cart can be viewed anytime by clicking the orange 'Sequence Cart' on the right. Sometimes, if sequences

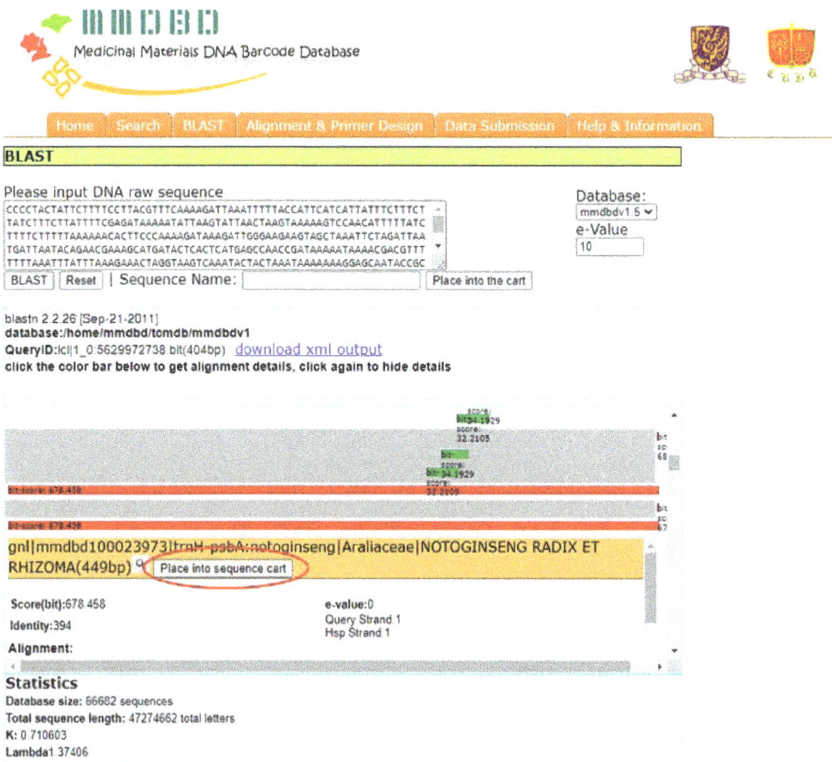

Fig. 4.15 BLAST function in MMDBD.

are stored in a reverse complement way, which cannot be aligned, they can be individually converted into complement, reverse or reverse complement sequences from 'Sequence Cart' (Figure 4.16).

5. Go to the 'Alignment & Primer Design' page, recall the 'Sequence Cart' panel on the right.
6. All the sequences in the cart can be submitted for Clustal Omega alignment by clicking 'Use all the sequence in cart' button, ensure 'DNA' sequence is selected, change parameters if necessary and select 'Submit' to run the alignment (Figure 4.17).
7. Alignment results will show the forensically informative nucleotide (FIN) sites or called nucleotide signatures, which

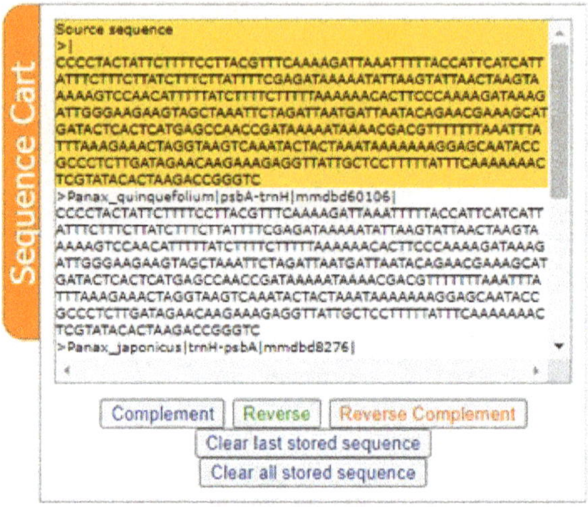

Fig. 4.16 Sequence cart in MMDBD.

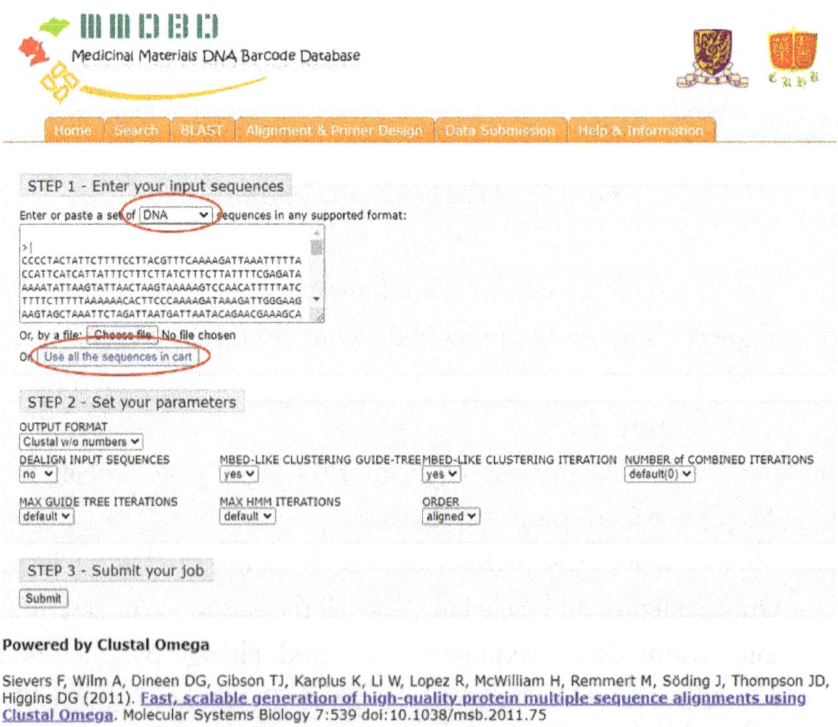

Fig. 4.17 Clustal Omega alignment function in MMDBD.

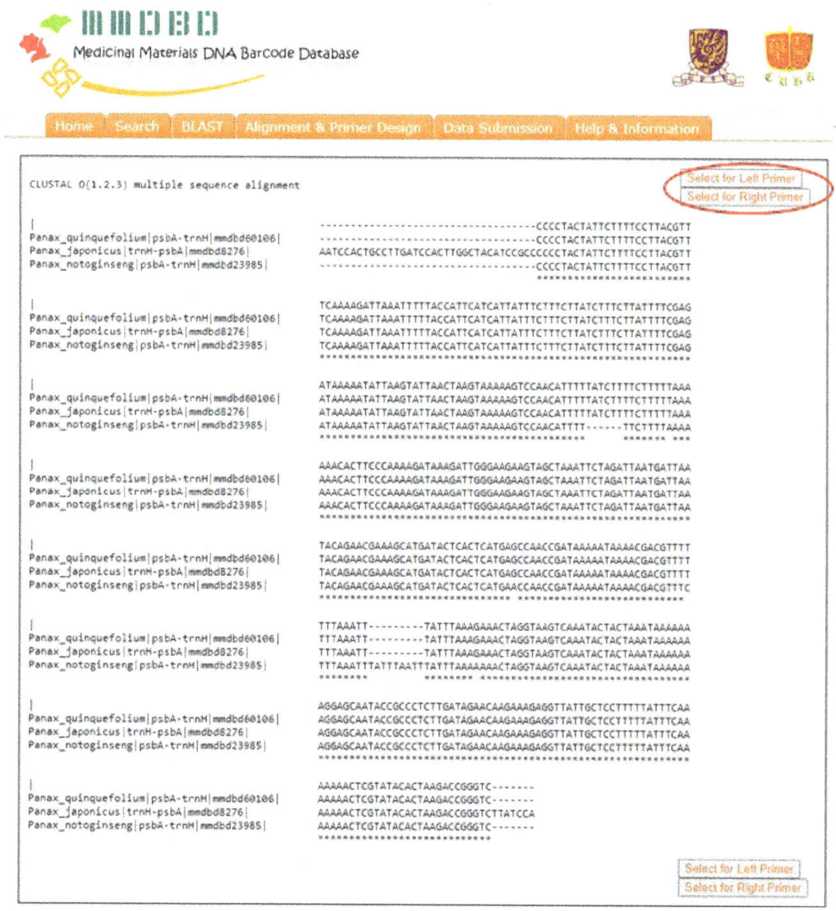

Fig. 4.18 Clustal Omega alignment results showing the FINs and primer selection function.

are species-specific nucleotides in a certain DNA region and can be used to discriminate the species from its common adulterants or closely related species (Figure 4.18). It is necessary to align different DNA regions of the target species and their adulterants/closely related species before carrying out any 'wet lab' experiment.

8. If FINs of the target species are found, the user may try to design species-specific primers with the FINs on the 3' end

of primers, or primers that flank the FINs for sequencing (Li, Zhang, But, & Shaw, 2011). This can be easily done by highlighting the potential primer sequence and clicking on the button 'Select for Left Primer' or 'Select for Right Primer' to transfer the highlighted DNA sequence to the interface of the 'Primer3'. The first DNA entry in the alignment will also be automatically loaded to 'Primer3' as the DNA template. To select the sequence for the opposite primer, close the Primer3 pop-up window, highlight the chosen sequence and click the 'Select for Left (or Right) Primer' button (Figure 4.18). Then both primer sequences will be entered to 'Primer3'.

9. Check the parameter in the primer design tool pop-up box and select 'Pick Primers'. Primer3 output can then be reviewed (Figure 4.19).

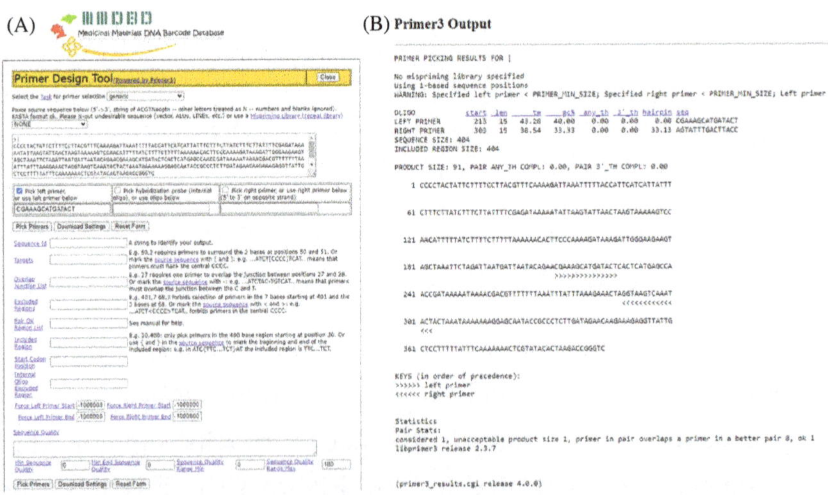

Fig. 4.19 Primer 3 (**A**) pop-up box and (**B**) output primer results.

4.4 Taxonomic Identification

Due to the incompleteness of DNA barcode reference libraries and inconsistencies in the use of Linnaean names, it is valuable and common practice to cluster DNA barcodes into Operational Taxonomic Units (OTU) (Casas *et al.*, 2018; Ratnasingham & Hebert, 2013; Sukantamala, Sing, Jaturas, Polseela, & Wilson, 2017). Among various clustering methods, the character-based method utilises nucleotide polymorphism features such as variable sites, sequence length variation, indel information and GC% content, etc., as tools for identification (Guo, Luo, Liu, & Wang, 2012; Kim *et al.*, 2015; Shaw, Lickey, Schilling, & Small, 2007; Tanee, 2012; Vu, Huynh, Tran, & Le, 2018). In genetic distance-based methods, intra- and inter-specific differences between query and reference sequences are compared based on the smallest genetic distances ('Nearest Distance') (Feng *et al.*, 2015) or the most similarity ('Best match' and 'Best close match') (Guo, Huang, Liu, & Wang, 2016; Meier, Shiyang, Vaidya, & Ng, 2006; Xiang, Hu, Wang, & Jin, 2011; Xu *et al.*, 2015).

One of the most widely used clustering method is the tree-based method, which is a simple and easily visualised approach, and is used in various classification studies (Asahina *et al.*, 2010; Chattopadhyay *et al.*, 2017; Ghorbani, Gravendeel, Selliah, Zarre, & de Boer, 2017; Givnish *et al.*, 2015; Guo *et al.*, 2016; H. M. Kim *et al.*, 2014; Parveen *et al.*, 2017; Poovitha, Stalin, Balaji, & Parani, 2016; Rajaram *et al.*, 2019; Tang *et al.*, 2015; Truong, Khanh, Ham, Duong, & Khoa, 2013; Wu *et al.*, 2012; Xiang *et al.*, 2011; Xu *et al.*, 2015). Tree-building algorithms attempt to examine all possible topologies and reconstruct the order in which sequence mutations accumulated as different lineages diverged from a common ancestor. Query sequence is compared against a 'backbone' tree, and the priori criterion is applied for species delimitation and flagging novel sequences as potentially new species. Two species are completely separated when all sequences of one species are clustered in a monophyletic branch (Meyer & Paulay, 2005). The tree constructed is presented in the way that the length of line represents the evolutionary distance. Roughly speaking, a higher in sequence identity suggests that the sequences in question have a comparatively young common ancestor, whereas low identity suggests that the divergence is more ancient. Thus, this approximation reflects the 'molecular clock' hypothesis. However, it should be stressed that the tree constructed is not technically 'phylogenetic' trees that should be constructed with the basis of synapomorphies, whereas this method produced phenetic trees based on sequence similarity. In addition, limited sequence information (400–800 bp) may not be enough to reflect the evolutional relationship.

In a tree-based method, Neighbour-joining (NJ), Maximum Likelihood (ML), Maximum Parsimony (MP), Bayesian (BA) or Unweighted Pair Group Method with Arithmetic Mean (UPGMA) are common phylogenetic algorithms inferred along with suitable models. In the NJ model, sequences with best matching sequences are linked as 'neighbours' that share common nodes in the tree. It builds a tree from the bottom up by comparing the evolutionary distance between pairs of DNA sequences. The chief advantage of this method is that it is simple, fast and computationally less intensive than other methods; it also always retrieves a single tree regardless of ambiguity in the data. On the other hand, the ML algorithm evaluates all possible trees and determines which is most likely to be produced by the observed data and gives a more accurate tree model.

To construct the tree, the Molecular Evolutionary Genetics Analysis (MEGA) program is a cross interface (graphical and command line) and cross platform (Microsoft Windows and Linux operating systems) software that includes a large repertoire of programs for assembling sequence alignments, inferring evolutionary trees, estimating genetic distance and diversities, inferring ancestral sequences, computing time trees and testing selection (Kumar,

Stecher, & Tamura, 2016). It is an extremely popular program for tree-building and is free to download from the program's website (Tamura, Stecher, Peterson, Filipski, & Kumar, 2013).

Steps of Analysis using MEGA Program

1. Open the MEGA program.
2. Select *File > Open A File/Session*, select the aligned query sequences in FASTA format (e.g., sequences_aligned.fasta).
3. Open the FASTA file and select 'Analyse'.
4. Ensure 'Nucleotide Sequences' is selected, select the correct genetic code.
5. Select the 'Phylogeny' button and phylogenetic algorithms in the dropdown menu for tree construction. It should be noted that an NJ tree is fast but not accurate enough, while the ML tree is slow but more accurate, and the MP tree is of medium speed and accuracy (Figure 4.20).

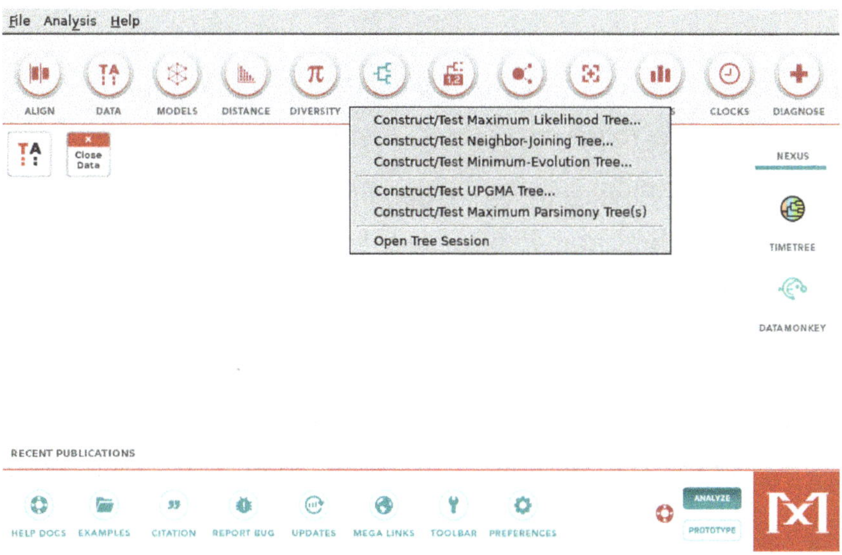

Fig. 4.20 Dropdown menu of 'Phylogeny' button in MEGA program.

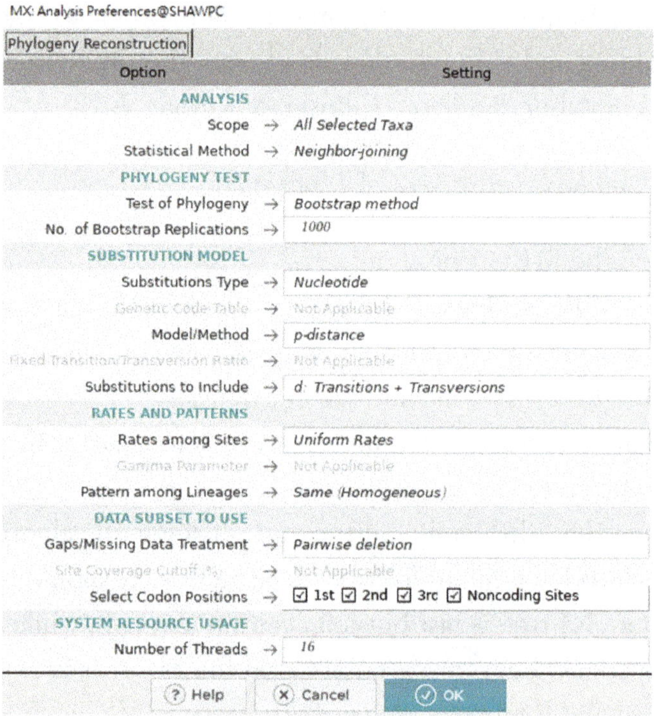

Fig. 4.21 Analysis preferences window options summary tab in MEGA program.

6. In the 'Analysis Preferences window Options Summary' tab, choose the following options (Figure 4.21):
   - Test of Phylogeny: Bootstrap method
   - No. of Bootstrap Replications: 1,000 (i.e., repeat 1,000 times)
   - Substitutions Type: Nucleotide
   - Model/Method: *p*-distance
   - Substitutions to Include: *d*: Transitions + Transversions
   - Gaps/Missing Data Treatment: Pairwise deletion
   - Specify the maximum number of cores to be deployed in the analysis

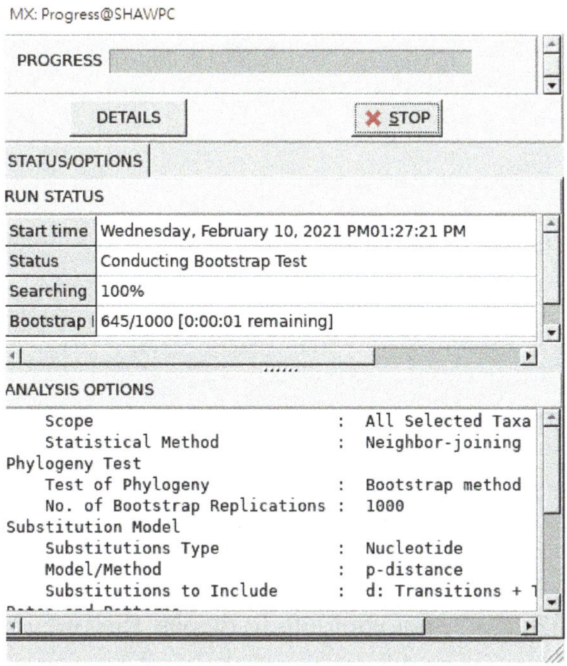

Fig. 4.22 Progress indicator in MEGA program.

7. Computation will then begin. A 'Progress indicator' will appear (Figure 4.22) during this process before the tree is displayed in the Tree Explorer.
8. The tree produced (Figure 4.23) can then be exported as a Newick (text) file (e.g., tree.nwk) by *File > Export Current Tree (Newick)*.
9. To select a branch, click on it with the left mouse button. If you click on a branch with the right mouse button, you will get a small options menu that will let you flip the branch or other operations on it. To edit the taxon labels, double click on them.
10. Change the branch style by *View > Tree/Branch Style*.

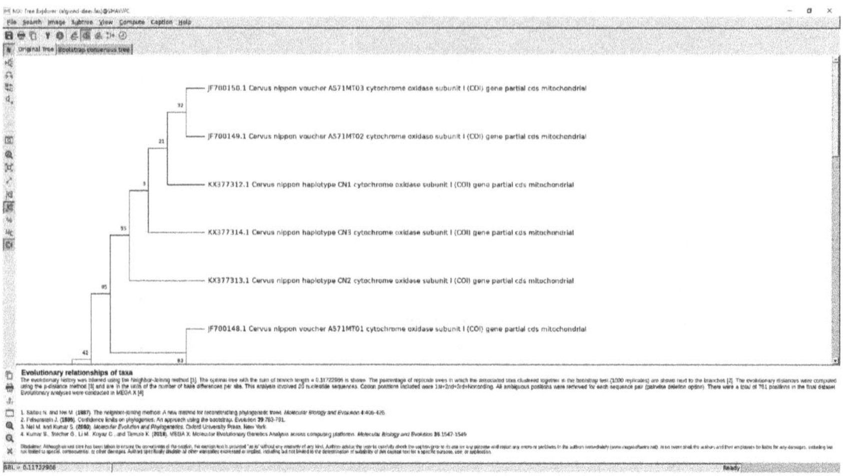

Fig. 4.23 Tree produced in MEGA program.

11. Select *View* > *Topology Only* to display the branching pattern (i.e., without actual branch lengths on the screen).
12. Edit your tree to create the image that you want to use in your publication or report. The tree can then be exported by *Image* > *Save as PDF file* or *Image/Save as PNG file*.

4.5 Conclusion

Correctly identified medicinal materials are the premise of research and applications. DNA authentication is an accurate method for the routine identification of medicinal materials. During this process, bioinformatics assists in: (1) providing a means for the storing, sorting, retrieving and analysing of experimental data; (2) providing computer programs for identifying the unknown sample by matching with the reference sequences and (3) aiding the design of appropriate testing procedures and identification tools. This chapter describes the application of bioinformatics in molecular authentication, introduces the databases and analytical tools, and provides guidelines to obtain high-quality DNA sequences for bioinformatics analysis and instructions on how to operate various software programs as well as the primer design. For molecular authentication of medicinal materials, a reliable database as reference for sequence comparison is of paramount importance. At present, many sequence data disposed in public databases have not been validated. Therefore, it is essential to exercise caution when using these public sequence data.

References

Asahina, H., Shinozaki, J., Masuda, K., Morimitsu, Y., & Satake, M. (2010). Identification of medicinal Dendrobium species by phylogenetic analyses using matK and rbcL sequences. *J Nat Med, 64*(2), 133–138. doi:10.1007/s11418-009-0379-8

Casas, P. A. S., Sing, K. W., Lee, P. S., Nuneza, O. M., Villanueva, R. J. T., & Wilson, J. J. (2018). DNA barcodes for dragonflies and damselflies (Odonata) of Mindanao, Philippines. *Mitochondrial DNA A DNA Mapp Seq Anal, 29*(2), 206–211. doi:10.1080/24701394.2016.1267157

Chattopadhyay, P., Banerjee, G., & Banerjee, N. (2017). Distinguishing orchid species by DNA barcoding: Increasing the resolution of population studies in plant biology. *OMICS J Integr Biol, 21*(12), 711–720. doi:10.1089/omi.2017.0131

Duong, T., Trung, K., Nghia, L., Thuy, N., Hien, P., Khoa, N., Dung, T. H., Trung, D. M., & Khanh, T. (2018). Identification of Vietnamese native Dendrobium species based on ribosomal DNA internal transcribed spacer sequence. *Adv Stud Biol, 10*, 1–12. doi:10.12988/asb.2018.7823

Feng, S., Jiang, Y., Wang, S., Jiang, M., Chen, Z., Ying, Q., & Wang, H. (2015). Molecular identification of Dendrobium species (Orchidaceae) based on the DNA barcode ITS2 region and its application for phylogenetic study. *Int J Mol Sci, 16*(9), 21975–21988. doi:10.3390/ijms160921975

Ghorbani, A., Gravendeel, B., Selliah, S., Zarre, S., & de Boer, H. (2017). DNA barcoding of tuberous Orchidoideae: A resource for identification of orchids used in Salep. *Mol Ecol Resour, 17*(2), 342–352. doi:10.1111/1755-0998.12615

Ginibun, F. C., Saad, M. R. M., Hong, T. L., Othman, R. Y., Khalid, N., & Bhassu, S. (2010). Chloroplast DNA barcoding of Spathoglottis species for genetic conservation. *Acta Hortic, 878*, 453-459.

Givnish, T. J., Spalink, D., Ames, M., Lyon, S. P., Hunter, S. J., Zuluaga, A., William, J. D. Iles, Clements, M. A., Arroyo, M. T. K., Leebens-Mack, J., Endara, L., Kriebel, R., Neubig, K. M., Whitten, W. M., Williams, N. H., & Cameron, K. M. (2015). Orchid phylogenomics and multiple drivers of their extraordinary diversification. *Proc Biol Sci, 282*(1814). doi:10.1098/rspb.2015.1553

Guo, Y. Y., Huang, L. Q., Liu, Z. J., & Wang, X. Q. (2016). Promise and challenge of DNA barcoding in venus slipper (Paphiopedilum). *PLoS One, 11*(1), e0146880. doi:10.1371/journal.pone.0146880

Guo, Y. Y., Luo, Y. B., Liu, Z. J., & Wang, X. Q. (2012). Evolution and biogeography of the slipper orchids: Eocene vicariance of the conduplicate genera in the old and new world tropics. *PLoS One, 7*(6), e38788. doi:10.1371/journal.pone.0038788

Kim, H. M., Oh, S. H., Bhandari, G. S., Kim, C. S., & Park, C. W. (2014). DNA barcoding of Orchidaceae in Korea. *Mol Ecol Resour, 14*(3), 499–507. doi:10.1111/1755-0998.12207

Kim, J. S., Kim, H. T., Son, S. W., & Kim, J. H. (2015). Molecular identification of endangered Korean lady's slipper orchids (Cypripedium, Orchidaceae) and related taxa. *Botany, 93*(9), 603–610. doi:10.1139/cjb-2014-0255

Kumar, S., Stecher, G., & Tamura, K. (2016). MEGA7: Molecular evolutionary genetics analysis version 7.0 for bigger datasets. *Mol Biol Evol, 33*(7), 1870–1874. doi:10.1093/molbev/msw054

Leray, M., Knowlton, N., Ho, S. L., Nguyen, B. N., & Machida, R. J. (2019). GenBank is a reliable resource for 21st century biodiversity research. *Proc Nat Acad Sci USA, 116*(45), 22651–22656. doi:10.1073/pnas.1911714116

Li, M., Zhang, K. Y., But, P. P., & Shaw, P. C. (2011). Forensically informative nucleotide sequencing (FINS) for the authentication of Chinese medicinal materials. *Chin Med, 6*, 42. doi:10.1186/1749-8546-6-42

Lou, S. K., Wong, K. L., Li, M., But, P. P., Tsui, S. K., & Shaw, P. C. (2010). An integrated web medicinal materials DNA database: MMDBD (Medicinal Materials DNA Barcode Database). *BMC Genomics, 11*, 402. doi:10.1186/1471-2164-11-402

Luscombe, N. M., Greenbaum, D., & Gerstein, M. (2001). What is bioinformatics? A proposed definition and overview of the field. *Methods Inf Med, 40*(4), 346–358. Retrieved from https://www.ncbi.nlm.nih.gov/pubmed/11552348

Meier, R., Shiyang, K., Vaidya, G., & Ng, P. K. (2006). DNA barcoding and taxonomy in Diptera: A tale of high intraspecific variability and low identification success. *Syst Biol, 55*(5), 715–728. doi:10.1080/10635150600969864

Meiklejohn, K. A., Damaso, N., & Robertson, J. M. (2019). Assessment of BOLD and GenBank — Their accuracy and reliability for the identification of biological materials. *PLoS One, 14*(6), e0217084. doi:10.1371/journal.pone.0217084

Meusnier, I., Singer, G. A., Landry, J. F., Hickey, D. A., Hebert, P. D., & Hajibabaei, M. (2008). A universal DNA mini-barcode for biodiversity analysis. *BMC Genomics, 9*, 214. doi:10.1186/1471-2164-9-214

Meyer, C. P., & Paulay, G. (2005). DNA barcoding: Error rates based on comprehensive sampling. *PLoS Biol, 3*(12), e422. doi:10.1371/journal.pbio.0030422

Parveen, I., Singh, H. K., Malik, S., Raghuvanshi, S., & Babbar, S. B. (2017). Evaluating five different loci (rbcL, rpoB, rpoC1, matK, and ITS) for DNA barcoding of Indian orchids. *Genome, 60*(8), 665–671. doi:10.1139/gen-2016-0215

Poovitha, S., Stalin, N., Balaji, R., & Parani, M. (2016). Multi-locus DNA barcoding identifies matK as a suitable marker for species identification in Hibiscus L. *Genome, 59*(12), 1150–1156. doi:10.1139/gen-2015-0205

Rajaram, M. C., Yong, C., Azlan, G. J., & Go, R. (2019). DNA barcoding of endangered Paphiopedilum species (Orchidaceae) of Peninsular Malaysia. *Phytotaxa, 387*(2), 94–104.

Ratnasingham, S., & Hebert, P. D. (2007). The barcode of life data system. *Mol Ecol Notes, 7*(3), 355–364. doi:10.1111/j.1471-8286.2007.01678.x

Ratnasingham, S., & Hebert, P. D. (2013). A DNA-based registry for all animal species: The barcode index number (BIN) system. *PLoS One, 8*(7), e66213. doi:10.1371/journal.pone.0066213

Santos, C., & Pereira, F. (2018). Identification of plant species using variable length chloroplast DNA sequences. *Forensic Sci Int Genet, 36*, 1–12. doi:10.1016/j.fsigen.2018.05.009

Shaw, J., Lickey, E. B., Schilling, E. E., & Small, R. L. (2007). Comparison of whole chloroplast genome sequences to choose noncoding regions for phylogenetic studies in angiosperms: The tortoise and the hare III. *Am J Bot, 94*(3), 275–288. doi:10.3732/ajb.94.3.275

Singh, H. K., Parveen, I., Raghuvanshi, S., & Babbar, S. B. (2012). The loci recommended as universal barcodes for plants on the basis of floristic studies may not work with congeneric species as exemplified by DNA barcoding of Dendrobium species. *BMC Res Notes, 5*, 42. doi:10.1186/1756-0500-5-42

Sukantamala, J., Sing, K. W., Jaturas, N., Polseela, R., & Wilson, J. J. (2017). Unexpected diversity of sandflies (Diptera: Psychodidae) in tourist caves in Northern Thailand. *Mitochondrial DNA A DNA Mapp Seq Anal, 28*(6), 949–955. doi:10.1080/24701394.2016.1214728

Tamura, K., Stecher, G., Peterson, D., Filipski, A., & Kumar, S. (2013). MEGA6: Molecular evolutionary Genetics Analysis version 6.0. *Mol Biol Evol, 30*(12), 2725–2729. doi:10.1093/molbev/mst197

Tanee, T. (2012). Genetic analysis for identification, genomic template stability in hybrids and barcodes of the Vanda species (Orchidaceae) of Thailand. *Afr J Biotechnol, 11*. doi:10.5897/AJB11.3992

Tanee, T., Chadmuk, P., Sudmoon, R., Chaveerach, A., & Noikotr, K. (2012). Genetic analysis for identification, genomic template stability in hybrids and barcodes of the Vanda species (Orchidaceae) of Thailand. *Afr J Biotechnol, 11*(55), 11772–11781.

Tang, Y., Yukawa, T., Bateman, R. M., Jiang, H., & Peng, H. (2015). Phylogeny and classification of the East Asian Amitostigma alliance (Orchidaceae: Orchideae) based on six DNA markers. *BMC Evol Biol, 15*, 96. doi:10.1186/s12862-015-0376-3

Truong, K., Khanh, T., Ham, L., Duong, T., & Khoa, T. (2013). Molecular phylogeny of the endangered Vietnamese Paphiopedilumspecies based on the internal transcribed spacer of the nuclear ribosomal DNA. *Adv Stud Biol, 5*(7), 337–346. doi:10.12988/asb.2013.3315

Vu, H. T., Huynh, P., Tran, H. D., & Le, L. (2018). In silico study on molecular sequences for identification of Paphiopedilum species. *Evol Bioinform, 14*, 1176934318774542. doi:10.1177/1176934318774542

Wong, T. H., But, G. W., Wu, H. Y., Tsang, S. S., Lau, D. T., & Shaw, P. C. (2018). Medicinal Materials DNA Barcode Database (MMDBD) version 1.5-one-stop solution for storage, BLAST, alignment and primer design. *Database (Oxford)*. doi:10.1093/database/bay112

Wu, C. T., Gupta, S., Wang, A., Lo, S. F., Kuo, C. L., Ko, Y. J., C. L. Chen, Hsieh, C. C., & Tsay, H. S. (2012). Internal transcribed spacer sequence based identification and phylogenic relationship of Herba Dendrobii. *J Food Drug Anal, 20*, 143–151. doi:10.38212/2224-6614.2051

Wu, C. T., Hsieh, C. C., Lin, W. C., Tang, C. Y., Yang, C. H., Huang, Y. C., & Ko, Y. J. (2013). Internal transcribed spacer sequence-based identification and phylogenic relationship of I-Tiao-Gung originating from Flemingia and Glycine (Leguminosae) in Taiwan. *J Food Drug Anal, 21*(4), 356–362. doi:https://doi.org/10.1016/j.jfda.2013.08.002

Wu, H. Y., Chan, K. T., But, G. W., & Shaw, P. C. (2021). Assessing the reliability of medicinal Dendrobium sequences in GenBank for botanical species identification. *Sci Rep, 11*(1), 3439. doi:10.1038/s41598-021-82385-z

Xiang, X. G., Hu, H., Wang, W., & Jin, X. H. (2011). DNA barcoding of the recently evolved genus Holcoglossum (Orchidaceae: Aeridinae): A test of DNA barcode candidates. *Mol Ecol Resour, 11*(6), 1012–1021. doi:10.1111/j.1755-0998.2011.03044.x

Xu, S., Li, D., Li, J., Xiang, X., Jin, W., Huang, W., Jin, X., & Huang, L. (2015). Evaluation of the DNA barcodes in Dendrobium (Orchidaceae) from mainland Asia. *PLoS One, 10*(1), e0115168. doi:10.1371/journal.pone.0115168

Yao, H., Song, J. Y., Ma, X. Y., Liu, C., Li, Y., Xu, H. X., Han, J. P., Duan, L. S. & Chen, S. L. (2009). Identification of Dendrobium species by a candidate DNA barcode sequence: The chloroplast psbA-trnH intergenic region. *Planta Med, 75*(6), 667–669. doi:10.1055/s-0029-1185385

Part III
DNA Fingerprinting-based Techniques for Molecular Authentication

Chapter 5

Authentication of Medicinal Materials and Their Formula by Randomly Primed Polymerase Chain Reaction

Hui Cao, Ying Zhang, Kur-Ta Cheng & Pang-Chui Shaw

5.1 Introduction

Polymerase chain reaction (PCR) is the enzymatic amplification of a specific DNA fragment. The target DNA fragment is flanked by two oligonucleotide primers that hybridise to opposite strands of the target sequence. The primers are oriented with 3′ ends pointing towards each other. Repeated cycles of heat denaturation of the template, annealed primers to their complementary sequences and extension of the annealed primers with a DNA polymerase result in the amplification of the segment defined by the 5′ ends of the PCR primers. Since the extension product of each primer can serve as a template for the other primer, each cycle essentially doubles the amount of the DNA fragments produced in the previous cycle. This results in the exponential accumulation of the specific target fragment, up to several million folds in a few hours (Mullis *et al.*, 1986).

The principle of randomly primed PCR (RP-PCR) is based on the selective amplification of genomic sequences that, by chance, are flanked by adequate matches to a randomly chosen primer. The development of a PCR process using only a single arbitrary oligonucleotide primer, known as arbitrarily primed PCR (AP-PCR) (Welsh & McCelland, 1990) and random amplified polymorphic DNA (RAPD) (Williams, Kubelik, Livak, Rafalski & Tingey, 1990), makes the amplification of random sequences in genomic DNA possible. The amplification technique of RP-PCR differs from that used in the conventional PCR. The annealing temperature in the reaction ranges from 36°C to 40°C, significantly lower than that commonly used in conventional PCR with 55°C and above. RAPD analysis, with low stringency, increases the probability of generating polymorphic products.

Generally, 10 nucleotides in RAPD, or 20 to 30 nucleotides in AP-PCR are used for enzymatic amplification of DNA instead of using two primers. The origin of these fragments is not defined but they presumably contain DNA sequences complementary to the 3′ end of the primer sequence. Moreover, the sequence of the primer used is not specifically designed to hybridise with a target sequence. Instead, the primer with arbitrary sequence used in RP-PCR is randomly chosen. An arbitrarily primed fingerprint is then generated by subjecting a small amount of template DNA to PCR at relaxed stringency. In RP-PCR, such a low-stringency condition is maintained only for the first two cycles. After the low-stringency condition is terminated, 30 to 40 thermal cycles with high-stringency condition are then followed. Therefore, the DNA fragments generated under the relaxed stringency condition act as a set of templates for the specific DNA amplification in the next 30 to 40 high-stringency thermal cycles. It should be noted that although the whole set of DNA generated in the first two cycles is under a relaxed stringency condition, the site of primer hybridisation is not random but specific. That is, although we cannot predetermine the amplification products of the first two thermal cycles, the whole set of DNA fragments generated in the first two cycles is a specific set of products under the same stated stringency condition (Figure 5.1). For RAPD, because of the short primer sequence, annealing at low temperature is used throughout the PCR process.

Therefore, the RP-PCR is a modification of PCR that provides an information-rich fingerprint of genomic DNA. If two template genomic DNA sequences are different, their RP-PCR products display different banding patterns (Figure 5.2).

Such differences can be exploited in ways largely analogous to the use of polymorphisms in genotypes that reflect the diversity in phenotypes among organisms. Also, these randomly amplified genomic sequences can in many cases be used as molecular markers and represent an arbitrarily chosen small sample of the template DNA. Over the years, several modifications of these basic methods have been made. These include primers containing a hairpin at the 5′ end, primers with tRNA gene motifs or with some degenerate bases. Sometimes, two primers are used. The pairwise combination enables the detection of more polymorphic bands.

Advantages of RP-PCR include (1) only a small quantity of DNA is needed; (2) a universal set of primers can be used and screened in a short period of time, and many samples can be tested per day; (3) no isolation of cloned DNA probes or preparation of hybridisation filters is required and (4) no sequence data are needed for reference. The genome sizes vary, mainly in the number of highly repetitive sequences, even between closely related species. RP-PCR markers that are specific to a taxonomic level or linked to a particular trait facilitate the identification of medicinal

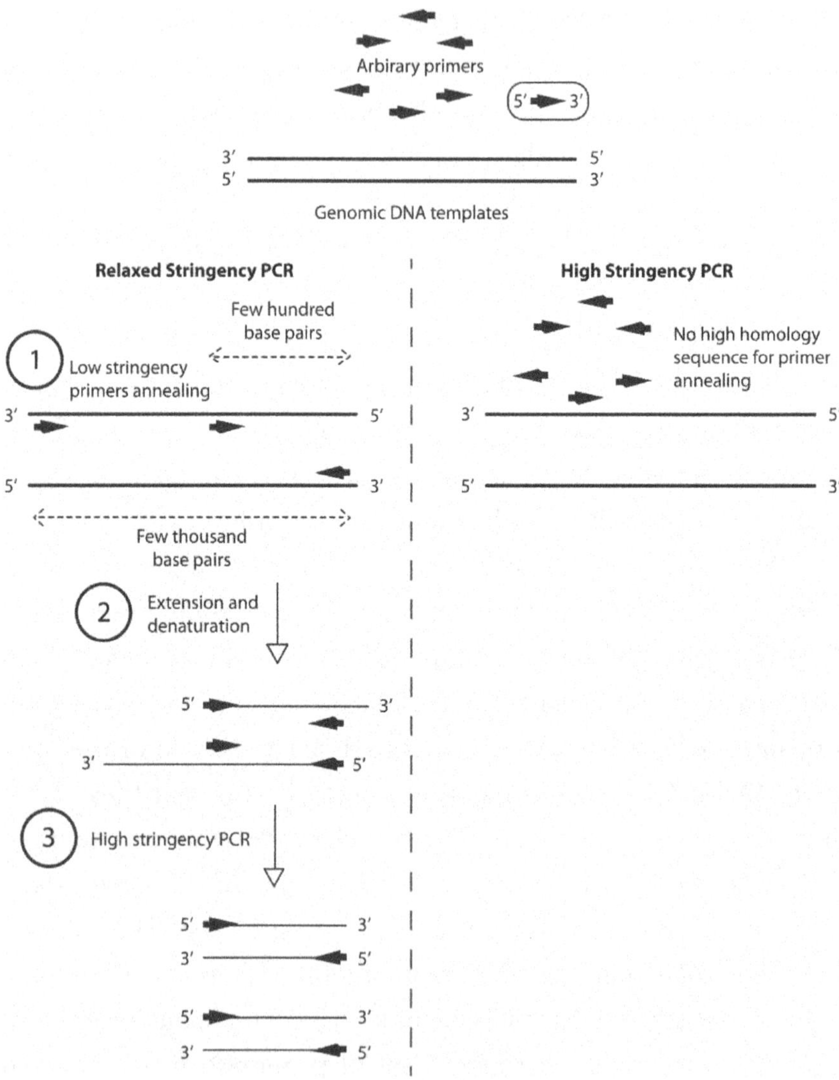

Fig. 5.1 Schematic diagram of RP-PCR. At a sufficiently low temperature, primers can be expected to anneal to many sequences with a variety of mismatches. Some of these will be within a few hundred base pairs of each other and on opposite strands. Sequences between these positions will become PCR amplifiable. The extent to which sequences amplified will depend on the efficiency of priming at each pair of primer annealing sites and the efficiency of extension. At early cycles, those that prime most efficiently will predominate. At later times, those that amplify most efficiently will predominate.

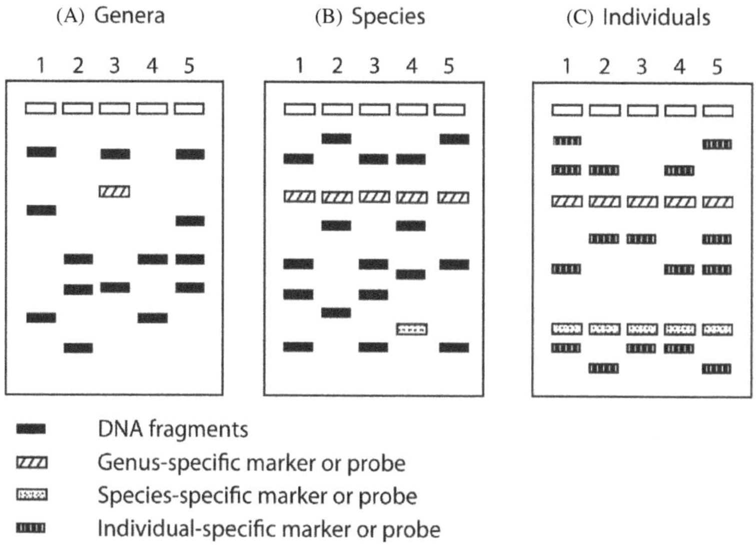

Fig. 5.2 Molecular characteristics of different taxonomic levels by RP-PCR markers. In gel A, a genus-specific marker is identified for genus 3. In gel B, a species-specific marker is identified for species 4. In gel C, different fingerprints are generated for the five individuals.

materials. In the analysis to identify the medicinal materials or the components in a Chinese medicine formula, a mixture of the DNA is used as the target template. The applied components are defined in terms of different species, genera or even families. The RP-PCR marker specific to each component is therefore obtained more easily.

5.2 Materials and Methods

5.2.1 Samples Studied

5.2.1.1 *Kudidan*

Nine species of plant samples and four commercial samples collected in different localities and markets of Mainland China, Hong Kong and Macau as well as Taiwan were used. All the voucher

Table 5.1 Collection Data of Kudidan and Its Substitutes from Various Localities and Markets

Name	Locality/market	Code
Elephantopus scaber	Hong Kong, China	Es
Elephantopus mollis	Hong Kong, China	Em
Pseudo-elephantopus spicatus	Hong Kong, China	Ps
Emilia sonchifolia	Hong Kong, China	Ea
Paraixeris denticulata	Hong Kong, China	Pd
Piloselloides hirsuta	Hong Kong, China	Ph
Pterocypsela indica	Hong Kong, China	Pi
Sonchus arvensis	Hong Kong, China	Sa
Taraxacum mongolicum	Hong Kong, China	Tm
Tugongying	Hong Kong, China	K1 (Es)
Didantou	Macau, China	K2 (Es)
Didancao	Fujian Province	K3 (Es)
Xiaobendengshuwu	Taiwan Province	K4 (Es)

specimens were deposited in the Shiu-Ying Hu Herbarium, The Chinese University of Hong Kong. (Table 5.1).

5.2.1.2 *Ginseng*

Dried or fresh root samples were obtained from various sources. The vouchers were stored in the Museum of Institute of Chinese Medicine, The Chinese University of Hong Kong (Table 5.2). The eight ginseng products were all from local markets (Table 5.3).

5.2.1.3 *Guanghuoxiang*

Fresh samples were collected from different geographical origins. Dried materials were purchased from various markets in the Guangdong province (Table 5.4).

Table 5.2 Characteristics of Ginseng and Related Samples and Their Source Locality

Sample	Code	Characteristics	Locality
Panax quinquefolius	Pq1	3-year-old dried root	Canada
P. quinquefolius	Pq2	4-year-old dried root	Canada
P. quinquefolius	Pq3	Dried root	United States
P. quinquefolius	Pq4	Dried root	United States
P. quinquefolius	Pq5	4-year-old dried root	China
P. quinquefolius	Pq6	4-year-old dried root	China
P. quinquefolius	Pq7	4-year-old dried root	China
P. ginseng	Pg1	Root without epidermis	China
P. ginseng	Pg2	Fresh root	China
P. ginseng	Pg3	Fresh root	China
P. Notoginseng	Pn	Dried root	China
Platycodon grandiflorum	Pl.g	Dried root	China
Mirabilis jalapa	Mj	Dried root	Hong Kong, China
Talinum paniculatum	Tp	Dried root	Hong Kong, China
Phytolacca acinosa	Ph.a	Dried root	Hong Kong, China

Table 5.3 Eight Commercial Ginseng Products

Sample	Code	Physical form
G 1	149-4	Ginseng tea
G 2	N.A.	Pills containing powder
G 3	148-3	Granular root
G 4	96007	Powder
G 5	96008	Powder
G 6	96009	Powder
G 7	96011	Powder
G 8	168	Ginseng root

Table 5.4 Guanghuoxiang Samples Collected from Different Localities and Markets

Sample code	Locality/market
G2	Huodao, Gaoyao, Guangdong
G3	Liantang, Gaoyao, Guangdong
G5	Luogang, Guangzhou
G8	Yingli, Leizhou, Guangdong
G9	Longmen, Leizhou, Guangdong
G10	Chengyue, Suixi, Guangdong
G11	Chengyue, Suixi, Guangdong
G12	Wancheng, Wanning, Hainan
G13	Xuwen, Guangdong
G16	Zhenwen, Wuchuan, Guangdong
G19	Longdong, Guangzhou
G20	Tissue culture sample (Generation I, 1 year), Luogang, Guangzhou
G21	Tissue culture sample (Generation I, 2 year), Luogang, Guangzhou
G22	Tissue culture sample (Generation II, 1 year), Luogang, Guangzhou
G23	Tissue culture sample (Generation II, 2 year), Luogang, Guangzhou
G24	Tissue culture sample with big leaves (Generation II), Luogang, Guangzhou
G26	Zhangpu, Wuchuan, Guangdong (furry leaves)
G27	Liantang, Gaoyao, Guangdong (furry leaves)
G28	Liantang, Gaoyao, Guangdong (furry-less leaves)
G29	Longdong, Guangzhou (green stem)
G30	Longdong, Guangzhou (purple stem)
G31	Longdong, Guangzhou (purple stem, in greenhouse)
G32	Longdong, Guangzhou (furry-less leaves)
PCH (*Pogostemon chinensis*)	Dafukeng village, Heping country, Guangdong
PAU (*Pogostemon auricularius*)	Institute of Chinese Materia Medica, Longdong, Guangzhou

5.2.1.4 *Yu-Ping-Feng San*

The dried Huangqi (*Astragalus membranaceus* var. *mongolicus*), Baizhu (*Atractylodes macrocephala*) and Fangfeng (*Saposhnikovia divaricata*), used to prepare the formula, were collected from the market. They were pulverised after surface sterilisation by ethanol. The powdered samples were prepared with various amounts of the three components. The composition of the sample was Huangqi:Baizhu:Fangfeng = 3:1:1. Other samples were as follows: (1) Huangqi, (2) Baizhu, (3) Fangfeng, (4) Huangqi:Baizhu: Fangfeng = 1:1:1, (5) Huangqi:Baizhu:Fangfeng = 6:2:1, (6) Huangqi:Baizhu:Fangfeng = 3:1:0. (7–16) Ten commercial patent formulae were purchased from stores in Taipei and Chiayi, Taiwan.

5.2.2 Methods

5.2.2.1 *Total Genomic DNA Preparation*

The genomic DNA was isolated by using a modified cetyltrimethylammonium bromide (CTAB) procedure (Rogers & Bendich, 1985). The concentration of DNA was estimated with a DNA DipStick™ Kit (Invitrogen, Waltham, MA).

5.2.2.2 *Arbitrarily Primed PCR*

Kudidan and Ginseng

The following method was a modification of the procedure of Welsh and McClelland (1990). Amplification reactions were performed in volumes of 25 µL containing 1× Taq buffer (Promega), 1.5 mmol/L $MgCl_2$ (Sigma-Aldrich, St. louis, MO), 0.2 mmol/L of each deoxynucleoside triphosphates (dNTPs) (Promega,

Table 5.5 The 11 Arbitrarily Chosen Primers Used for DNA Fingerprinting by AP-PCR

Primer name	Sequence (5′ to 3′)
M13 For	CGC CAG GGT TTT CCC AGT CAC GAC
M13 Rev	AGC GGA TAA CAA TTT CAC ACA GGA
Gal K	TAC GGT GGC GGA GCG CAG CA
Seq 2	CTG GTC AAG GCA CAA GAG AT
SH1133	CAT CGG ATC CAC CAC GTC
TCS-back	GGT GGA TCC CTA AGC ATC AAC ATT GGT
MB2F	TAA TTA ACA AGT ACA AGC GG
#4	GCT TCT CAA GCA GGA CCT
#13	ATG AGC CAT GGC AGT GAG TAT CGC
#18	CAT CGG ATC ACC ACG TC
#20	GCC TCA ACG ATT CTC CCT TTA

Madison, WI), 2 mmol/L primer, 2.5 U AmpliTaq polymerase (PerkinElmer, Waltham, MA) and 100 to 200 ng template DNA. The reaction mixture was pipetted into a 0.5-mL microcentrifuge tube. Different primers (17–27 mers) were used in the present study (Table 5.5).

Light mineral oil (Sigma) was overlaid onto the mixture and the tube was placed into the Thermolyne Thermocycler (Barnstead/Thermolyne Corp., Ramsey, MN). The mixture was then subjected to the following thermal cycles with a 'hot start' step (heat the mixture at 94°C for 10 min before adding polymerase) in order to minimise non-specific amplification. Two cycles of low-stringency amplification: 94°C for 5 min, 35°C for 5 min and 72°C for 5 min; 40 cycles of high-stringency amplification: 94°C for 1 min, 55°C for 1 min and 72°C for 1 min; 1 cycle of high-stringency amplification with longer primer extension time: 94°C for

1 min, 55°C for 1 min and 72°C for 10 min. The experiment was repeated. The amplified products were kept at 4°C for further analysis. Agarose gel electrophoresis was carried out for the amplified product. About 10 µL of the AP-PCR product was analysed by agarose gel electrophoresis with 1× TBE buffer system in which 2.5% agarose gel was stained with ethidium bromide, followed by ultraviolet (UV) illumination. 100 bp DNA size marker (Takara Bio Inc., Kusatsu, Japan) was used as a size marker.

5.2.2.3 *Random Amplified Polymorphic DNA*

Kudidan and Ginseng

The method was a modification of the procedure of Williams *et al.* (1990). About 25 ng template DNA were used in 1× buffer, 2 mmol/L $MgCl_2$, 0.1 mmol/L of each dNTP with 0.2 mol/L primer and 0.5 U AmpliTaq polymerase in a final volume of 25 µL. The mixture was not covered with light mineral oil and the tube was placed in FTS-960 Microplate Fast Thermal Sequencer (Corbett Research Co., Manchester, UK). The reaction was programmed as follows: 1 min at 94°C, 1 min at 36°C and 2 min at 72°C for 45 cycles. A 'hot start' step (addition of the enzyme at 94°C) was also used. Random 10-mers primers were from many sets of kit (Operon Technologies, Louisville, KY). The specific primers and their sequences are listed in Table 5.6.

Guanghuoxiang

About 10 to 40 ng of DNA template was amplified in 25 µL PCR mixture consisting of 1× PCR buffer (Takara Bio, Japan), 0.2 mmol/L dNTP, 1.0 µmol/L primer and 1.0 U *Taq* polymerase (Takara Bio). For DNA amplification, a ABI 9700 DNA thermocycler

Table 5.6 List of the Primers Used in RAPD Amplification

Primer name	Sequence (5′ to 3′)	% G+C Content
OPC-05	GAT GAC CGC C	70
OPC-06	GAA CGG ACT C	60
OPC-19	GTT GCC AGC C	70
OPC-20	ACT TCG CCA C	60
S42	GGA CCC AAC C	70
S43	GTC GCC GTC A	70
S224	CCC CTC ACG A	70
S227	GAA GCC AGC C	70
OPP-10	TCC CGC CTA C	70

was programmed for 3 cycles of 94°C for 30 s, 40°C for 1 min and 72°C for 1 min; followed by 42 cycles of 94°C for 20 s, 45°C for 40 s and 72°C for 50 s.

Yu-Ping-Feng San

About 1 ng of the DNA template was amplified in 25 µL PCR mixture consisting of 1× PCR buffer (Boehringer Mannheim, Germany), 0.2 mmol/L dNTP, 0.8 to 4.0 µmol/L primer and 0.625 U *Taq* polymerase (Boehringer Mannheim). A Perkin-Elmer Cetus 2400 DNA thermocycler was programmed for three cycles of 94°C for 30 s, 40°C for 1 min and 72°C for 1 min; followed by 42 cycles of 94°C for 20 s, 45°C for 40 s and 72°C for 50 s.

5.2.2.4 *Data Analysis*

Gel images were stored as TIF files and sizes of AP-PCR or RAPD products were analysed by the ImageQuant program (Cytiva, Marlborough, MA). The Similarity Indexes (SI) of fingerprints were calculated for each possible pairwise comparison between samples by the program DNA SIMDEX. DNA band patterns of the species were compared in a pairwise manner using the following equation:

$$Sxy = \frac{2nxy}{nx} + ny$$

where Sxy = the similarity index between samples in lane x and y
nxy = the number of bands common to both lane x and y
nx = the number of bands in lane x
ny = the number of bands in lane y

5.3 Results

5.3.1 Kudidan

Genomic DNA fingerprints of all fresh specimens were successfully generated. The representative DNA profiles of the genomic fingerprints by AP-PCR using random long primers and by RAPD using arbitrary short primers are presented in Figures 5.3 and 5.4.

DNA fingerprinting of AP-PCR and RAPD, which use random primers, usually results in the detection of a large number of fragments. These fragments tend to become progressively more crowded with diminishing size. Thus, the larger ones, 0.8 to 1.2 kb, are relatively easy to score, whereas fragments smaller than 0.2 to 0.3 kb are almost impossible to evaluate unambiguously. The number of useful fragments detected usually ranges between 5 and 15 in the present study. The SI values for each of the seven primers used for comparing all species and commercial samples tested are calculated in Table 5.7.

This assumption was validated by calculating the SI values for each of the three primers used for comparing Kudidan with the nine Compositae species tested. The SI values of these

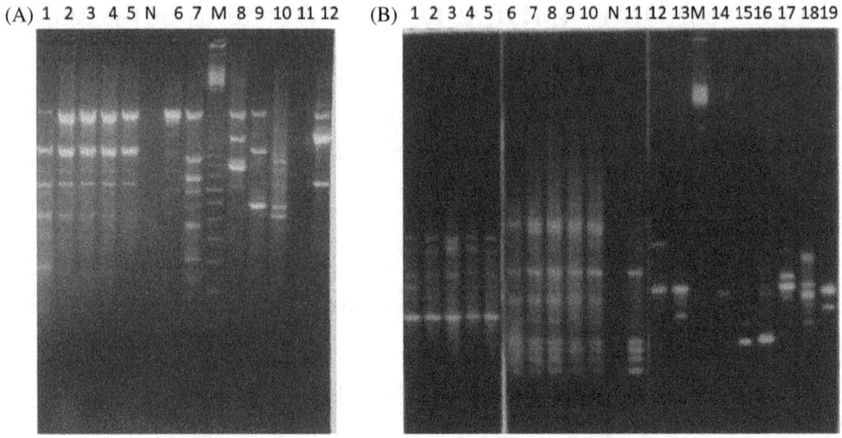

Fig. 5.3 AP-PCR fingerprinting of Kudidan and its substitutes using (A) primer M13 Rev. Lane 1: Em; lane 2: Es; lane 3–6: K1–K4 (Es); lane 7: Ps; lane 8: Ph; lane 9: Ea; lane 10: Sa; lane 11: Tm; lane 12: Pi. (B) Primer Gal K. Lane 1: Es; lane 2–5: K1–K4 (Es); lane 6–11: Em; lane 12–13: Ps; lane 14: Ea; lane 15: Sa; lane 16: Tm; lane 17: Pi; lane 18: Pd; lane 19: Ph. N: negative control, Lane M: 100 bp DNA size marker.

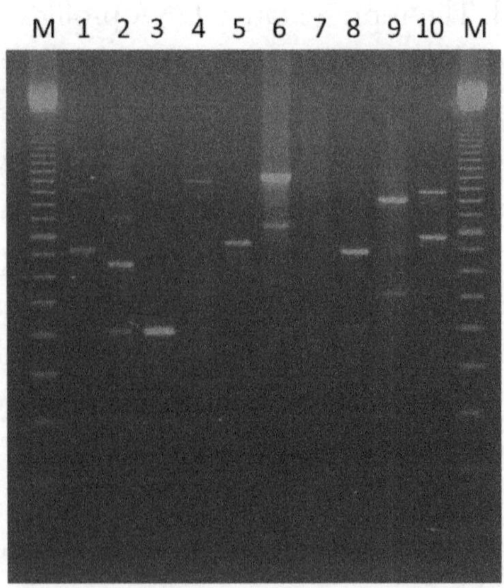

Fig. 5.4 RAPD pattern of Kudidan and its substitutes using primer OPC-06. Lane 1: Es; lane 2: Em; lane 3: Ps; lane 4: Ea; lane 5: Sa; lane 6: Tm; lane 7: Pi; lane 8: Pd; lane 9: Ph; lane 10: K1 (Es); lane M: 100 bp DNA size marker.

Table 5.7 SI Values of Commercial Samples of Kudidan to Nine Species Deduced by RP-PCR

Sample \ Primer	M13 For	Gal K	OPC-06	Average SI*
K vs. Es	0.61	0.36	0.67	0.55
K vs. Ea	0.12	0.25	0.40	0.26
K vs. Em	0.19	0.20	0.33	0.24
K vs. Pd	0.18	0.33	0.40	0.31
K vs. Ph	0.21	0.19	0.25	0.22
K vs. Pi	0.32	0.20	0.40	0.31
K vs. Ps	0.26	0.20	0.22	0.23
K vs. Sa	0.43	0.17	0.50	0.37
K vs. Tm	0.21	0.18	0.33	0.24

*The SI values were calculated from pairwise comparison done between a representative species from Figures 5.3 and 5.4.

fingerprints were calculated and summarised in Table 5.7. The degree of similarity among these genomic DNA fingerprints confirmed that the commercial samples of Kudidan (K1–K4 [Es]) are more closely related to *Elephantopus scaber* L. (Es) than to other species.

5.3.2 Ginseng

Distinctive profiles were generated among the three *Panax* species and their adulterants (Figure 5.5). Basically, these patterns were not influenced by the source or age of materials. The SI values of the *Panax* species were calculated and summarised in Table 5.8. *P. ginseng* and *P. quinquefolius* had the highest SI value, which implied that they are closely related. This result matches the conclusion based on morphological study.

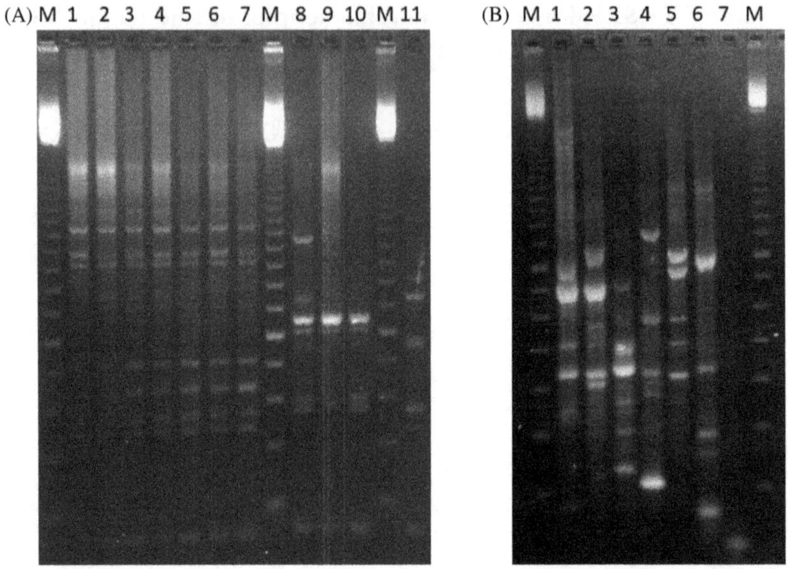

Fig. 5.5 (A) RAPD fingerprints of *P. quinquefolius* and *P. ginseng* as well as their adulterants generated by OPC-05. Lane 1–7: Pq1–Pq7; lane 8–10: Pg1–Pg3; lane 11: Pn. (B) AP-PCR fingerprints using TCS-back primer. Lane 1: *P. quinquefolius*; lane 2: *P. ginseng*; lane 3: *Platycodon grandiflorum*; lane 4: *Mirabilis jalapa*; lane 5: *Talinum paniculatum*; lane 6: *Phytolacca acinose*; lane 7: negative control (without template DNA). Lane M: 100 bp DNA size marker.

Table 5.8 SI Values of Three *Panax* Species Deduced by RP-PCR

	Primer				
Sample	**OPC-05**	**OPC-20**	**Seq 2**	**TCS-back**	**Average SI**
Pg vs. Pq	0.47	0.53	0.80	0.57	0.59
Pq vs Pn	0.25	0.27	0.50	0.13	0.29
Pg vs. Pn	0.31	0.43	0.56	0.38	0.42

Six AP-PCR primers were used to authenticate eight commercial ginseng products (Table 5.3). Each reaction was repeated at least twice, and the results are summarised in Table 5.9. The identity of ginseng in most samples could be found by comparing the characteristic bands in the samples to those of the reference

Table 5.9 RP-PCR Analysis of the Eight Ginseng Product Samples

Ginseng sample number	Primer						Conclusion	Identity by HPLC*
	#13	#18	#20	TCS-back	Gal K	MB2F		
G1	—	—	—	AG	—	—	AG	AG
G2	AG	AG	AG	AG	—	AG	AG	AG
G3	—	AG	—	—	—	AG	AG	AG
G4	G	—	G	G	G	G	G	G
G5	—	—	G	G	G	G	G	G
G6	AG	AG	AG	AG	—	AG	AG	AG
G7	AG	AG	AG	AG	AG	AG	AG	AG
G8	AG	AG	AG	AG	—	AG	AG	AG

AG or G indicate that the sample contained American ginseng or Oriental ginseng, respectively.
'—' indicates that the sample identification did not give a definite outcome.
*The identity of the samples was revealed by the high performance liquid chromatography (HPLC) ginsenoside profile.

ginsengs. For ginseng sample 1, only one primer provided a species-specific DNA fingerprint. As this sample was an instant ginseng tea bag, extensive DNA degradation occurred during manufacturing and this might adversely affect the analysis.

5.3.3 Guanghuoxiang

Genomic DNA fingerprints of all 23 *Pogostemon cablin* samples and 2 substitutes: *P. chinesis* (PCH) and *P. auricularius* (PAU), were successfully generated (Figure 5.6). The five primers (S42, S43, S224, S227 and OPC-19) were found to give distinctive DNA bands of RAPD markers. The results showed the RAPD markers of two substitutes PCH and PAU were much different from *P. cablin*. There are significant differences among samples of *P. cablin* obtained from different localities by the RAPD assay. The

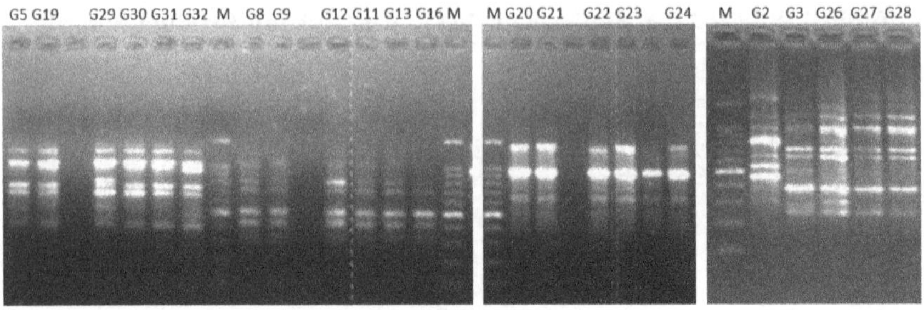

Fig. 5.6 RAPD fingerprints of *Pogostemon cablin* generated by S227 primer. Sample codes are shown in Table 5.4. Lane M: 100 bp DNA size marker.

clustering trees based on RAPD markers revealed that PCH and PAU had lower coefficients with samples of *P. cablin*. Among the 23 samples of *P. cablin*, G2, G3, G5, G19, G20, G21, G22, G23, G24, G26, G27, G28, G29, G30, G31 and G32 are assembled as one group, showing Paixiang (G5, G19, G29–G32), which include tissue culture samples (G20–G24) from Guangzhou and Zhaoxiang (G2–G3, G27–28) from Gaoyao were closely related. G8, G9, G10, G11, G12, G13 and G16 are assembled as another group, showing Zhanxiang (G8–G11, G13, G16) from Zhanjiang and Qiongxiang (G12) from Hainan were in close relationship, which indicates a good correlation between the genotype and distribution of *P. cablin* (Figure 5.7).

5.3.4 Yu-Ping-Feng San

In this study, 40 arbitrary decamer primers were screened. Whichever primer simultaneously generated the distinguishable component-specific RAPD markers in the formula was then selected for further use. Only one primer, OPP-10, was suitable for the identification of the components in the formula (Figure 5.8). In the OPP-10 reaction, a 200 bp RAPD band was generated in the *Astragalus membranaceus* var. *mongbolicus* (Huangqi) sample. Two major bands, 440 bp and 380 bp, were produced in *Saposhnikovia*

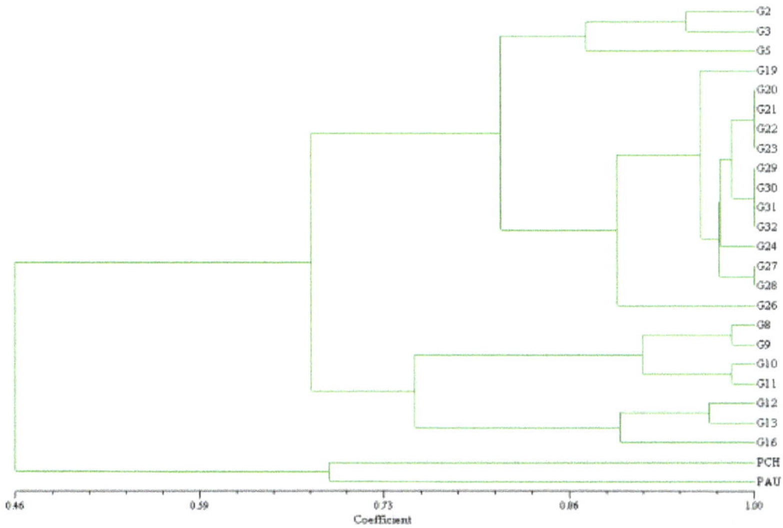

Fig. 5.7 Cluster tree of RAPD marker with five combined primers of *Pogostemon cablin*. Sample codes are shown in Table 5.4.

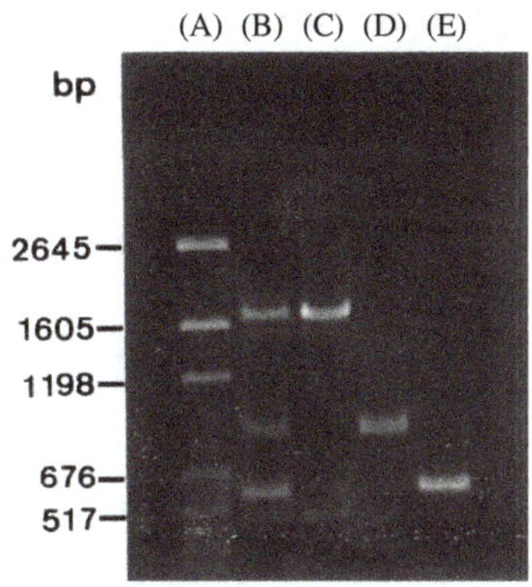

Fig. 5.8 RAPD fingerprints generated by primer OPP-10 from the samples. Lanes: (A) molecular weight marker, (B) Yu-Ping-feng San, (C) *Astragalus membranaceus* var. *mongbolicus*, (D) *Atractylodes macrocephala* and (E) *Saposhnikovia divaricata*.

divaricata (Fangfeng) sample, and one 500 bp band was produced in the *Atractylodes macrocephala* (Baizhu) sample. The 380 bp of the *Saposhnikovia divaricata*-specific marker was absent in the RAPD pattern of the formula. The 200 bp, 440 bp and 500 bp bands were therefore used as component-specific markers. The 440 bp marker disappeared in the RAPD fingerprint when the amount of *Saposhnikovia divaricata* in the formula was reduced by half. All the 10 commercial products purchased from the stores showed the three markers simultaneously, but the *Saposhnikovia divaricata*–specific marker showed varying fragment lengths among the samples.

5.4 Discussion

In this study, we used RP-PCR to authenticate *Panax* species, their adulterants (Cheung, Kwan & But, 1994; Shaw & But, 1995) and a traditional Chinese medicine (TCM) formula (Cheng Tsay, Chen & Chou, 1998). In addition, we found that this approach is effective in authenticating commercial ginseng products on the market (Ngan, Wang & But, 1997). We further applied RAPD and AP-PCR to authenticate various species of Kudidan *(Elephantopus)* and Pugongying (*Taraxacum*) and their substitutes and adulterants (Cao, But & Shaw, 1996a; 1996b).

In Kudidan, evidence for the genomic material in nine Compositae species was obtained using the RP-PCR (including AP-PCR and RAPD) fingerprinting technique. In AP-PCR and RAPD fingerprints, the degree of similarity of the commercial samples of Kudidan retailed in Hong Kong, Macau, Taiwan and Fujian markets, and authentic plant specimens confirm that the commercial samples of Kudidan (K1–K4 [Es]) are more closely related to *Elephantopus scaber* L. than other species.

In Ginseng, distinctive and reproducible genomic fingerprints from the DNA of the ginseng samples were generated with PCR from long (17–27 mer) and short (10 mer) random-chosen primers. It is evidenced that RP-PCR is able to distinguish samples of different genera and species. It is not restricted to the source and age of materials. The identity of commercial samples and substitutions could be detected by these techniques. The three *Panax* species can be easily distinguished by their fingerprints. Moreover, adulterants of *P. ginseng* and *P. quinquefolius* can also be differentiated. These adulterants do not have the pharmacological effects of Ginseng and may be poisonous. For example, *Phytolacca acinosa* has caused intoxication. This method may be further explored to detect the DNA content of some commercial ginseng products.

In Guanhuoxiang, the samples in different localities have different RAPD markers. Moreover, there is a good correlation between the genotype and distribution of samples. Based on the clustering analysis, samples G2, G3, G27 and G28 have a nearer genetic relationship to G19; this discovery well confirms the traditional viewpoint that the quality of Zhaoxiang is close to Paixiang. Besides, the genotypes of samples G16 and G26 are also nearer to sample G12, and morphological similarities have been observed, which may be caused by the introduction of germplasm resources in Zhanjiang to Hainan.

For Yu-Ping-Feng San, 40 decamer primers were screened; only primer OPP-10 was selected for identification purposes because it revealed the simplest fingerprints, and the marker for each component showed different lengths. In the mixed components, RAPD reaction resulted in the three markers, 200, 440 and 500 bp, which were generated simultaneously.

RP-PCR compares the differences at the genome level. With the appropriate primer, it is, in principal, possible to differentiate closely related species and even one individual from another. The advantages of the approach include the limited amount of DNA required and procedure simplicity, and without the need of isotopes or prior genetic information. The goal of RP-PCR analysis is to get reproducible and polymorphic markers. The simpler the RP-PCR pattern, the more efficient the analysis. On the other hand, the reaction conditions should be stringently controlled so as to obtain high reproducibility. The reproducibility is affected by DNA quality, primer concentration, different thermocyclers and the brand of DNA polymerase. Medicinal materials contain secondary metabolites such as alkaloids, polysaccharides, saponins and flavonoids. These compounds may decrease the PCR efficiency and reproducibility. In addition, the treatment of medicinal materials such as air-drying or drying in an oven at 50°C to 60°C may lead to DNA degradation. Also, the RP-PCR fingerprinting techniques may not be applicable if the formula is prepared from the extract of the medicinal materials. To increase the accuracy of authentication for closely related species, it may be essential to add another molecular approach, e.g., gene loci sequencing (ITS, 5S rRNA, 18S rRNA from nrDNA, *trnK*, *matK*, *rbcL* from cpDNA, *cytb*, 12SrRNA from mtDNA), which looks for the differences in a definite region of the genome that may have a higher rate of genetic change.

5.5 Conclusion

In this study, we applied RP-PCR to authenticate Kudidan (Elephantopin Herba) and Guanghuoxiang (Pogostemonis Herba), rare medicinal materials, including Ginseng and American ginseng, and a traditional Chinese formula Yu-Ping-Feng San consisting of the three components (Astragali Radix, Atractylodis Macrocephalae Rhizoma and Saposhnikoviae Divaricatae Radix). We conclude that RP-PCR is a useful tool for the molecular authentication of a wide range of medicinal materials.

References

Cao, H., But, P. P. H., & Shaw, P. C. (1996a). Authentication of the Chinese drug 'Ku-Di-Dan' (Herba Elephantopi) and its substitutes using random primed polymerase chain reaction (PCR). *Acta Pharm Sin, 31*(7), 543–553.

Cao, H., But, P. P. H., & Shaw, P.C. (1996b). A molecular approach to identification of Chinese drug 'Pu-Gong-Ying' (Herba Taraxaci) by DNA fingerprinting using random primed PCR. *J Chin Pharm Sci, 5*,186–194.

Cheng, K. T., Tsay, H. S., Chen, C. F., & Chou, T. W. (1998). Determination of the components in a Chinese prescription, Yu-Ping-Feng San, by RAPD analysis. *Planta Med, 64*(6), 563–565. doi:10.1055/s-2006-957515

Cheung, K. S., Kwan, H. S., & But, P. P. H. (1994). Pharmacognostical identification of American and Oriental ginseng roots by genomic fingerprinting using arbitrarily primed polymerase chain reaction (AP-PCR). *J Ethnopharmacol, 42*(1), 67–69. doi:10.1016/0378-8741(94)90025-6

Mullis, N. B., Faloona, F., Scharf, S., Saiki, R., Horn, G., & Erlich, H. (1986). Specific enzymatic amplification of DNA *in vitro*: The polymerase chain reaction. *Cold Spring Harb Symp Quant, 51*(1), 263–273. doi:10.1101/sqb.1986.051.01.032

Ngan, F. N., Wang, J., But, P. P. H. (1997). Application of arbitrarily primed polymerase chain reaction (AP-PCR) in commercial ginseng products. 5th International Congress of Plant Molecular Biology, Singapore.

Rogers, S. O., & Bendich, A. J. (1985). Extraction of DNA from milligram amounts of fresh, herbarium and mummified plant tissues. *Plant Mol Biol, 5*(2), 69–76. doi:10.1007/BF00020088

Shaw, P. C., & But, P. P. H. (1995). Authentication of *Panax* species and their adulterants by random-primed polymerase chain reaction. *Planta Med, 61*(5), 466–469. doi:10.1055/s-2006-958138

Welsh, J., & McClelland, M. (1990). Fingerprinting genomes using PCR with arbitrary primers. *Nucleic Acids Res, 18*(24), 7213–7218. doi:10.1093/nar/18.24.7213

Williams, J. G. K., Kubelik, A. R., Livak, K. J., Rafalski, J. A., & Tingey, S. V. (1990). DNA polymorphisms amplified by arbitrary primers are useful as genetic markers. *Nucleic Acids Res, 18*(22), 6531–6535. doi:10.1093/nar/18.22.6531

Chapter 6

Authentication of Medicinal Materials by Amplified Fragment Length Polymorphism

Hui Cao, Ying Zhang & Pang-Chui Shaw

6.1 Introduction

Amplified Fragment Length Polymorphism (AFLP) technology is a powerful fingerprint technique that combines the technologies of restriction fragment length polymorphism (RFLP) and polymerase chain reaction (PCR) (Vos *et al.*, 1995). The schematic outline of the AFLP technique is illustrated in Figure 6.1.

There are three major steps in AFLP analysis. The first step is the restriction of the genomic DNA with two different restriction enzymes: a 'rare-cutter' *Eco*RI that recognises GAATTC, and a 'frequent-cutter' *Mse*I that recognises AATT. The 'frequent-cutter' generates short fragments that amplify well and are in the optimal size range for separation on denaturing gel. Then, the number of fragments to be amplified is limited by using the 'rare-cutter', since only the rare-cutter/frequent-cutter fragments are amplified. This reduces the number of nucleotides required for selective amplification. After that, the use of two restriction enzymes makes it possible to selectively label one strand of the double-stranded

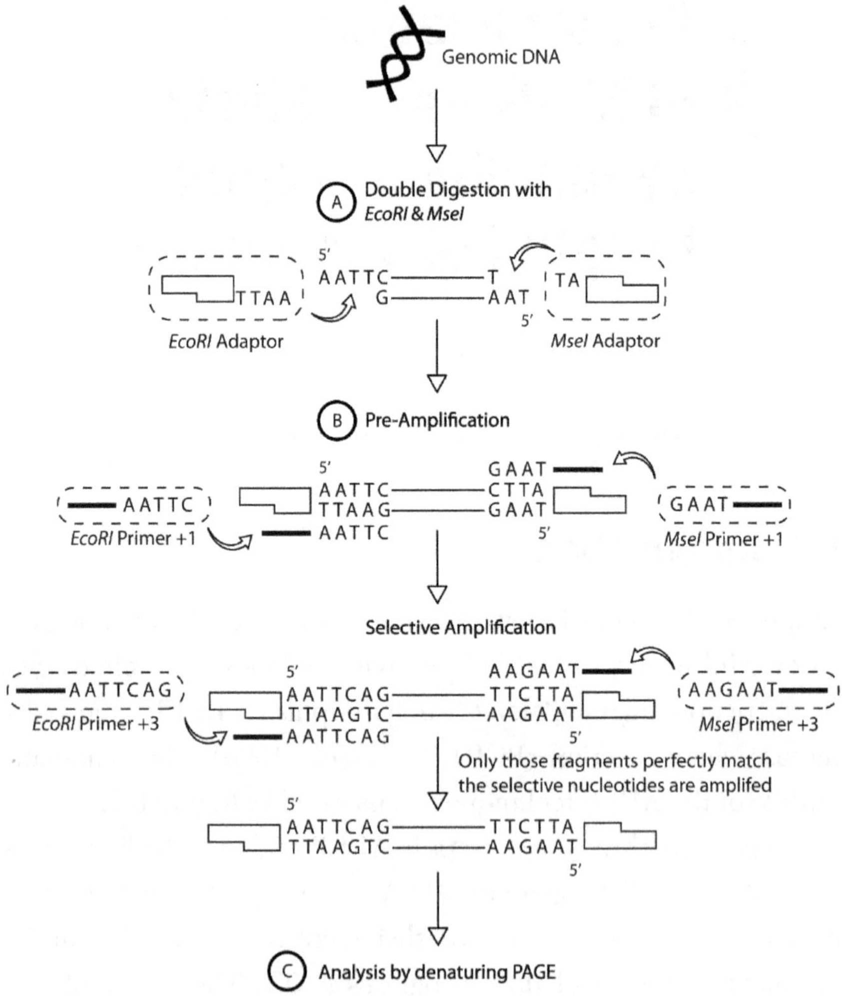

Fig. 6.1 The three major steps of the AFLP procedure. (A) Genomic DNA is restricted to produce *Eco*RI-*Mse*I fragments, which are subsequently ligated with the ds-adaptors. (B) Ligated DNAs are then amplified by pre-amplification and selective amplification. (C) Fragments of various lengths are generated and displayed on polyacrylamide gel electrophoresis (PAGE).

PCR products (Figure 6.1A). After digestion, the double-stranded adaptors *Eco*RI and *Mse*I (Figure 6.2A) are ligated to the ends of the restricted fragments. Adaptors consist of a core sequence (CORE) and an enzyme-specific sequence (ENZ) with cohesive

EcoRI Adaptor (17nt)

5′ CTCGTAGACTGCGTACC
CATCTGACGCATGGTTAA 5′
CORE ENZ

MseI Adaptor (16nt)

5′ GACGATGAGTCCTGAG
TACTCAGGACTC AT 5′
CORE ENZ

(A)

EcoRI Primer

5′ GACTGCGTACC AATTC NNN
CORE ENZ EXT

MseI Primer

5′ GATGAGTCCTGAG TAA NNN
CORE ENZ EXT

(B)

Fig. 6.2 (A) AFLP adaptor sequences. Both the *Eco*RI-adaptor and the *Mse*I-adaptor consist of a core sequence (CORE) and an ENZ. (B) AFLP primer sequences. Both the *Eco*RI-adaptor and the *Mse*I-adaptor consist of a core sequence (CORE), an ENZ and a selective nucleotide sequence (EXT) at the 3′ ends. By changing the number or combination of selective nucleotides (N), altered AFLP fingerprints are generated.

ends at 5′, which serve as a primer-binding site in the subsequent amplification steps.

The second step of the AFLP procedure is the amplification of subsets of restriction fragments using selective AFLP primers (Figure 6.1B). The primers used are complementary to the adaptor and restriction site sequences and have additional selective nucleotides (EXT) at their 3′ ends (Figure 6.2B). The addition of selective nucleotides to the AFLP primers limits the number of bands, at an approximately fourfold reduction with each additional selective base. These 3′ extensions assure that only a subset of the restriction fragments that match the 3′ primer extensions is amplified. A two-step amplification strategy is employed, to reduce background 'smears' in fingerprint patterns that frequently occur during direct AFLP, and to save the primary amplified template for subsequent amplification. In the pre-amplification step, one selective nucleotide at the ends of both primers is used. The appropriate portion of the amplified products is used in selective amplification, with primers having two additional selective nucleotides. At this step, for the detection of polymorphic bands, the *Eco*RI primer is chosen and labelled with γ-^{33}P-ATP at the 5′ end.

The final step of the AFLP technique is the resolution of fingerprints using denaturing PAGE, which provides well separation of the bands (Figure 6.1C). For plants with genomes ranging in size from 5×10^8 to 6×10^9 bp, such as the tomato, corn, soybean, cucumber, lettuce, barley, cotton, oilseed, rape, potato, sunflower, pepper and brassica, approximately 50 to 100 bands are produced.

6.2 Materials and Methods

6.2.1 Samples Studied and DNA Extraction

Dried or fresh roots of *Panax* species were obtained from the following sources: *P. ginseng* samples from China (Ji'an county of Jilin province and Xingbing county of Liaolin province) and Korea (Kangwon, Pochon, Kanghwa, Kumsan and Kimpo); *P. quinquefolius* samples from farms in Ontario, British Columbia and Wisconsin. Samples were identified and deposited in the Institute of Chinese Medicine, The Chinese University of Hong Kong. DNA was extracted using the Potassium Acetate/Sodium Dodecyl Sulphate (SDS) method (please refer to Chapter 2 for a detailed discussion).

6.2.2 Choice of Primers and Radiolabelling

Primer labelling was performed by phosphorylating the 5′ end of *Eco*RI primers with γ^{32}P- or γ^{33}P-ATP and T4 polynucleotide kinase. The choice of primer pairs is listed in Table 6.1. The primer was mixed with 90 μL *Mse*I primer containing dNTPs to produce a primer/deoxynucleoside triphosphates (dNTP) mix for subsequent selective amplification.

Table 6.1 AFLP Primer Combinations

***Eco*RI primer (E)**	***Mse*I primer (M)**
E-AAA	M-CTT
E-AAC	M-CTT
E-AAG	MC-AA
E-AAT	M-CTT
E-ACA	M-CTT
E-ACC	M-CAA
E-ACG	M-CAA
E-ACT	M-CTT
E-AGC	M-CAT
E-AGG	M-CTA
E-AGG	M-CAA
E-ATA	M-CTT

6.2.3 AFLP Assay

A GIBCO BRL AFLP Analysis System II was used in accordance with the manufacturer's instructions. In brief, 125 ng of genomic DNA was digested in 1× reaction buffer (50 mmol/L Tris-HCl [pH 7.5], 50 mmol/L magnesium acetate and 250 mmol/L potassium acetate), 15 units of *Eco*RI and *Mse*I in a 12.5 μL reaction volume. The reaction mixture was mixed and placed into a MJ

PTC-100™ PCR thermocycler at 37°C for 2 h, then 70°C for 15 min to inactivate the restriction enzyme, and left standing at 4°C. The mixture was then ligated with a 12 μL adaptor/ligation solution containing *Eco*RI and *Mse*I adaptors and 0.5 unit ligase in a final volume of 25 μL. After incubation of the ligation mixture at 20°C for 2 h, it was diluted 10-fold with TE buffer by mixing 10 μL of the mixture with 90 μL TE buffer. The pre-amplification reaction was carried out in a volume of 25 μL containing 5 μL of the 10-fold PCR buffer plus Mg^{2+} (200 mmol/L Tris-HCl [pH 8.4]), 15 mmol/L $MgCl_2$ and 500 mmol/L KCl), 20 μL pre-amp primer mix (AFLP primer *Eco*RI + A, *Mse*I + C and dNTPs), 0.5 U *Taq* DNA polymerase and overlaid with a drop of mineral oil. PCR amplification was performed in the MJ PTC-100™ thermocycler using the following cycling profile: 20 cycles of 94°C for 30 s, 56°C for 1 min and 72°C for 1 min. A 20-fold dilution was done by diluting 10 μL of the pre-amplification DNA mixture with 190 μL TE buffer. In selective amplification, the reaction was performed in a 10 μL volume containing 2.5 μL of diluted template DNA, 1× PCR buffer with magnesium ions, 0.25 U *Taq* DNA polymerase, 2.5 μL primer/dNTPs mix and overlaid with a drop of mineral oil. PCR amplification was performed in the thermocycler using the following 'touch down' cycling profile: 1 cycle of 94°C for 30 s, 65°C for 30 s and 72°C for 1 min; 12 cycles of subsequently lowering the annealing temperature (65°C) by 0.7°C per cycle; 23 cycles of 94°C for 30 s, 56°C for 1 min and 72°C for 1 min; and left to soak at 4°C. Following PCR, an equal volume (10 μL) of formamide dye (98% formamide, 10 mmol/L ethylenediaminetetraacetic acid [EDTA], bromophenol blue, xylene cyanol) was added to each reaction. Electrophoresis of AFLP products was then conducted and sequencing reaction product of M13 DNA was run parallel to AFLP samples as a marker of fragment size.

6.2.4 Similarity Index Analysis of AFLP Profile

Gel image was stored as a TIF file and sizes of the AFLP product were analysed by the ImageQuant program (Molecular Dynamics, Solon, OH, United States). The similarity index (SI) value of fingerprints was calculated for each possible pairwise comparison between samples by the program DNA SIMDEX (Archer & Leung, 1998). DNA band patterns of the species were compared in a pairwise manner using the SI (please refer to Chapter 5 for a detailed discussion).

6.2.5 Reamplification and Cloning of Polymorphic DNA Fragments Isolated from the Dried Sequencing Gel

The elution of DNA from the dried sequencing gel was done in accordance with procedures mentioned in Chapter 3. With 1 μL of the DNA eluant as the template, PCR amplification was performed in a volume of 20 μL using the same conditions as in the selective AFLP amplification (Section 6.2.3), with the exception that 75 ng of unlabelled AFLP primers was used. The reamplified products were fractionated on 2% TAE agarose gel, followed by bands excision and DNA purification using the GENECLEAN® III Kit (Bio 101 Inc, Piscataway, NJ, United States). The AFLP fragments purified were then cloned and sequenced (please refer to Chapter 3 for a detailed discussion).

6.2.6 Conversion of AFLP Marker into Directed Amplification of Minisatellite-Region DNA Polymorphism Marker

Based on the sequence data found in the *P. ginseng* polymorphic bands, an oligonucleotide corresponding to the sequence of 22 bp minisatellite 5′-AGG ACT CAT CAC ATT GTT ACT C-3′

was designed for direct amplification of the minisatellite region. Directed amplification of the minisatellite-region DNA (DAMD) was performed in a 20-μL volume containing 40 ng plant DNA, 1× *Taq* buffer (10 mmol/L Tris-HCl, pH 8.3; 50 mmol/L KCl; 0.001% gelatin), 0.125 mmol/L dNTPs, 2.5 mmol/L $MgCl_2$ and 40 picomoles of primer. The reaction was carried out in the thermocycler with addition of 1 U of *Taq* DNA polymerase, using the cycling profile: 30 cycles of 94°C for 45 s, 55°C for 45 s and 72°C for 30 s. After the amplification, the products were resolved using 2% TBE agarose gel. The result was visualised through staining with ethidium bromide and photographed upon an ultraviolet (UV) transilluminator.

6.3 Results

Combinations of various primers were used to detect polymorphism between the two *Panax* species. Primer pair E-AGG/M-CAA was able to generate significant polymorphism and was employed to examine more samples from various localities. The fingerprint profiles of *P. ginseng* and *P. quinquefolius* are shown in Figures 6.3 and 6.4, respectively. Polymorphic bands are indicated by light arrows and the common bands shared between the two species are represented by dark arrows. Individual polymorphisms are also observed. By calculating the SI, the relatedness of the two *Panax* species from different localities can be estimated. Samples of *P. ginseng* from different farms in China and Korea show a high SI (0.88–0.99) (Table 6.2). However, *P. quinquefolius* from different farms appears to have a heterogeneous genetic makeup, with the SI between 0.64 and 0.96 (Table 6.3). A comparison of the sequence of polymorphic

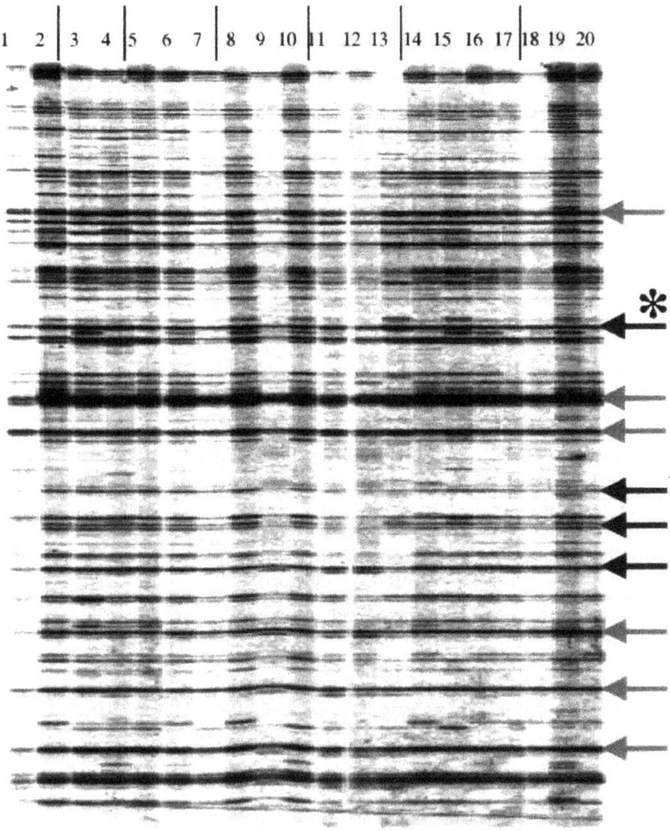

Fig. 6.3 AFLP profile of *P. ginseng* obtained using primer pair E-AGG/M-CAA. Two to four individuals from each locality were examined. Lanes 1 and 2 are samples from Ji'an county of Jilin province; lanes 3 and 4, from Xingbing county of Liaolin province; lanes 5–7, from Kangwon; lanes 8–10, from Pochon; lanes 11–13, from Kanghwa; lanes 14–17, from Kumsan and lanes 17–20, from Kimpo. Dark arrows are polymorphic bands unique to *P. ginseng*. Light arrows represent the common bands of two *Panax* species. The asterisk indicates that the sequence contains the minisatellite repeat that is used for DAMD analysis.

bands reveals that one of the sequenced polymorphic bands obtained in *P. ginseng* (Kanghwa) shows eight repeats of the 22 bp minisatellite in the 200 bp fragment (Figure 6.5). The minisatellite repeating sequence was not found to match any

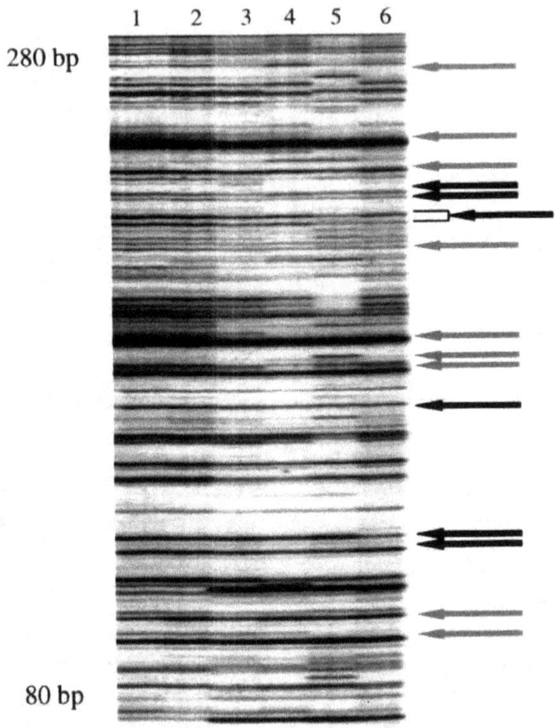

Fig. 6.4 AFLP profile of *P. quinquefolius* obtained using primer pair E-AGG/M-CAA. Lane 1 is a sample from Ontario; lanes 2 and 3, from two farms in British Columbia; lane 4, from a farm in Canada; lane 5, from a farm in the United States and lane 6, from Wisconsin. Dark arrows are polymorphic bands unique to *P. quinquefolius*. Light arrows represent the common bands of two *Panax* species.

entries in GenBank. Using the 22 bp minisatellite sequence as the primer for a PCR amplification from genomic DNA of two *Panax* species, a multiple fingerprint was obtained. Relatively large fragments were amplified and ranged from 0.8 to 1.8 kb. Polymorphic bands are shown by white arrows (Figure 6.6).

Table 6.2 SI Value of *P. ginseng* Based on the E-AGG/M-CAA AFLP Profile

	1	2	3	4	5	6	7	8	9	10	11	12	13	14	15	16	17	18	19
2	0.93																		
3	0.91	0.97																	
4	0.93	0.92	0.93																
5	0.96	0.93	0.92	0.93															
6	0.95	0.94	0.89	0.94	0.95														
7	0.95	0.93	0.90	0.95	0.95	0.92													
8	0.96	0.92	0.91	0.93	0.96	0.96	0.95												
9	0.95	0.92	0.90	0.89	0.93	0.93	0.89	0.95											
10	0.93	0.92	0.93	0.95	0.94	0.88	0.91	0.93	0.95										
11	0.95	0.92	0.90	0.92	0.96	0.96	0.95	0.98	0.96	0.97									
12	0.95	0.92	0.90	0.92	0.96	0.96	0.95	0.98	0.96	0.95	0.99								
13	0.94	0.94	0.93	0.97	0.98	0.90	0.90	0.95	0.95	0.96	0.98	0.98							
14	0.96	0.93	0.91	0.94	0.96	0.96	0.95	0.97	0.94	0.97	0.96	0.96	0.99						
15	0.93	0.92	0.92	0.93	0.95	0.93	0.92	0.95	0.93	0.95	0.96	0.96	0.95	0.96					
16	0.95	0.93	0.95	0.95	0.96	0.91	0.91	0.95	0.94	0.95	0.92	0.94	0.96	0.95	0.93				
17	0.95	0.92	0.94	0.95	0.97	0.92	0.90	0.95	0.92	0.95	0.95	0.95	0.96	0.97	0.94	0.96			
18	0.96	0.92	0.91	0.94	0.96	0.95	0.95	0.97	0.94	0.89	0.96	0.96	0.95	0.96	0.95	0.98	0.95		
19	0.96	0.93	0.91	0.94	0.97	0.95	0.94	0.96	0.93	0.89	0.96	0.96	0.95	0.96	0.96	0.97	0.96	0.96	
20	0.95	0.93	0.95	0.94	0.96	0.94	0.95	0.96	0.92	0.90	0.95	0.95	0.96	0.94	0.95	0.95	0.95	0.97	0.96

Table 6.3 SI Value of *P. quinquefolius* Based on the E-AGG/M-CAA AFLP Profile

	1	2	3	4	5
2	0.96				
3	0.89	0.88			
4	0.76	0.95	0.75		
5	0.72	0.75	0.72	0.72	
6	0.87	0.85	0.70	0.82	0.64

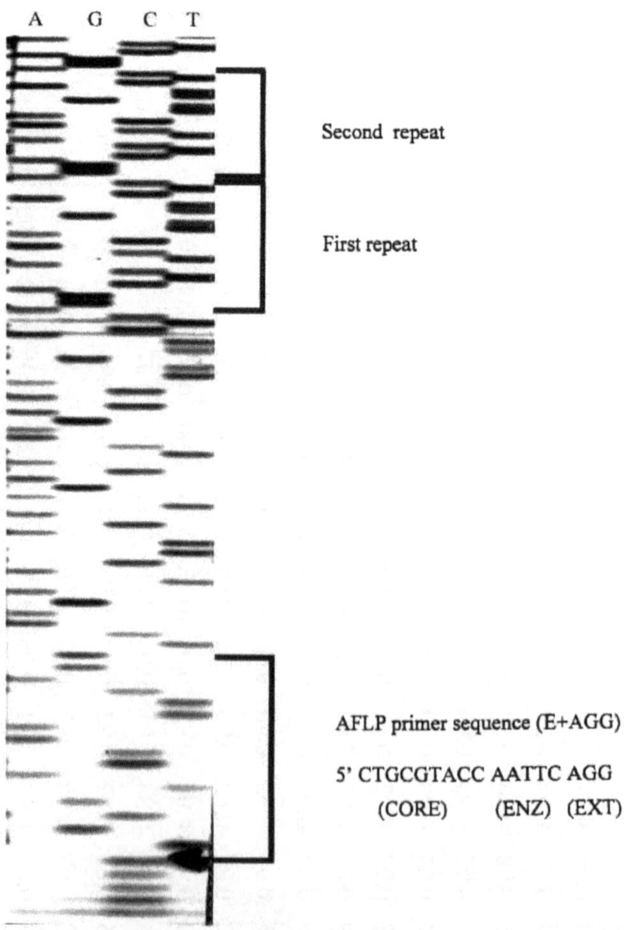

Fig. 6.5 Minisatellite sequence of the *P. ginseng* polymorphic band. The first and second repeats of 5′-AGG ACT CAT CAC ATT GTT ACT C-3′ are shown.

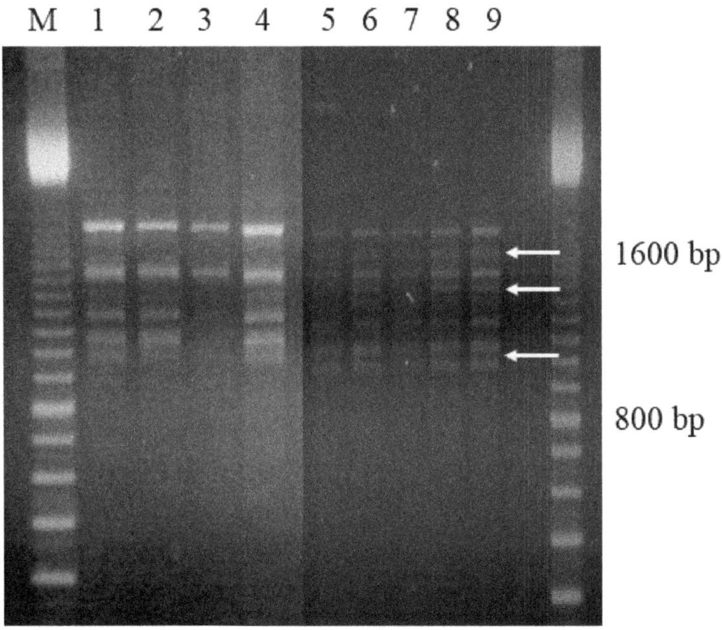

Fig. 6.6 DAMD analysis of two *Panax* species using the 22 bp minisatellite as the primer. Lanes 1–4 are *P. ginseng* from Ji'an county of Jilin province; Xingbing county of Liaolin province; Kanghwa and Kimpo, respectively. Lanes 5–9 are *P. quinquefolius* from two farms in British Columbia, Ontario, Wisconsin and a farm in the United States, respectively. Arrows indicate the polymorphic bands. M is the 100 bp DNA size marker (Pharmacia).

6.4 Discussion

The AFLP technique has two key characteristics. First, the template DNA are restriction fragments. Second, AFLP primers contain a variable selective nucleotide at the 3′ end, allowing selective amplification of a distinct set of restriction fragments. The number of nucleotides included in the 3′ end of the AFLP primer is flexible. By altering the numbers of selective nucleotides, an AFLP fingerprint with desired complexity can be generated. For example, a primer with one or no selective nucleotide was used for molecular typing of bacteria (Lin, Kuo & Ma, 1996) and a primer having seven to eight selective nucleotides was used for organisms with large-sized genome, e.g., *Alstroemeria* spp. (Han, van Eck, De Jeu & Jacobsen, 1999). The technique is reliable because optimal primer selectivity is obtained by using a 'touch down' PCR cycle in which the annealing temperature is lowered gradually to a level in which efficient primer binding is maintained for the rest of the PCR cycles. It is also reproducible, as indicated by reproducibility testing of AFLPs by a network of European laboratories (Jones & Harrower, 1998). Among the seven European laboratories, AFLP profiles were identical and highly reproducible. This technique is suitable for applications such as biodiversity studies, analysis of germplasm collections and genetic relationship studies.

Most plant DNAs are AT-rich and if the genome size is large, it is better to use AT-poor primers to limit the number of bands (Qi & Lindhout, 1997). Using primer pair E-AGG/M-CAA, optimal numbers of fragments, about 70 to 95, can be obtained and distinct AFLP fingerprint can be generated (Figures 6.3–6.4). Bands with different intensity can be observed. Faint bands are caused by poor amplification efficiency and may be due to a secondary structure that causes the blockage of enzymatic reactions, or a lower copy number than that of a strong one. Polymorphisms detected by AFLP may be caused by a single nucleotide change when either the restriction site itself or nucleotides adjacent to the restriction sites are affected, resulting in the AFLP primers mispairing at the 3′ end and failing to amplify. Deletions, insertions and rearrangements lead to polymorphisms as well. One of the polymorphic bands found in *P. ginseng* from Kanghwa (Figure 6.5) contained eight repeats of a 22 bp minisatellite. Minisatellite is a tandem repeat of a basic motif, approximately 10 to 60 bp long. They are not randomly dispersed throughout the genome, but rather are located mainly at the telomeric region of the chromosomes. They are highly polymorphic in regard to the number of repeats at a particular locus. Possible mechanisms for the presence of minisatellites include replication slippage, transposition, recombinational events and/or unequal crossover between sister chromatids at mitosis or meiosis, or between homologous chromosomes at meiosis, and gene conversion (Jeffreys, Wilson & Thein, 1985). Minisatellite tandem repeats can serve as a probe for hybridisation-based fingerprinting in order to detect many highly variable loci simultaneously, or they can be used as a primer for PCR.

Our discovery of the 22 bp minisatellite in one of the *P. ginseng* polymorphic bands impels its use as a rapid and easy method for authentication of *Panax* species. DAMD, the single step PCR amplification, was first reported by Heath and collaborators (Heath, Iwama & Devlin, 1993). Using a minisatellite as a single primer in PCR, the fragments amplified showed little variation within a species, but distinctive differences between species. When the amplified fragments were used as probes for genomic Southern blots, they revealed hypervariable single-locus or few-locus patterns in fish, birds and humans (Heath *et al.*, 1993). Minisatellites occur in many diverse species of plants and animals, and the orientation of a portion of a minisatellite array may become inverted, due to local inversions or other chromosomal rearrangements. Furthermore, if inversions have taken place in such a way that a single copy of DNA is present between them, then PCR, using a single minisatellite for the primer, may amplify the sequence historically adjacent to highly variable loci. DAMD thus produces random amplified polymorphic DNA (RAPD)-like fingerprints, but with much higher reproducibility. DAMD-PCR has been applied in the identification of wheat cultivars, rice, oilseed and mushroom species (Barroso, Sonnenberg, Van Griensven & Labarere, 2000; Bebeli, Zhou, Somers & Gustafson, 1997; Somers & Demmon, 2002; Zhou, Bebeli, Somers & Gustafson,

1997). Using this technique, multiple banding patterns were produced in all samples of *P. ginseng* and *P. quinquefolius* that are differentiated by three polymorphic bands (Figure 6.6).

The major advantage of AFLP is that it does not require a prior investment in sequence analysis, primer synthesis or characterisation of probes. Primers with different selective nucleotide combinations at the 3′ end of the core sequence allow the generation of different patterns and fingerprints from samples of any origin or complexity. AFLP is different from other PCR-based fingerprinting methods, because it is more reproducible due to the stringent reaction conditions used for the annealing of primers. Also, the band patterns are not affected by further thermal cycling because the radiolabelled *Eco*RI primer is a limiting factor, even though the unlabelled primer is in excess. Once the labelled primer is exhausted, the amplification reaction stops. AFLP fingerprinting is insensitive to the template DNA concentration. AFLP fingerprint patterns are very similar even when using template quantities that range 1,000-fold, i.e., from 25 pg to 25 ng, although the fingerprints vary significantly in terms of intensity and some bands may be absent when the template DNA is below 25 pg (Vos *et al.*, 1995).

Although AFLP has numerous advantages, it has also a number of limitations. First, informative fingerprints should be derived from complete digestion of genomic DNA. This requires that the digested fragments be examined on agarose gel to assure digestion has been completed. In fingerprints generated from partial digestion, the shift to a greater number of larger fragments is evident. Second, AFLP fingerprints share very few common fragments when the sequence homology is <90% (Janssen *et al.*, 1996). Third, high-quality DNA, especially high molecular weight DNA, is required. This is the major limitation in applying AFLP to the analysis of dried or processed medicinal materials, as intact genomic DNA are difficult to acquire.

6.5 Conclusion

AFLP is a PCR-based technique that utilises the differences in restriction fragment length caused by nucleotide polymorphism that create or abolish restriction endonuclease recognition sites. Restriction fragments from the total digestion of genomic DNA is selectively amplified by PCR to produce characteristic DNA fingerprinting. In this chapter, two medicinal materials, *P. ginseng* and *P. quinquefolius*, can be effectively differentiated using AFLP. AFLP markers are well suited for the use as molecular markers for the assessment of the botanical origin of medicinal materials.

References

Archer, E. S., & Leung, F. C. (1998). Computer program for automatically calculating similarity indexes from DNA fingerprints. *BioTechniques, 25*(2), 252–254. doi:10.2144/98252bc01

Barroso, G., Sonnenberg, A. S., Van Griensven, L. J., & Labarere, J. (2000). Molecular cloning of a widely distributed microsatellite core sequence from the cultivated mushroom Agaricus bisporus. *Fungal Genet Biol, 31*(2), 115–123. doi:10.1006/fgbi.2000.1239

Bebeli, P. J., Zhou, Z., Somers, D. J., & Gustafson, J. P. (1997). PCR primed with minisatellite core sequences yields DNA fingerprinting probes in wheat. *Theor Appl Genet, 95*(1), 276–283. doi:10.1007/s001220050560

Han, T. H., van Eck, H. J., De Jeu, M. J., & Jacobsen, E. (1999). Optimization of AFLP fingerprinting of organisms with a large-sized genome: A study on Alstroemeria spp. *Theor Appl Genet, 98*(3), 465–471. doi:10.1007/s001220051093

Heath, D. D., Iwama, G. K., & Devlin, R. H. (1993). PCR primed with VNTR core sequences yields species specific patterns and hypervariable probes. *Nucleic Acids Res, 21*(24), 5782–5785. doi:10.1093/nar/21.24.5782

Janssen, P., Coopman, R., Huys, G., Swings, J., Bleeker, M., Vos, P., Zabeau, M., Kersters, K. (1996). Evaluation of the DNA fingerprinting method AFLP as an new tool in bacterial taxonomy. *Microbiology (Reading), 142 (Pt 7)*, 1881–1893. doi:10.1099/13500872-142-7-1881

Jeffreys, A. J., Wilson, V., & Thein, S. L. (1985). Hypervariable 'minisatellite' regions in human DNA. *Nature, 314*(6006), 67–73. doi:10.1038/314067a0

Jones, J. T., & Harrower, B. E. (1998). A comparison of the efficiency of differential display and cDNA-AFLPs as tools for the isolation of differentially expressed parasite genes. *Fundam Appl Nematol, 21*(1), 81–88.

Lin, J. J., Kuo, J., & Ma, J. (1996). A PCR-based DNA fingerprinting technique: AFLP for molecular typing of bacteria. *Nucleic Acids Res, 24*(18), 3649–3650. doi:10.1093/nar/24.18.3649

Qi, X., & Lindhout, P. (1997). Development of AFLP markers in barley. *Mol Gen Genet, 254*(3), 330–336. doi:10.1007/s004380050423

Somers, D. J., & Demmon, G. (2002). Identification of repetitive, genome-specific probes in crucifer oilseed species. *Genome, 45*(3), 485–492. doi:10.1139/g02-006

Vos, P., Hogers, R., Bleeker, M., Reijans, M., van de Lee, T., Hornes, M., Friters, A., Pot, J., Paleman, J., Kuiper, M., & Zabeau, M. (1995). AFLP: A new technique for DNA fingerprinting. *Nucleic Acids Res, 23*(21), 4407–4414. doi:10.1093/nar/23.21.4407

Zhou, Z., Bebeli, P. J., Somers, D. J., & Gustafson, J. P. (1997). Direct amplification of minisatellite-region DNA with VNTR core sequences in the genus Oryza. *Theor Appl Genet, 95*(5), 942–949. doi:10.1007/s001220050645

Chapter 7

Authentication of Medicinal Materials by Polymerase Chain Reaction–Restriction Fragment Length Polymorphism

Hui Cao, Ying Zhang, Ping Li & Katsuko Komatsu

7.1 Introduction

Restriction fragment length polymorphism (RFLP) is a classical technique in which organisms can be differentiated by analysing the patterns derived from cleavage of their DNA. Simply, it is a technique that exploits variations in homologous DNA sequences. RFLP is defined by the existence of alternative alleles associated with restriction fragments that differ in size from each other. Thus, it occurs when the length of a detected fragment varies between individuals. Polymerase chain reaction-restriction fragment length polymorphism (PCR-RFLP) analysis, also known as cleaved amplified polymorphic sequence (CAPS), is a popular technique for genetic analysis. It has been applied for the detection of intraspecific as well as interspecific variation. The PCR-RFLP method is based on the digestion of PCR amplicons with appropriate restriction enzymes to produce distinct polymorphic fragments used as markers for species identification (Wolf, Rentsch & Hübner, 1999,

Wolf, Burgener, Hübner & Lüthy, 2000). PCR-RFLP consists of several separate steps including primer design, identification of an appropriate restriction enzyme, amplification, restriction enzyme treatment of amplified products and electrophoresis to resolve the restriction fragments (Figure 7.1).

7.2 Materials and Methods

7.2.1 Samples Studied

7.2.1.1 *Beimu*

Beimu (*Fritillaria* spp.) is a famous folk medicine that has been widely used to remove internal heat, nourish the lung, relieve cough and eliminate phlegm, and is indicated for the treatment of colds and acute bronchitis. Based on the evidence of previous *in vivo* or *in vitro* studies, Beimu exerts a series of biological activities, including antitussive, expectorant, analgesic, anticancer, anti-inflammatory, and antioxidative activities. Ten species of *Fritillaria* plant specimens (R1–R10) collected from different localities in China were used. Dried commercial samples (S1–S12) collected from various markets were also used (Tables 7.1–7.2). The samples were deposited in the Herbarium of China Pharmaceutical University, China.

7.2.1.2 *Daihuang*

Daihuang (*Rheum* spp.) is usually used to drain heat, relax the bowels, cool the blood, resolve toxicity, dispel blood stasis and unblock menstruation. It is indicated for the treatment of constipation and intestinal obstruction, bleeding, carbuncles and furuncles, burns and scalds, and even autoimmune diseases (Chen *et al.*, 2021). Forty-seven plant specimens of *Rheum palmatum*, *R. tanguticum* and

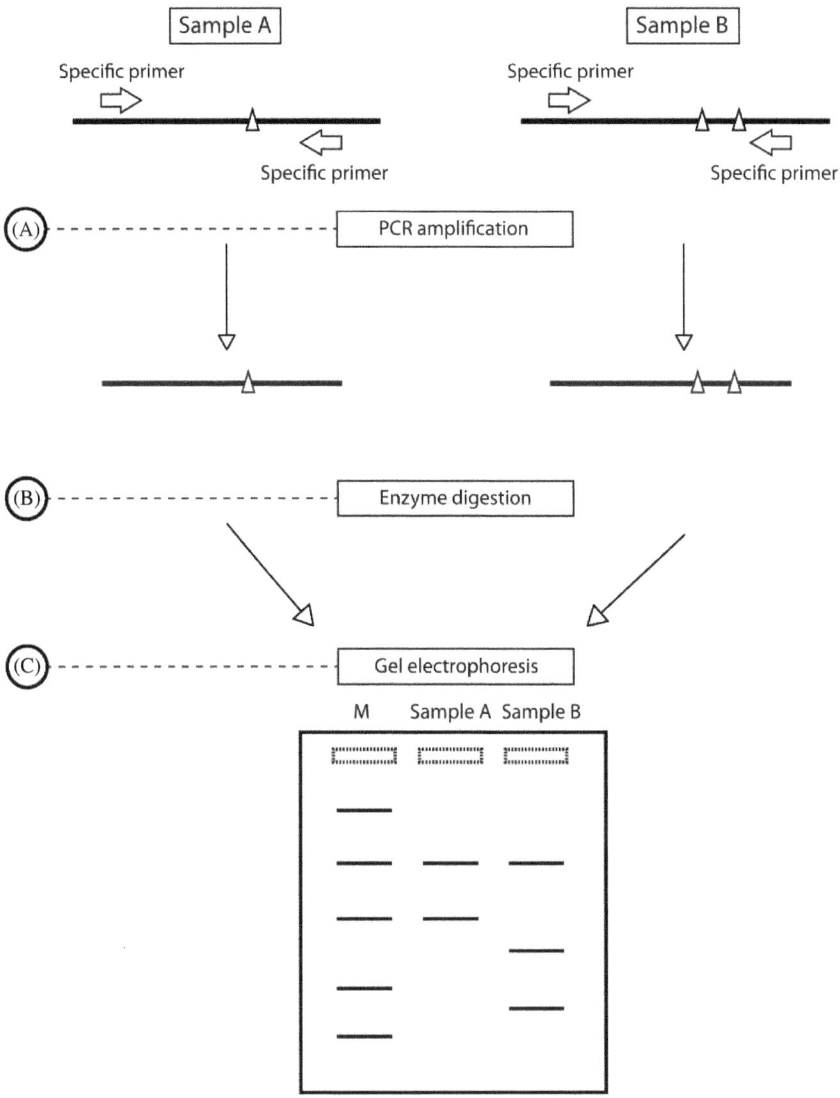

Fig. 7.1 Schematic outline of the RFLP technique. There are several main steps in RFLP analysis. First, the DNA from the target is isolated, the DNA-specific sequences are amplified, then the PCR amplification products are purified. Second, the purified PCR amplification products are cleaved by a restriction enzyme to produce specific DNA fragments. Third, DNA fragments are separated based on the sizes by gel electrophoresis. Differences in the DNA pattern between samples create polymorphism. (A) DNA-specific sequences are amplified by specific primers, and the triangle symbol represents the site identified by the restriction enzyme. There is one site in Sample A and two sites in Sample B. (B) PCR amplification products are purified and digested by the restriction enzyme. (C) The digested DNA fragments are separated by gel electrophoresis.

Table 7.1 Ten Species of *Fritillaria* Specimens Used in this Study

No.	Chinese name	Latin name	Habitat/source
R1	Anzibeimu	*Fritillaria. unibracteata* Hsiao et K.C. Hsia	Mao county, Sichuan
R2	Gansubeimu	*F. przewalskii* Maxim.	Yeduo, Qinghai
R3	Juanyebeimu	*F. cirrhosa* D. Don	Kangding, Sichuan
R4	Suoshabeimu	*F. delavayi* Franch.	Luding, Sichuan
R5	Taibaibeimu	*F. taipaiensis* P. Y. Li	Chengkou, Chongqing
R6	Wabubeimu	*F. unibracteata* Hsiao et K. C. Hsia var. *wabuensis* (S. Y. Tang et S. C. Yue) Z. D. Liu	Songpan, Sichuan
R7	Hubeibeimu	*F. hupehensis* Hsiao et K. C. Hsia	NICPBP
R8	Pingbeimu	*F. ussuriensis* Maxim.	NICPBP
R9	Yibeimu	*F. pallidiflora* Schrenk	NICPBP
R10	Zhebeimu	*F. thunbergii* Miq.	NICPBP

NICPBP: National Institute for the Control of Pharmaceutical and Biological Products.

Table 7.2 Twelve Commercial Samples of Beimu Used in this Study

No.	Chinese name	Habitat/source
S1	Hubeibeimu	Hubei
S2	Pingbeimu	Heilongjiang
S3	Pingbeimu	Jilin
S4	Yibeimu	Xinjiang
S5	Yibeimu	Zhejiang
S6	Zhebeimu	Gansu
S7	Chuanbeimu (Songbei)	Gansu
S8	Chuanbeimu (Qingbei)	Anhui
S9	Chuanbeimu (Lubei)	Yunnan
S10	Chuanbeimu (Qingbei)	NICPBP
S11	Chuanbeimu (Lubei)	Sichuan
S12	Chuanbeimu (Songbei)	Sichuan

NICPBP: National Institute for the Control of Pharmaceutical and Biological Products.

R. officinale, and eight specimens of *R. rhaponticum*, *R. franzenbachii*, *R. undulatum*, *R. przewalskyi* and *R. kialense* were used in this study (Table 7.3). Twenty-two commercial samples of Daihuang were purchased from Chinese markets near the *Rheum* fields, from Uchida Wakanyaku Co., Ltd. (Tokyo, Japan) and Tochimoto Tenkaido Co., Ltd. (Osaka, Japan) (Table 7.4). Both plant specimens and commercial samples were deposited in the Museum of Materia Medica, Institute of Natural Medicine, Toyama University (TMPW).

7.2.2 Total Genomic DNA Preparation

Total DNA was extracted from 100 to 200 mg of bulbs or leaves of Beimu samples, using the DNA Plant Mini Kit (Beijing Sanbo Yuanzhi Bio-Tech Co., China). The total DNA was dissolved in TE buffer and stored at 4°C for PCR. Total DNA was extracted from 50 to 100 mg of dried or fresh leaves of Daihuang samples using the DNeasy™ Plant Mini Kit (Qiagen, Germany), and from 0.1 to 1 g of Rhei Rhizoma samples using the cetyltrimethylammonium bromide (CTAB) method.

7.2.3 Choice of Primers

Specific primers were designed for these two medicinal materials (Table 7.5). For Beimu, the primers P1–P2 of internal transcribed spacer (ITS) were based on rice rDNA sequences (Takaiwa, Oono & Sugiura, 1985). An antisense primer P3 was designed according to the nrDNA 5.8S homologous sequences of sibling species (Wang, Li, Ding, Peng & Yuan, 2007, Xu, Li, Li, Zhang, & Wang, 2010). All the primers were synthesized by Shanghai Sangon Co. Ltd. (China). The whole nrDNA ITS region (ITS1,

Table 7.3 Fifty-five Species of *Rheum* Specimens Used in this Study

Species	Locality of voucher		Statement	Code no.	Clade[a]	GenBank accession no.
Section Palmata A.						
Rheum palmatum L.	Qinghai Prov., China	Banma (班瑪) Co.	cult.	Pq1, 2	RPI	AB115669
		Dongqingou (東傾溝)	cult.	Pq3	RPI	AB115670
	Sichuan Prov., China	Heping (和坪), Shimian (石棉) Co.	cult.	Ps4	RPII	AB115672
		Heping, Shimian Co.	cult.	Ps5	RPI	AB115671
		Caoke (草科), Shimian Co.	cult.	Ps6	RPIII	AB115676
		Caoke, Shimian Co.	cult.	Ps7	RPIII	AB115677
		Zheduo (折多山), Kangding (康定) Co.	wild	Ps8, 9, 10	RPIII	AB115678
		Geka (葛卡), Daofu (道孚) Co.	cult.	Ps11	RPI	AB115670
		Geka, Daofu Co.	cult.	Ps12	RPIII	AB115679
		Tagong (塔公), Kangding Co.	cult.	Ps13	RPIII	AB115680
		Xinduqiao (新都橋), Kangding Co.	wild	Ps14	RPIII	AB115680
		Xinlong (新隆) Co.	wild	Ps15	RPI	AB115671
		Yulong (玉隆), Dege (德格) Co.	cult.	Ps16, 17	RPI	AB115670
		Shiqu (石渠) Co.	cult.	Ps18	RPIII	AB115680
	Yunnan Prov., China	Heqing (鶴慶), Dali (大理) Co.	cult.	Ps19, 20, 21, 22	RPIII	AB115681

		Heqing, Dali Co.	cult.	Ps23	RPII	AB115673
		Heqing, Dali Co.	cult.	Ps24	RPII	AB115673
	Gansu Prov., China	Li (禮) Co.	cult.	Ps25	RPII	AB115673
		Gezigou (格子溝), Li (禮) Co.	cult.	Ps26	RPII	AB115673
		Quanshui (銓水), Li (禮) Co.	cult.	Ps27	RPIII	AB115677
		Quanshui, Li Co.	cult.	Ps28	RPIII	AB115677
		Nanyang (南陽), Dangchang (宕昌) Co.	cult.	Ps29	RPII	AB115673
		Nanyang, Dangchang Co.	cult.	Ps30	RPIII	AB115677
		Chengjiao (城郊), Min (岷) Co.	cult.	Ps31, 32	RPII	AB115673
		Chengjiao, Min Co.	cult.	Ps33	RPIII	AB115677
		Hanban (憨班), Zhouqu (舟曲) Co.	cult.	Ps34	RPII	AB115674
		Baidian(白點山), Zhouqu Co.	wild	Ps35, 36, 37	RPII	AB115675
R. tanguticum MAXIM. ex BALF.	Qinghai Prov., China	Qunjia (群加), Huangzhong (湟中) Co.	cult.	T1	RT	AB115682
		Mashidang (麻什當), Huangnan (黄南) Co.	wild	T2	RT	AB115682
		Reshui (熱水), Dulan (都蘭) Co.	wild	T3, 4	RT	AB115683
R. officinale BAILLON	Sichuan Prov., China	Fengtong (蜂桶), Wanyuan (萬源) Co.	cult.	O1, 2, 3	ROC	AB115684
		Piwo (皮窩), Wanyuan Co.	cult.	O4	ROC	AB115685
		Piwo, Wanyuan Co.	wild	O5, 6	ROC	AB115686

(Continued)

Table 7.3 (*Continued*)

Species	Locality of voucher		Statement	Code no.	Clade[a]	GenBank accession no.
Section Rhapontica A. LOS.						
R. rhaponticum L.	Qinghai Prov., China	Dulan (都蘭) Co.	cult.	R	RR	AB115688
R. franzenbachii M_{UNT}	Hebei Prov., China	Anguo (安國)	cult.	F	RR	AB115689
R. undulatum L.	Ulaanbaatar, Mongolia	Hairthaan	wild	U1	RR	AB115690
	Ovorhangay, Mongolia	Gandyn Had	wild	U2	RR	AB115690
	Bayanhongor, Mongolia	Suuj Teeg Uul	wild	U3	RR	AB115691
Section Spiciformia A. LOS.						
R. przewalskyi A. LOS.	Qinghai Prov., China	Xidatan (西大灘), Geermu (格爾木)	wild	S1	RS	AB115693
	Qinghai Prov., China	Reshui (熱水), Dulan (都蘭) Co.	wild	S2	RS	AB115694
Section Acuminata C. Y						
R. kialense FRANCH.	Sichuan Prov., China	Yulong (玉隆), Dege (德格) Co.	wild	K	RK	AB115692

[a]Each clade was determined on the basis of phylogenetic analysis of the *matK* gene sequence.

Table 7.4 Twenty-two Commercial Samples of Rhei Radix et Rhizoma Used in this Study and their Botanic Origins

Sample name	Market	Production area	TMPW no.[a]	Code no.	Botanic origin (group)[c]
Daihuang (大黃)[b]	Banma (班瑪) County, Qinghai (青海), China	Banma County, Qinghai	20061	D1	*Rheum palmatum* (I)
Daihuang[b]	Tongren (同仁) County, Qinghai, China	Huangnan County, Qinghai	20065	D2	*R. tanguticum*
Daihuang	Tongren County, Qinghai, China	Huangnan County, Qinghai	20066	D11	*R. tanguticum*
Daihuang	Dulan (都蘭) County, Qinghai, China	Dulan County, Qinghai	20107	D12	*R. tanguticum*
Daihuang	Dulan County, Qinghai, China	Dulan County, Qinghai	20108	D13	*R. tanguticum*
Daihuang	Dulan County, Qinghai, China	Dulan County, Qinghai	20109	D14	*R. tanguticum*
Daihuang	Ganzi (甘孜) County, Sichuan (四川), China	Ganzi County, Sichuan	20218	D15	*R. palmatum* (I)
Daihuang[b]	Kangding (康定) County, Sichuan, China	Jiulong County, Sichuan	20216	D3	*R. palmatum* (III)
Yin-huang (陰黃)	Yaan (雅安) County, Sichuan, China	Litang County, Sichuan	20574	D16	*R. palmatum* (III)
Yin-kang-huang (陰康黃)	Yaan County, Sichuan, China	Shimian County, Sichuan	20573	D17	*R. palmatum* (III)
Daihuang	Wanyuan (萬源) County, Sichuan, China	Wanyuan County, Sichuan	20266	D18	*R. palmatum* (II)
Daihuang[b]	Wanyuan County, Sichuan, China	Wanyuan County, Sichuan	20267	D4	*R. officinale*
Mati-daihuang (馬蹄大黃)	Wanyuan County, Sichuan, China	Wanyuan County, Sichuan	07422	D19	*R. palmatum* (II)
Daihuang[b]	Zhongdian (中甸) County, Yunnan (雲南), China	Zhongdian County, Yunnan	19535	D5	*R. palmatum* (II)

(*Continued*)

Table 7.4 (*Continued*)

Sample name	Market	Production area	TMPW no.[a]	Code no.	Botanic origin (group)[c]
Ba-cheng-ji (八成吉)[b]	Li (禮) County, Gansu (甘肅), China	Li County, Gansu	20926	D6	*R. palmatum* (II)
Tong-huo (統貨)[b]	Li County, Gansu, China	Li County, Gansu	20928	D7	*R. palmatum* (II)
Daihuang[b]	Min (岷) County, Gansu, China	Diebu County, Gansu	20931	D8	*R. palmatum* (II)
Daihuang	Zhouqu (舟曲) County, Gansu, China	Zhouqu County, Gansu	20932	D20	*R. palmatum* (III)
Daihuang[b]	Uchida Wakanyaku Co., Ltd., Tokyo, Japan	Shimian County, Sichuan	19928	D9	*R. palmatum* (III)
Liu-cheng-ji (六成吉)[b]	Uchida Wakanyaku Co., Ltd., Tokyo, Japan	Li County, Gansu	19927	D10	*R. palmatum* (II)
Ya-huang (雅黄)	Tochimoto Tenkaido Co., Ltd., Osaka, Japan	Sichuan	19948	D21	*R. palmatum* (I)
Bao-huang (包黄)	Tochimoto Tenkaido Co., Ltd., Osaka, Japan	Qinghai	19949	D22	*R. tanguticum*

[a] The specimen reference number of the Museum of Materia Medica, Institute of Natural Medicine, TMPW.
[b] The botanic origins of D1–D10 have been identified by sequence analysis.
[c] (I) (II) and (III) represent different clades of R. palmatum determined on the basis of phylogenetic analysis of the *matK* gene sequence.

Table 7.5 Primers Used in this Study

Sample	Primer name	Sequence (5′ to 3′)
Beimu	ITS-P1	CGT AAC AAG GTT TCC GTA GGT GAA
	ITS-P2	TTA TTG ATA TGC TTA AAC TCA GCG GG
	ITS-P3	GCT ACG TTC TTC ATC GAT
Daihuang	*mat*KAF	CTA TAT CCA CTT ATC TTT CAG GAG T
	*mat*K191F	TAG TTA TTC GAA TGT ATC AAC AG
	*mat*K367CR	GAT CGT AAA TTT TGA TAT TTT TTG AG
	*mat*K367TR	GAT CGT AAA TTT TGA TAT TTT TTG AA
	*mat*K646F	TCC TAC GTG TGT GAA TGC G
	*trn*K1544R	GGA TAA CCC CAG AAT GCT TAG
	*mat*K937CR	ATA TAG ATT CTT TGC AAC CAG AG
	*mat*K937TR	GAT ATA GAT TCT TTG CAA CCA GAA
	*mat*K8R	AAA GTT CTA GCA CAA GAA AGT CGA

5.8S, ITS2) was amplified with ITS-P1 and ITS-P2, whereas the nrDNA ITS1 region was amplified with ITS-P1 and ITS-P3. For Daihuang, the primers of *matK* were the same as the previous study as described in (Yang, Fushimi, Cai & Komatsu, 2004).

7.2.4 PCR-RFLP Assay

7.2.4.1 *Beimu*

Amplification was carried out in an Eppendorf Mastercycler Gradient programmed for pre-denaturalization of 3 min at 95°C and 30 cycles of 30 s at 95°C, 30 s at 53°C and 30 s at 72°C, followed by one cycle of 5 min at 72°C. PCR products were fractionated by 2% agarose gel electrophoresis. The resulting DNA fragments were visualised by ultraviolet (UV) transillumination using the Gel Doc 2000 System. Sequences were determined using the PCR products with the two primers (ITS-P1 and ITS-P3). Automated DNA sequencing was run on an ABI 3700 Sequencer (Wang *et al.*, 2007, Xu *et al.*, 2010).

Restriction maps of the ITS1 sequences were generated using the software Primer-Premier. From the restriction maps, *Sma*I was selected as a suitable candidate for discrimination between Chuanbeimu and non-Chuanbeimu samples. Digestion with *Sma*I (Promega, Madison, WI) was performed in a total volume of 20 μL containing 5–10 μL PCR products, 5 U of *Sma*I enzyme and 2 μL 10 × digestion buffer as recommended by the manufacturer; incubation was at 30°C for 2 h. The DNA was fractionated by 2% agarose gel electrophoresis and visualised by ethidium bromide staining under UV. Ten reference drugs of Beimu were analysed with the PCR-RFLP method. Based on the standard electrophoresis diagram, 12 commercial samples of Beimu were identified by this method.

7.2.4.2 *Daihuang*

For each primer set, PCR amplification was carried out in a Thermal Controller PTC 100 (MJ Research, Inc., Hercules, CA) with the following cycling condition: hot start at 94°C for 1 min, followed by 40 cycles of 94°C for 1 min, 50°C for 1 min, 72°C for 2 min and a final extension at 72°C for 30 min. The 1/10 volume of the resulting PCR product was detected by 1.0% agarose gel electrophoresis and visualised by ethidium bromide staining under UV. In the case of commercial samples, a semi-nested PCR method was applied: the first PCR product amplified with a pair of primers, *mat*KAF and *mat*K8R under the abovementioned cycling condition was purified with a QIAquick PCR Purification Kit (Qiagen). Using this product as a template, the second PCR amplification was performed using a pair of primers, *mat*K191F and *mat*K8R.

The resulting PCR products from all materials were digested with 5 units of restriction enzyme, *Bgl*II (BioLabs, Inc., New York, NY) at 37°C for 1.5 h. Moreover, the PCR products from the materials derived from *R. palmatum* were digested with 5 units of restriction enzyme *Nsi*I or *Dra*I (BioLabs, Inc.). The fragments obtained were detected by 2.0% agarose gel electrophoresis and visualised by ethidium bromide staining under UV. In the case of sample D21 in Table 7.4, as a PCR product of the partial *matK* gene was not obtained, two regions (1 and 2) were amplified separately using *mat*K191F and *trn*K1544R, and *mat*K646F and *mat*K8R, respectively, together with the total DNA as a template. The cycling condition was the same as mentioned earlier except for the annealing temperature, which was adjusted to 53°C. The PCR product of region 1 was digested with restriction enzyme *Bgl*II, whereas that of region 2 was digested with restriction enzymes *Nsi*I or *Dra*I.

The PCR amplification was performed using total DNAs from all materials as template in 25 μL of reaction mixture composed of 10 mmol/L Tris-HCl (pH 9.0), 50 μmol/L KCl, 0.1% Triton X-100, 1.5 mmol/L $MgCl_2$, 0.2 mmol/L dNTP, 0.25 μ mol/L forward primer, 0.125 μmol/L reverse primer and 1.5U *Taq* Polymerase (Promega). The optimal cycling condition for primer set A was established as follows: hot start at 94°C for 1 min, followed by 40 cycles at 94°C for 1 min, 52°C for 1 min, 72°C for 2 min and a final extension at 72°C for 15 min. For primer sets B and C, the annealing temperature and time were changed to 59°C for 50 s and 58.5°C for 50 s, respectively, and the extension time was also changed to 1 min and 50 s. About 5 μL of the resulting product was analysed by 2.0% agarose gel electrophoresis.

7.3 Results

7.3.1 Beimu

Using the primers ITS-P1 and ITS-P3, a single PCR product about 0.7 kb was observed and then sequenced. For the PCR-RFLP analysis with primer pairs of ITS-P1 and ITS-P3, the PCR products from the reference Chuanbeimu species amplified included the complete nrDNA ITS1 region, partial 18S and 5.8S nrDNA regions: each showed two bands in the electrophoresis profile, approximately 100–200 bp in length. There was a single band in the electrophoresis profile of the reference medicinal materials of the non-Chuanbeimu, approximately 300 bp in length (Figure 7.2).

PCR-RFLP analysis for 12 commercial Beimu samples was also carried out using *Sma*I. The results of two fragments (190 bp and 118 bp) indicated that PCR products from six samples, each purchased from markets in Gansu, Anhui, Yunnan and Sichuan provinces (S7–S12), could be digested by *Sma*I, and these results were successfully repeated. The six samples were authenticated as

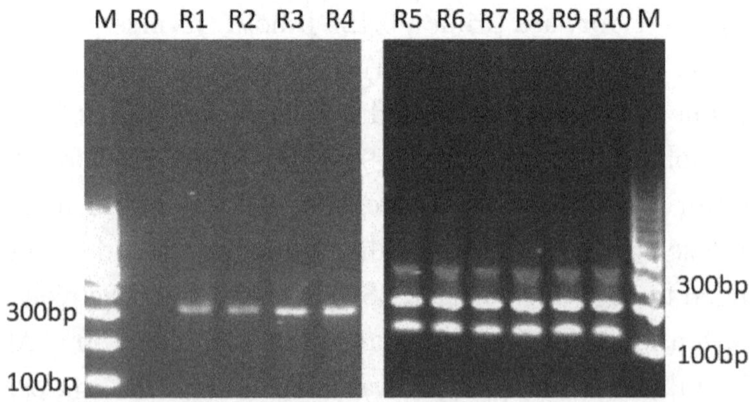

Fig. 7.2 PCR-RFLP electropherograms of reference medicinal materials. M: 100 bp DNA size marker; R0: Blank control; R1–R10: See also at Table 7.1.

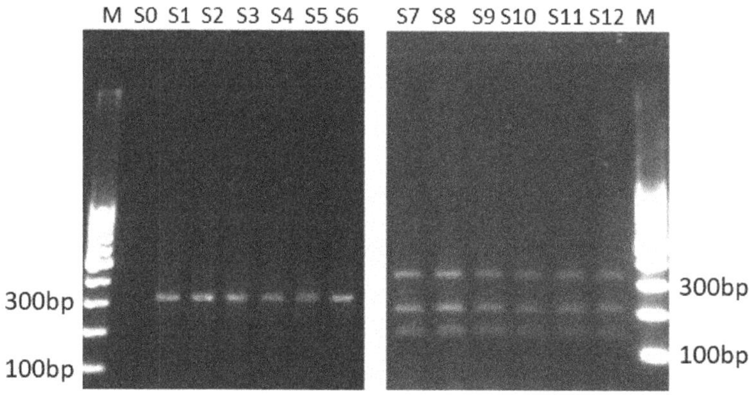

Fig. 7.3 PCR-RFLP electropherograms of commercial medicinal materials. M: 100 bp DNA size marker; S0: Blank control; S1–S12: See also at Table 7.2.

Chuanbeimu, including two Songbei samples, two Qingbei samples and two Lubei samples. The ITS1 fragments from other six commercial samples purchased from Hubei, Heilongjiang, Jilin, Xinjiang and Zhejiang provinces (S1–S6) could not be digested by *Sma*I, and these results indicated that they were not Chuanbeimu (Figure 7.3).

7.3.2 Daihuang

On the basis of the nucleotide substitutions at positions 367 and 937 among the three official Daihuang species on the *matK* gene, at each position two kinds of reverse primers, *mat*K367CR & *mat*K367TR and *mat*K937CR & *mat*K937TR with complementary 3′ terminal nucleotide, were designed. To enhance the specificity, a destabilizing mismatch was incorporated at the third nucleotide from the 3′ terminus in each reverse primer. Three sets of primers were prepared, each consisting of two kinds of reverse primers, *mat*K367CR or *mat*K367TR and *mat*K937CR or *mat*K937TR, and one forward primer, *mat*K191F (Figures 7.4 and 7.5).

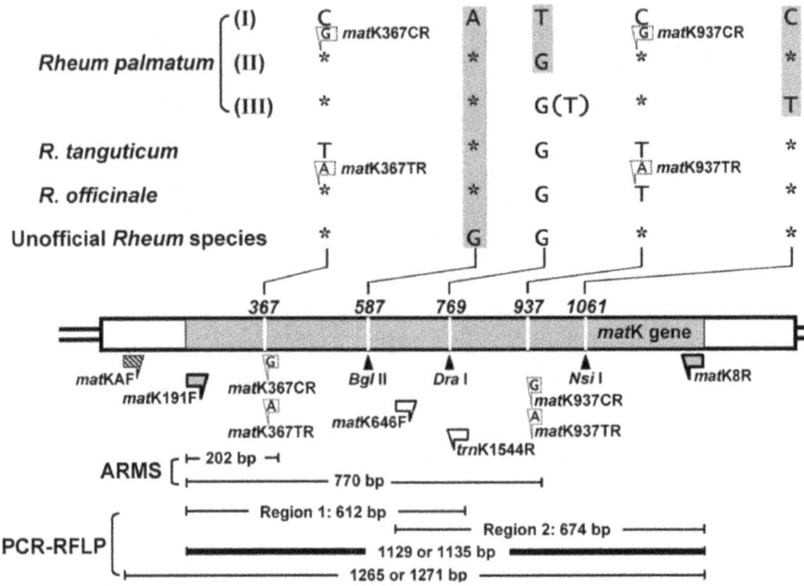

Fig. 7.4 Positions of marker nucleotides, PCR primers for PCR-RFLP and amplification-refractory mutation system (ARMS) analyses, and restriction enzyme sites on the *matK* gene. ARMS is a simple method for detecting any mutation involving a single base change or small deletion. It is based on the use of sequence-specific PCR primer that allows amplification of test DNA only when the target allele is within the sample. Marker nucleotides used in this study are indicated by numerals in italics above the *matK* gene; nucleotide substitutions with shadows at positions 587, 769 and 1061 were applied to PCR-RFLP analysis, and those at positions 367 and 937 to ARMS analysis. PCR primers for PCR-RFLP analysis are indicated by solid half-arrows and those for ARMS analysis by dotted half-arrows, mapped below the diagram. The lengths of the resulting PCR products are shown at the bottom. For PCR-RFLP analysis, PCR products of 1,129 bp (or 1,135 bp) obtained from PCR or semi-nested PCR methods were used. The PCR product of 1,265 bp was used as a template in semi-nested PCR. The PCR products of regions 1 and 2 were used for PCR-RFLP analysis of sample D21. Important restriction enzyme sites of *Bgl*II, *Nsi*I and *Dra*I used for identifying section Palmata and the distinction of the three groups of *R. palmatum* are indicated by sharp arrows.

The PCR products of *R. przewalskyi* and *R. kialense* amplified with *mat*K191F and *mat*K8R had the size of 1,129 bp in length. The PCR products of the other six Rheum species had the length of 1,135 bp (Figure 7.4). The restriction enzyme *Bgl*II, which recognizes the sequence of 5′-AGA TCT-3′, was found to

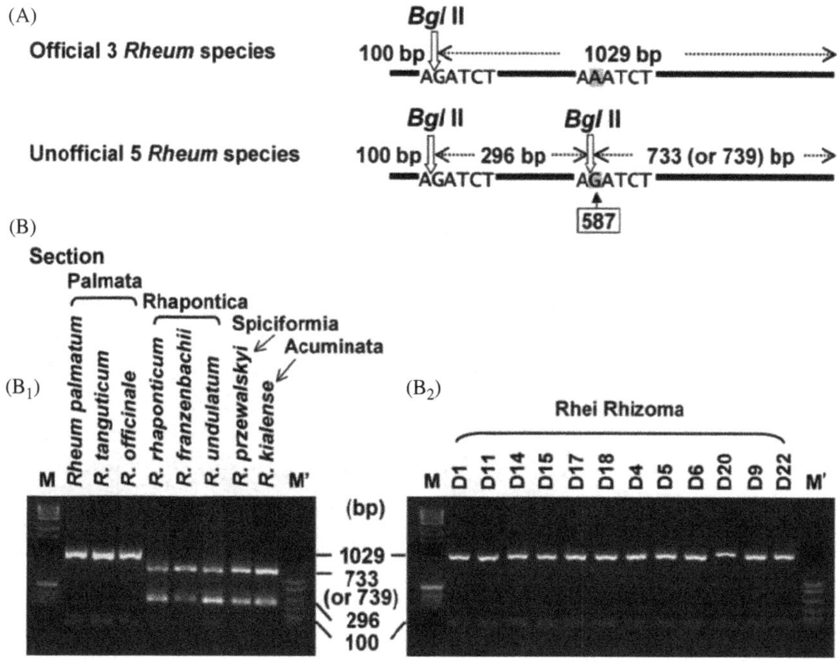

Fig. 7.5 PCR-RFLP analysis using the restriction enzyme *Bgl*II on the partial *matK* gene. (A) *Bgl*II restriction sites in three official *Rheum* species and five other species; nucleotides with shadows indicate the defined identification marker at position 587. (B) Agarose gel electrophoretograms of PCR products digested with *Bgl*II. (B_1) Eight *Rheum* species, and (B_2) commercial samples of Rhei Radix et Rhizoma. Codes of commercial samples are shown in Table 7.4. Lane M, 1 kb DNA size marker; M', pBR 322DNA-*Msp*I digestion.

give diagnostic fragments among the eight species. The *matK* gene of five species, excluding the three official species, had a *Bgl*II restriction site at the nucleotide position 586–591 (Figure 7.4). The PCR products of these five species digested with *Bgl*II showed three fragments of 100 bp, 296 bp and 733 bp or 739 bp (Figure 7.5), while the three official species showed two fragments of 100 bp and 1,029 bp (Figure 7.5B_1).

Three sets of primers (Primer set A, B and C in Figure 7.6) were used for the amplification (Figure 7.6A). When the primer set A was used, one fragment of 202 bp was observed in *R. palmatum*,

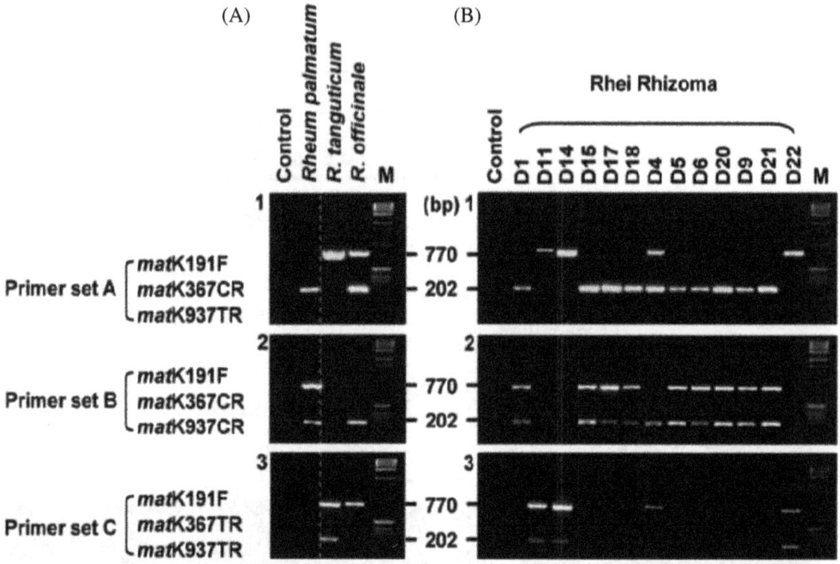

Fig. 7.6 ARMS analysis using three sets of primers on the partial *matK* gene. PCR amplification with primer sets A, B and C was carried out using the DNA of each material as template. (A) Three official *Rheum* species; (B) Commercial samples of Rhei Radix et Rhizoma derived from the official species; codes of samples are shown in Table 7.4. Resulting in the 1, 2 and 3 fragment patterns when using primer sets A, B and C, respectively. Control, blank without DNA template; Lane M, 1 kb DNA size marker.

one fragment of 770 bp in *R. tanguticum* and both fragments in *R. officinale* (Figure 7.6A_1). When primer set B was used, two fragments of 202 and 770 bp were observed in *R. palmatum*, one fragment of 202 bp in *R. officinale* and no fragment in *R. tanguticum* (Figure 7.6A_2). When primer set C was used, two fragments were observed in *R. tanguticum*, one fragment of 770 bp in *R. officinale*, and no fragment in *R. palmatum* (Figure 7.6A_3). By observing these three kinds of fragment profiles, the three official species could be authenticated.

The restriction enzymes, *Nsi*I and *Dra*I, which recognize the sequence of 5′-ATG CAT-3′ and 5′-TTT AAA-3′, respectively, were found to give diagnostic fragments among the three groups of *R. palmatum* (I, II and III). The *matK* gene of groups I and

II had an *Nsi*I restriction site at position 1058–1063. Moreover, that of group I had a *Dra*I restriction site at the position 768–773 (Figure 7.7A, Figure 7.7C). The PCR products of groups I and II digested with *Nsi*I showed two fragments of 263 and 866 bp, whereas that of group III showed one fragment of 1,129 bp (Figure 7.7B_1). On the other hand, digestion of the PCR products with *Dra*I resulted in the formation of three fragments of 247, 333 and 549 bp in group I, and two fragments of 247 and 882 bp in group II (Figure 7.7D_1).

Twenty-two commercial samples (Table 7.4) were analysed by using the above-mentioned PCR-RFLP and ARMS methods. Their PCR products, amplified with *mat*K191F and *mat*K8R, in a semi-nested PCR method, were 1,129 bp in length. Sample D21 did not give a PCR product. Digestion of the PCR products with restriction enzyme *Bgl*II resulted in the formation of two fragments of 100 and 1,029 bp (Figure 7.5B_2), suggesting that the samples were derived from the official *Rheum* species of section Palmata. In the ARMS method using three sets of primers, six commercial samples from Qinghai Province (D2, D11, D12, D13, D14 and D22) showed the same fragment patterns as those of *R. tanguticum* (D11, D14 and D22). One sample from Wanyuan County, Sichuan Province, had fragment patterns as those of *R. officinale* (D4) and remnants as those of *R. palmatum*, respectively (Figure 7.6B). As for the last 15 samples, their PCR products were digested with the restriction enzyme *Nsi*I or *Dra*I (Figure 7.7). The PCR products of five drug samples (D3, D16, D17, D9 and D20), mostly from Sichuan Province, digested with *Nsi*I showed one fragment (D17, D20 and D9), whereas those of the other 10 samples showed two fragments, which suggested that the former originated from group III and the latter from group I (D1, D15 and D21) or group II (D18, D19, D5, D6, D7, D8 and D10) of *R. palmatum*, respectively (Figure 7.7B_2).

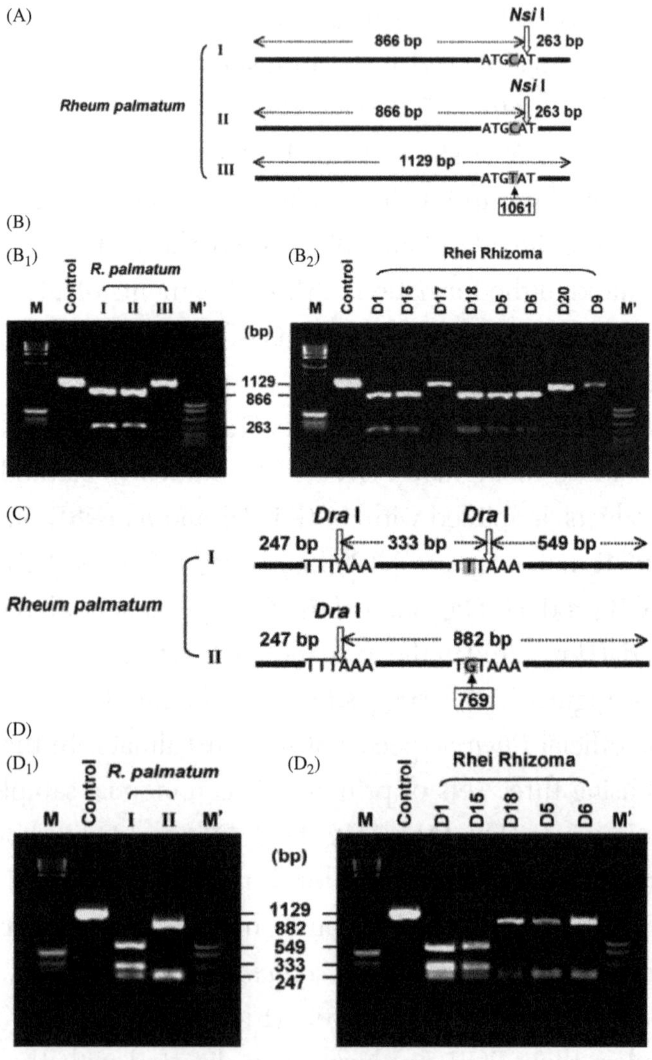

Fig. 7.7 PCR-RFLP analysis using the restriction enzyme *Nsi*I or *Dra*I on the partial *matK* gene. (A) *Nsi*I restriction site in three groups of *Rheum palmatum*; nucleotides with shadows indicate the defined identification marker at position 1061. (B) Agarose gel electrophoretograms of PCR products digested with *Nsi*I; B_1: three groups of *R. palmatum*; B_2: drug samples of Rhei Rhizoma; codes of drug samples are shown. (C) *Dra*I restriction sites in two groups of *R. palmatum*; nucleotides with shadows indicate the identification marker at position 769. (D) Agarose gel electrophoretograms of PCR products digested with *Dra*I; D_1, two groups of *R. palmatum*; D_2, commercial samples of Rhei Radix et Rhizoma. Lane M, 1 kb DNA size marker; M', pBR322DNA-*Msp*I digestion.

The digestion of the PCR products of the latter samples with *Dra*I resulted in the formation of three fragments in three samples from Banma County, Qinghai Province, Ganzi County, Sichuan Province and Sichuan Province (D1 and D15), and two fragments in samples from mostly Gansu and Yunnan Provinces, suggesting that the former originated from group I and the latter from group II of *R. palmatum*, respectively (Figure 7.7D_2).

Upon PCR amplification of regions 1 and 2 of the partial *matK* gene (Figure 7.4), the PCR products of 612 and 674 bp were obtained, respectively. The PCR product of region 1 digested with *Bgl*II showed two fragments of 100 and 512 bp, which was the same as in the three official *Rheum* species (Figure 7.8A). The

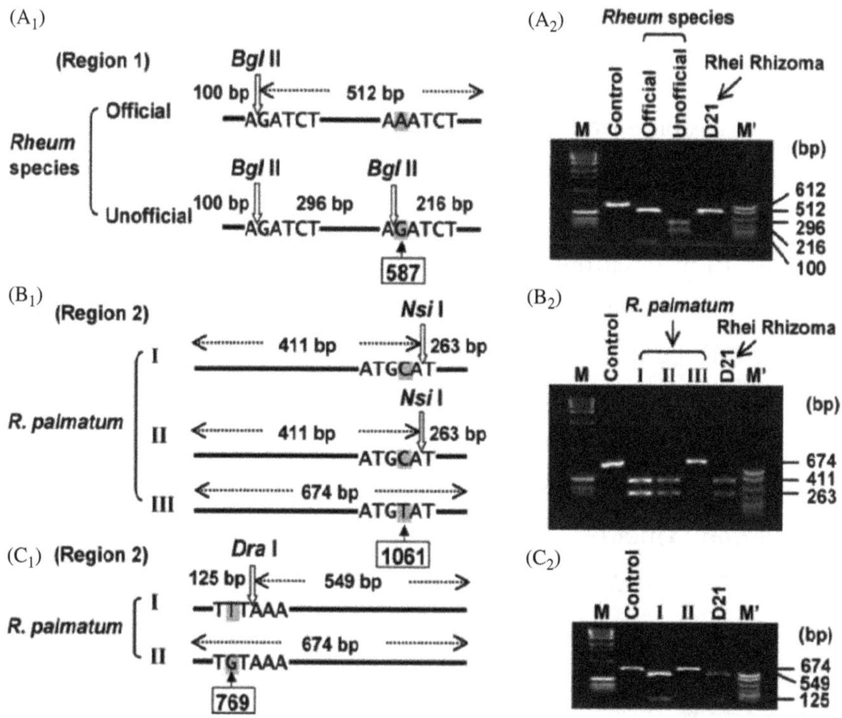

Fig. 7.8 PCR-RFLP analysis of a drug sample (D21) using the restriction enzyme *Bgl*II, *Nsi*I or *Dra*I on the partial *matK* gene.

result of ARMS analysis suggested that this sample was derived from *R. palmatum* (Figure 7.6B). Then, the PCR product of region 2 was digested with *Nsi*I or *Dra*I. Two fragments of 263 and 411 bp and those of 125 and 549 bp were observed in the digestion with *Nsi*I and *Dra*I, respectively, which were the same as in group I of *R. palmatum* (Figure 7.8B–C).

7.4 Discussion

7.4.1 Beimu

Medicinal products have become popular among many consumers. However, a study on their safety usage is an important issue that both the government and researchers must address (Chrubasik, Pittler & Roufogalis, 2005; Yoo *et al.*, 2005). Chuanbeimu is a commonly used medicinal materials in China because of its characteristic low toxicity among Beimu species. There are authentication methods using physical and chemical approaches. However, it is difficult to distinguish Chuanbeimu from other species of Beimu because they are similar in appearance and microscopic characteristics, the chemical constituents are not stable, and the results are not reproducible. For developing a simple and efficient method for the detection of Chuanbeimu, we sequenced the nrDNA ITS regions of nine species and one variety of the *Fritillaria* genus. It enabled the identification of Chuanbeimu from others such as Pingbeimu, Yibeimu, Zhebeimu and Hubeibeimu. In this study, we found an identical mutation site in the nrDNA ITS1 regions of the four species of Chuanbeimu, and the endonuclease analyses displayed that *Sma*I can recognise this site in these species and not in others.

Some PCR products of the ITS1 regions from Chuanbeimu could not be completely digested and, consequently, the fragment of 308 bp existed with two other digested fragments (Figures 7.2 and 7.3). Improper reaction conditions were not the reason for the under-digestion because we tested many reaction conditions such as increasing the quantity of enzyme and prolonging the reaction time. The activity of enzyme *Sma*I is affected by CG methylase. However, because there is no methylase in the PCR reaction system, the partial digestion is probably due to hybridisation between related species, and similar results were found in some bacteria (Hong *et al.*, 1999) and fungi (Thomas, Harold & Mark, 1996). Nevertheless, partial digestion did not disturb the identification of Chuanbeimu for the PCR products from other species, which could not be digested at all.

7.4.2 Daihuang

We investigated the phylogenetic relationship of the *Rheum* species, especially of *R. palmatum*, *R. tanguticum* and *R. officinale* of section Palmata, used as Rhei Radix et Rhizoma officially on the basis of their *matK* gene sequences. The phylogenetic tree suggested that *R. tanguticum* and *R. officinale* were monophyletic, but *R. palmatum* was mainly composed of three groups (I, II and III), which were related to the production area. In general, specimens from the southeast part of Qinghai Province and northwestern part of Sichuan Province belonged to group I, those from Gansu Province to group II and those from the central to southern part of Sichuan Province to group III. By sequence comparison, we determined marker nucleotides to identify the three official species and distinguish the three intraspecies groups of *R. palmatum*. In the present study, on the basis of five marker nucleotides at positions 367, 587, 769, 937 and 1061, PCR-RFLP and ARMS analyses were designed. PCR-RFLP methods using restriction enzymes *Bgl*II, and *Nsi*I or *Dra*I were developed for identifying section Palmata and the three groups of *R. palmatum*, respectively. For the identification of the three official species, the ARMS method was developed using three sets of primers, each having two kinds of species-specific reverse primers designed on the basis of nucleotide differences at positions 367 and 937. The plant specimens were analysed using the PCR-RFLP and ARMS methods to give the expected products in an electrophoretogram. For the plant specimen identified as group I of *R. palmatum*, two fragments were observed in the digestion of the PCR product with *Bgl*II; both 202 and 770 bp fragments were detected in the ARMS method using primer set B; and two and three fragments were observed in the digestion of the PCR product with *Nsi*I and *Dra*I, respectively. These methods were also applied to drug samples of Rhei Rhizoma. The ARMS method was found to be valuable in identifying the species of the drug samples. However, the PCR-RFLP method failed at first in most samples, since PCR products of the partial *matK* gene were not detected. When a semi-nested PCR method was performed using these PCR products as a template, the expected products were obtained except for one sample (D21). For sample D21, upon PCR amplification of dividing two regions of the partial *matK* gene, PCR products of 612 and 674 bp were obtained, respectively. It was understood that a semi-nested PCR method was required to obtain PCR products from drug samples, and a region shorter than 700 bp was suitable for amplification. After obtaining the PCR products, using the PCR-RFLP method, the groups of *R. palmatum* were identified.

We investigated 22 more commercial samples to identify their botanic origins by using PCR-RFLP and ARMS methods. Thereafter, 6 out of the 12 samples were selected to determine the partial *matK* gene sequences to validate the accuracy of the identification, then sequencing results were found to be completely consistent with those demonstrated in our present method. All 22 samples were found to be derived from the official *Rheum* species. Their botanic origins almost corresponded with those deduced from information about their production areas, as previously described. However, two drug samples (D18 and D19) from Wanyuan County, Sichuan Province, were found to be derived from group II of *R. palmatum*, not as expected from *R. officinale*. Although most Rhei Rhizoma derived from group II of *R. palmatum* is produced in Gansu Province, these samples were thought to be produced in Sichuan Province, since the partial *matK* gene sequence was identical to that of the plant specimen from Sichuan Province. On the other hand, one drug sample named 'Ya-huang' (D21), which is available in the Japanese market, was found to be derived from group I of *R. palmatum*, not as expected from group III. Although the 'Ya-huang' samples imported from China have been known to be produced in Jiulong and Shimian Counties, the central part of Sichuan Province, their production areas have been moved recently to the northwestern part. In fact, the partial *matK* gene sequence was found to be identical to that of wild plants from Xinlong County, in the northwestern part of Sichuan Province. In the present study, the PCR-RFLP and ARMS methods were established as convenient tools for identifying Rhei Radix et Rhizoma derived from *Rheum* species. After obtaining two kinds of PCR products from two regions of the *matK* gene, the combination of PCR-RFLP and ARMS are shown to be useful for identifying drug samples. Also, the *matK* gene sequences of drug samples are expected to be useful for the quality control of Rhei Radix et Rhizoma, and for predicting their production areas.

7.5 Conclusion

RFLP, as a molecular marker, is specific to a single clone/restriction enzyme combination. Labelled probe with DNA sequence that hybridises with one or more fragments of the digested DNA sample after they were separated by gel electrophoresis reveals a unique fingerprint. Short, single- or low-copy genomic DNA or cDNA can be used as RFLP probes. With PCR, a minute amount of DNA in a particular DNA region that contains the restriction site can be amplified, so there is no need to reveal the fingerprint using a radioactive probe. This study shows that the PCR-RFLP is a powerful tool for the identification of Chuanbeimu and Daihuang. Indeed, PCR-RFLP for Chuanbeimu authentication has been first recorded in the *Chinese Pharmacopoeia* (2015 edition).

References

Chen, Q. Y., Fu, C. M., Luo, R. F., Lin, M. S., Liao, W., & Gao, F. (2021). Research progress of effect of Rhei. Radix et Rhizoma and its anthraquinone in treatment of autoimmune diseases. *Zhongguo Zhong Yao Za Zhi, 46*, 15–23.

Chrubasik, S., Pittler, M. H., & Roufogalis, B. D. (2005). Zingi-beris rhizoma: A comprehensive review on the ginger effect and efficacy profiles. *Phytomedicine 12*, 684–701.

Hong, D., Tsute, C., Floyd, E. D., Robert, D. F., Claire, M. F., & Margaret, J. D. (1999). Genomic loci of the Porphyromonas gingivalis insertion element IS1126. *Infect Immun, 67*, 3416–3423.

Takaiwa, F., Oono, K., & Sugiura, M. (1985). Nucleotide sequence of the 17S-25S spacer region from rice rDNA. *Plant Mol Biol, 4*, 355–364.

Thomas, J. V., Harold, H. B., & Mark, T. B. (1996). Armillaria nabsnona, a new species from western North America. *Mycologia, 88*, 484–491.

Wang, C. Z., Li, P., Ding, J. Y., Peng, X., & Yuan, C. S. (2007). Simultaneous identification of *Bulbus Fritillariae cirrhosae* using PCR-RFLP analysis. *Phytomedicine, 14*, 628–632.

Wolf, C., Rentsch, J., & Hübner P. (1999). PCR–RFLP analysis of mitochondrial DNA: A reliable method for species identification. *J Agric Food Chem, 47*, 1350–1355.

Wolf, C., Burgener, M., Hübner, P., & Lüthy, J. (2000). PCR-RFLP analysis of mitochondrial DNA: Differentiation of fish species. *LWT-Food Sci Technol 33*, 144–150.

Xu, C. L., Li, H. J., Li, P., Zhang, Y., & Wang, S. (2010). Molecular method for the identification of Bulbus Fritilariae Cirhosae. *J China Pharm Univ, 41*, 226–230.

Yang, D. Y., Fushimi, H., Cai S. Q., & Komatsu, K. (2004). Polymerase chain reaction-restriction fragment length polymorphism (PCR-RFLP) and amplification refractory mutation system (ARMS) analyses of medicinally used Rheum species and their application for identification of Rhei Rhizoma. *Biol Pharm Bull, 27*(5), 661–669.

Yoo, J. H., Lee, E. J., Kwak, C. K., Sohn, E. H., Koh, B. H., Song, I. B., & Lee, K. S. (2005). Clinical trial of herbal formula on weight loss in obese Korean children. *Am J Chin Med, 33*, 713–722.

Chapter 8

Authentication of Medicinal Materials by Sequence Characterised Amplified Region

Grace Wing-Chiu But, Jun Wang, Wai-Yan Ha,
Forrest Chung-Fai Yau, Paul Pui-Hay But & Pang-Chui Shaw

8.1 Introduction

Sequence characterised amplified region (SCAR) is to amplify a specific region of the genomic DNA that is distinctive to the target species. Polymorphic bands generated from a random-primed polymerase chain reaction (RP-PCR) method (e.g., random amplified polymorphic DNA [RAPD], arbitrarily primed PCR [AP-PCR]) are a good starting point for searching SCAR. Species-specific bands are isolated and sequenced (Figure 8.1). Pairs of oligonucleotide primers of 20 to 25 bp specific to the sequence of the bands are designed and used to amplify the characterised regions from genomic DNA, under conditions more stringent than those in random-primed PCR. As these bands are only shared among the members of focal species or linked members of the same biological trait, the specific primers should only amplify PCR products of a defined size. The SCAR generated can be dominant or codominant. Dominant polymorphism refers to the presence or

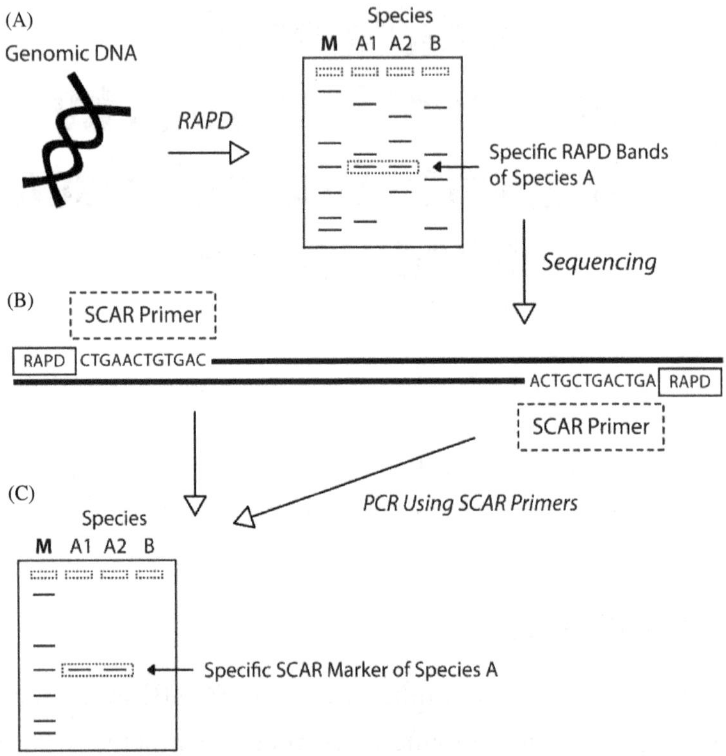

Fig. 8.1 SCAR procedures. The technique is divided into three steps: (A) RAPD fingerprint is prepared from the sample. (B) The specific RAPD bands are sequenced. (C) The RAPD band is turned into a species-specific SCAR marker.

absence of bands. Codominant polymorphism may either be displayed as length polymorphism or restriction fragment polymorphism of PCR products (Nair, Kumar, Srivastava & Mohan, 1996). Comparing to the RAPD method, SCAR only or the combination of RAPD with the SCAR method allow simple, easy and rapid detection with high reproducibility, high specificity and straightforward data interpretation.

SCAR analysis has successfully led to the mapping and tagging of a number of diseases or pest resistance genes, e.g., detection of resistance genes (Paran & Michelmore, 1993; Giovannelli, Farnham & Wang, 2002; Huaracha, Xu & Korban, 2004; Venter &

Botha, 2000), and mapping of the resistance gene, e.g., *Gm4t* in rice (Mohan, Sathyanarayanan, Kumar, Srivastava & Nair, 1997). Genetic maps have been constructed based on various markers including SCAR in pedunculate oak (*Quercus robur* L.), for studying the molecular organisation of genomic regions involved in interspecific and intraspecific differentiation, and for the identification of 'Quantitative Traits Locus' for adaptive traits (Barreneche *et al.*, 1998). SCAR markers have also been used in the pea (*Pisum sativum* L.) to identify markers linked to genes affecting plant architecture (Rameau *et al.*, 1998; Srivastava, Mishra, Singh & Mohapatra, 2012). SCAR markers facilitate efficient selection of desirable breeding characters and plants with resistance, e.g., DNA markers linked to the locus that controls flower doubleness in carnations (*Dianthus caryophyllus* L.) (Scovel, Ben-Meir, Ovadis, Itzhaki & Vainstein, 1998); the seedlessness in grapes (Lahogue, This & Bouquet, 1998); the aluminium tolerance gene Alt 1 in rye (*Secale cereale* L.) (Gallego, Calles & Benito, 1998), the markers linked to the male sex in dioecious hemp (*Cannabis sativa* L.) (Mandolino, Carboni, Forapani, Faeti & Ranalli, 1999), discrimination of Thai jasmine rice mutants (*Oryza sativa* L.) (Semsang, Chundet & Phanchisri, 2013), early sexual identification in *Idesia polycarpa* Maxim. for breeding and marker-assisted selection of the rose gum tree (*Eucalyptus grandis* W. Hill) with resistance to the plant pathogen *Puccinia psidii* (Laia *et al.*, 2015), and the SCAR marker as a complementary tool to distinguish high-artemisinin producer species under the genus Artemisia for antimalarial medication (Asghari, Naghavi, Hosseinzadeh, Ranjbar & Poorebrahim, 2015).

For the authentication of medicinal materials, SCAR markers have been widely developed on species identification targeting a wide range of medicinal materials from their close relatives or adulterants, e.g., Cordyceps (*Ophiocordyceps sinensis* [Berk.]) and its common adulterants (Lam *et al.*, 2015; Moon, Kim, Park, Sung & Noh, 2018), different generic-closely-related *Ganoderma* spp. and their cultivars (Chao, Tang, Zhang, Yu & Honda, 2018; Fu *et al.*, 2015; Khan, Cheng, Mei, Wei & Fu, 2016), Angelicae Sinensis Radix (*Angelica sinensis* (Oliv.)) and its common adulterants (Zhang *et al.*, 2015), Angelicae Dahuricae Radix (*Angelica dahurica* [Fisch. ex Hoffm.]) (Noh, Kim, Yang, Park & Moon, 2018) and *Lonicera japonica* Thunb. (Fu, Yang, Khan & Mei, 2013; Yang *et al.*, 2014). Other than identification using SCAR with a single marker, multiplex SCAR markers have also been developed for targeting several DNA regions simultaneously and allow different species identification in a shorter time, e.g., Angelicae Pubescentis Radix (*Angelica biserrata* [R.H. Shan & C.Q. Yuan]) and its closely related *Angelica* spp. (Kim *et al.*, 2016), Pinelliae Tuber (*Pinellia ternate* [Thunb.]) and its common adulterants (Lee *et al.*, 2016), kiwifruit cultivar (*Actinidia* spp.) (Cho *et al.*, 2020). Although conventional thermal cycler is commonly used to obtain rapid and easy identification with quantitative results, a real-time PCR method in conjunction with SCAR markers are also applied for differentiating medicinal materials from its closely related species, e.g., Cordyceps (*Cordyceps sinensis* (BerK.) Sacc.) and its common adulterants (Moon *et al.*, 2018), *Zanthoxylum schinifolium* and its congeneric species (Kim *et al.*, 2019) and quantity detection, e.g., *Catharanthus roseus* L. Don. (Chaudhary, Yadav, Jamil & Asil, 2013).

8.2 Materials and Methods

8.2.1 Materials

Dried or fresh roots of *Panax* species were obtained from the following sources: *P. ginseng* C. A. Mey. samples from China (Ji'an county of Jilin province, Xingbing county and Xinkiahe county of Liaolin province) and Korea (Kangwon, Pochon, Kanghwa, Kumsan and Kimpo); *P. quinquefolius* L. samples from farms in Ontario, British Columbia and Wisconsin; *P. notoginseng* (Burk.) F. H. Chen from China; *P. major* (Burkill) from China; *P. japonicus* C. A. Mey. from Japan and *P. trifolius* L. from the United States. Samples of adulterants *Mirabilis jalapa* L. and *Phytolacca acinosa* Roxb. were obtained from Hong Kong. Samples were identified and have been deposited in the Museum of the Institute of Chinese Medicine, The Chinese University of Hong Kong.

8.2.2 Methods

8.2.2.1 *Total Genomic DNA Preparation*

To obtain DNA samples, cetyltrimethylammonium bromide (CTAB) extraction method was used according to Chapter 2.

8.2.2.2 *RAPD Reaction*

Equipment

- Thermocycler

Reagents

- Deoxynucleoside triphosphates (dNTPs), 2.5 mmol/L
- $MgCl_2$, 25 mmol/L
- 10× *Taq* buffer
  - 0.01% Gelatin
  - 0.5 M KCl
  - 0.1 M Tris-HCl, pH 8.3
- *Taq* DNA polymerase, 5 U/μL
- OPC-20 primer, 10 μmol/L

Procedures

1. Prepare and mix well the RAPD reaction mixture as follows:

Ingredient	Final volume per reaction	Final concentration
Taq buffer	2.5 µL	1×
$MgCl_2$	1.5 µL	1.5 mM
dNTPs	1 µL	0.1 mM
OPC-20 primer	0.5 µL	0.2 µM
Taq polymerase (5 U/µL)	0.1 µL	0.5 U
Template DNA (10.0 ng/µL)	1.0 µL	
ddH_2O	18.4 µL	
Total	25 µL	

2. Perform RAPD reaction in a T-100 Thermo Cycler with PCR cycles consisting of an initial denaturation at 94°C for 3 min, 45 cycles of 1 min at 94°C, 2 min at 36°C and 2 min at 72°C, followed by a final extension at 72°C for 5 min.
3. RAPD-PCR products are visualised in 2% TBE agarose gel (refer to Chapter 3).
4. Purify the desired DNA band with a GENECLEAN® III Kit (MP Biomedicals, United States, Irvine, CA).
5. The 3′ end of the desired DNA band is modified to facilitate blunt-end cloning to a pUC19 vector and the recombinant plasmid is transformed to *Escherichia coli* (refer to Chapter 3).

8.2.2.3 *SCAR Procedures*

Equipment

- Thermocycler

Reagents

- dNTPs, 2.5 mmol/L
- $MgCl_2$, 25 mmol/L

- 10× *Taq* buffer
  - 0.01% Gelatin
  - 0.5 M KCl
  - 0.1 M Tris-HCl, pH 8.3
- *Taq* DNA polymerase, 5 U/μL
- Upstream primer, 10 μmol/L
- Downstream primer, 10 μmol/L

Procedures

1. Based on the sequence of the original RAPD fragment (RAPDAG) amplified by primer OPC-20 (5′-ACT TCG CCA C-3′) from *P. quinquefolius* (Figure 8.2), specific SCAR primers were synthesised (Table 8.1).

```
   (SCAR.F2)10          20          30(SCAR.F1)40          50          60
5' TTCGCCACCC GGAGCAGCAT TGAGATCCGC CAAGTCAACT GCAGGGGTTA AGAAGCCCTT
          70          80          90         100         110         120
   AAAAATCCAG TGAAGTTTCC TTGGTCTGCT TCATTGCTTC TCAATTCGAT CATCGGTGTG
         130         140         150         160         170         180
   AGCTCGTCAA CCTTTTGTCA GTCAAAGTCC TCACCCACTC CTGCCCATTG AAAATTCCAC
         190         200         210         220         230         240
   CTTCCCCGCC CATTGAAAAT TTTGCCAACT TATTTAATAC ACTTCTCCTT CCATTCGGCT
         250         260         270         280         290         300
   ATAAAGGCAG CTAAGCATAA GGATCAAATA CACCAGCAAC AATACGTACT CCCATCCTAG
         310         320         330         340         350(SCAR.R1)360
   AGAGGAAAAG AGAAAGGGAG AGAAAAGCTT TTGTAAAGCT TTAGAAAAAT AGAGAGAGAA
         370         380         390         400         410  (SCAR.R2)
   AGATAGTTCA AATAAAAGGG TGTTTTATTT GGGTTCCATC ACATAGTTAT TGTGGCGAA 3'
```

Fig. 8.2 Sequence of RAPDAG from *Panax quinquefolius*. Total length of the fragment is 419 bp. Sequences of the OPC-20 RAPD primer are indicated in bold. Internal PCR primers (SCAR.F1 and SCAR.R1) are underlined. The sequences of SCAR.F2 and SCAR.R2, which include RAPD OPC-20, are indicated by a dashed line.

Table 8.1 SCAR Primers for Identification of *Panax ginseng* and *P. quinquefolius*

Primer name	Sequence (5′ to 3′)	Nucleotide position of primer (bp)	Amplicon size (bp)
SCAR.F1	CAA GTC AAC CTG CAG GGG TTA AGA A	31–51	350
SCAR.R1	CCC TTT TAT TTG AAC TAT CTT TCT CTC TC	352–380	
SCAR.F2	TTC GCC ACC CGG AGC AGC ATT G	1–22	419
SCAR.R2	TTC GCC ACA ATA ACT ATG TGA TGG AAC	393–419	

2. Prepare and mix well the SCAR reaction mixture as follows:

Ingredient	Final volume per reaction	Final concentration
Taq buffer	2.5 µL	1×
$MgCl_2$	2 µL	2 mM
dNTPs	1 µL	0.1 mM
Upstream primer	2.5 µL	1 µM
Downstream primer	2.5 µL	1 µM
Taq polymerase (5 U/µL)	0.2 µL	1 U
Template DNA (10.0 ng/µL)	4.0 µL	
ddH_2O	12.8 µL	
Total	25 µL	

3. Perform SCAR reaction in a T-100 Thermo Cycler with PCR cycles consisting of an initial denaturation at 94°C for 3 min, 40 cycles of 1 min at 91°C, 1 min at 50°C or 56°C (for primers SCAR.F1 and SCAR.R1) or 60°C (for primers SCAR.F2 and SCAR.R2) and 1 min 30 s at 72°C, followed by a final extension at 72°C for 5 min.

4. SCAR-PCR products are visualised in 2% TBE agarose gel (refer to Chapter 3).

8.3 Results

RAPD fingerprints from samples of *P. ginseng* and *P. quinquefolius* amplified using OPC-20 primer (5′-ACT TCG CCA C-3′) are shown in Figure 8.2. The polymorphic band of *P. quinquefolius* (RAPDAG), indicated by an arrow (Figure 8.3), was subsequently cloned and sequenced. No match to RAPDAG was found

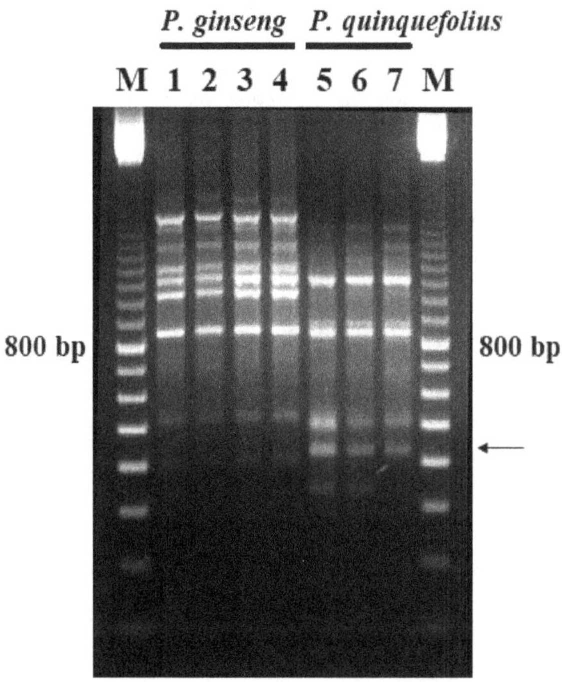

Fig. 8.3 RAPD analysis of *Panax ginseng and Panax quinquefolius* using the OPC-20 primer. Lane M: 100 bp DNA size marker, 1: *P. ginseng* from Ji'an county of Jilin province, 2: Xingbing county of Liaolin province, 3: Xingbing county of Kangwon, 4: Xingbing county of Pochon, 5-6: *P. quinquefolius* from Canada, 7: *P. quinquefolius* from the United States. The arrow indicates the polymorphic band (RAPDAG), which was consequently cloned and sequenced (Figure 8.2) from *P. quinquefolius* and used for a SCAR study.

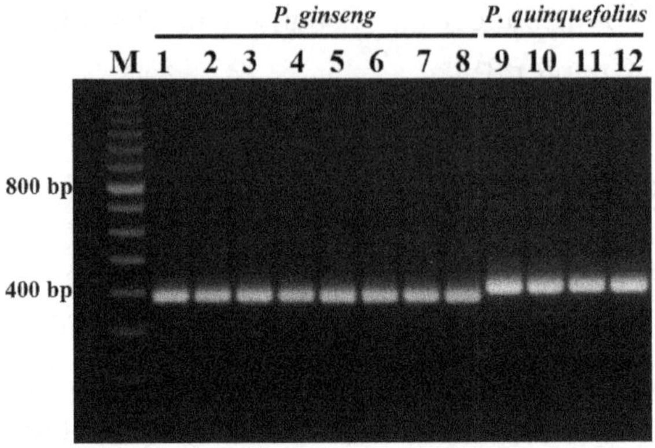

Fig. 8.4 SCAR analysis using primers SCAR.F2 and SCAR.R2. Lane M: 100 bp DNA size marker, 1: *Panax ginseng* from Ji'an county of Jilin province, 2: Xingbing county of Liaolin province, 3: Xingbing county of Kangwon, 4: Xingbing county of Pochon, 5: Xingbing county of Kanghwa, 6: Xingbing county of Kumsan, 7: Xingbing county of Kimpo, 8: Xingbing county of Xinkiahe, 9: *Panax quinquefolius* from British Columbia, 10: *P. quinquefolius* from Ontario, 11: *P. quinquefolius* from Wisconsin and 12: *P. quinquefolius* from the United States.

among the entries of the GenBank. Primer SCAR.F2 and SCAR.R2 (Table 8.1), which are corresponding to positions 1 to 22 and 393 to 419 bp of the RAPDAG sequence, were used to amplify the DNA from eight samples of *P. ginseng* and five samples of *P. quinquefolius* (Figure 8.4). Single PCR product band was amplified for all 13 samples. The SCAR bands in the five *P. quinquefolius* samples are in the expected size (419 bp), the same as the original RAPDAG marker. The SCAR bands in the eight *P. ginseng* samples were found to be around 390 bp, which is 25 to 30 bp shorter than those from the *P. quinquefolius* samples.

Similar result was obtained with amplification using primers SCAR.F1 and SCAR.R1 (Table 8.1). Shown in Figure 8.5, clear amplification was found in an expected size of 350 bp for *P. quinquefolius* samples, whereas amplification with *P. ginseng* samples was found to be around 330 bp, which is also 25 to 30 bp shorter

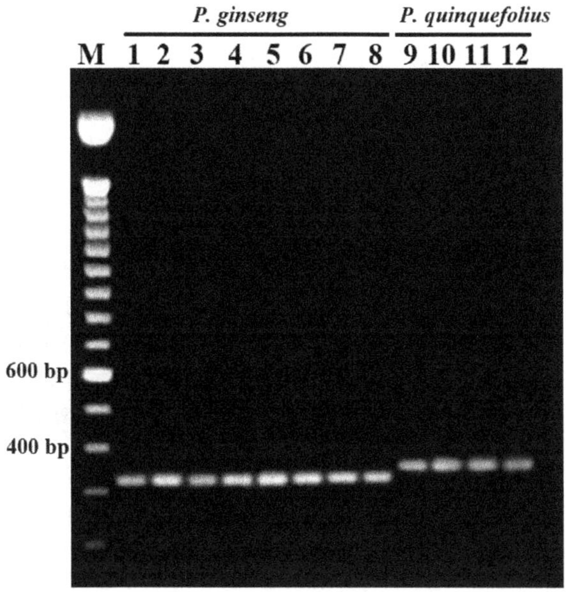

Fig. 8.5 SCAR analysis using internal primers SCAR.F1 and SCAR.R1. Lane M: 100 bp DNA size marker, 1: *Panax ginseng* from Ji'an county of Jilin province, 2: Xingbing county of Liaolin province, 3: Xingbing county of Kangwon, 4: Xingbing county of Pochon, 5: Xingbing county of Kanghwa, 6: Xingbing county of Kumsan, 7: Xingbing county of Kimpo, 8: Xingbing county of Xinkiahe, 9: *Panax quinquefolius* from British Columbia, 10: *P. quinquefolius* from Ontario, 11: *P. quinquefolius* from Wisconsin and 12: *P. quinquefolius* from the United States.

than those from the *P. quinquefolius* samples. DNA sequencing and sequence alignment of the SCAR fragments from *P. ginseng* and *P. quinquefolius* indicate that the difference in fragment size was because of a 25 bp insertion in *P. quinquefolius*, or a 25 bp deletion in *P. ginseng* (Figure 8.2).

To further investigate the ability of SCAR markers developed, samples of other *Panax* species and their common adulterants were amplified using primers SCAR.F1 and SCAR.R1 (Figure 8.6). The results clearly demonstrated that the bands generated from *P. ginseng* and *P. quinquefolius* are distinct from the other *Panax* species tested, including *P. japonica*, *P. major*,

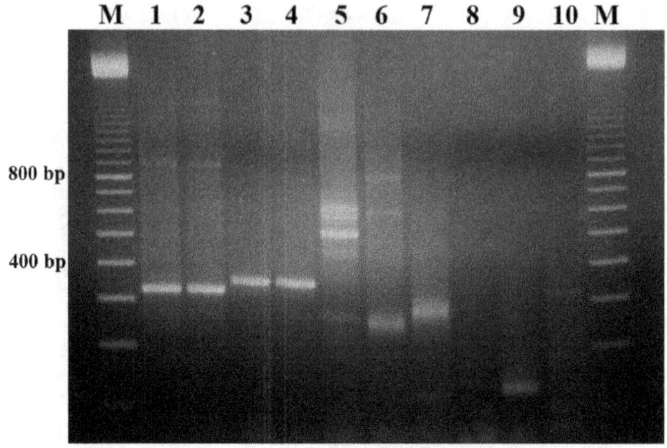

Fig. 8.6 SCAR analysis using primer SCAR.F1 and SCAR.R1. Lane M: 100 bp DNA size marker, 1: *Panax ginseng* from Ji'an county of Jilin province, 2: Ji'an county of Kimpo, 3: *Panax quinquefolius* from Ontario, 4: *P. quinquefolius* from Wisconsin, 5: *Panax japonica*, 6: *Panax major*, 7: *Panax trifolius*. 8: *Panax notoginseng*, 9: *Mirabilis jalapa* L. and 10: *Phytolacca acinosa* Roxb.

P. trifolius, *P. notoginseng* and from those of two adulterants, *Mirabilis jalapa* L. and *Phytolacca acinosa* Roxb. This shows that primers SCAR.F1 and SCAR.R1 could be used for the discrimination of *P. ginseng* and *P. quinquefolius* from other common adulterants and related congeneric *Panax* spp.

8.4 Discussion

The RAPD technique has been widely adopted to characterise the DNA of plants and other organisms (Williams, Kubelik, Livak, Rafalski & Tingey, 1990). The technique has numerous advantages. It is rapid and simple. It does not use radioactive material and can be readily scaled up to analyse large numbers of samples. However, because of the non-stringent amplification conditions used, the amplified markers or patterns often vary between different DNA preparations, and RAPD usually does not allow for the detection of a single locus (Mohan *et al.*, 1997; William, Pande, Nair, Mohan & Bennett, 1991; Williamson, Ho, Wu, Miler & Kaloshian, 1994; Yang & Korban, 1996). Furthermore, the RAPD marker is usually dominant, and therefore is not suitable for differentiating heterozygotes from homozygotes (Kumar & Gurusubramanian, 2011; Ohmori, Murata & Motoyoshi, 1996).

To circumvent these problems, RAPD markers are converted into the more reliable SCAR markers. SCAR markers have several advantages over RAPD markers. As the annealing conditions are more stringent for SCAR than for RAPD, only one locus is amplified by SCAR primers. Also, the use of longer oligonucleotide primers for SCAR secures a robust and reliable result (Paran & Michelmore, 1993). SCAR can also be converted into codominant markers, which are useful for genetic studies in differentiating heterozygotes from homozygotes (Ohmori *et al.*, 1996).

In this study, RAPD fingerprints were first generated from *P. ginseng* and *P. quinquefolius*. One of the resultant polymorphic bands was sequenced and specific primers corresponding to its sequence were designed targeting on specific DNA fragments. Primers designed based on the RAPDAG sequence, e.g., SCAR.F1 and SCAR.R1 have a long size of 24 and 29 bp, respectively. This allows the generation of a single distinctive band for all the *Panax* species and adulterants tested. This study is the first to use SCAR for the authentication of medicinal materials. This work shows that SCAR is applicable to differentiate ginseng and American ginseng from their related *Panax* species and adulterants.

Pros and cons of using the SCAR approach

In comparison to the RAPD approach, SCAR has a higher stability and specificity with high reproducibility. SCAR is also a method with high sensitivity: a nanogram of DNA sample is sufficient for amplification since a small region of DNA is amplified, and the quality of DNA is less important for generating the required fragment. Other than its specificity and sensitivity, the SCAR method is also easy to perform, which allows screening of samples in large scale. Furthermore, the result of SCAR-PCR amplification only depends on the presence or absence of a SCAR band, which makes the interpretation of results more straightforward. By the conversion of several RAPD markers to SCAR markers, multiplex SCAR markers can also be developed for the identification of different species and different DNA regions simultaneously.

On the other hand, in comparison to AP-PCR and RAPD, SCAR requires the investment of more time and effort at the beginning, in order to screen suitable primer pairs and optimise the primer ratio, which are necessary to generate robust polymorphic SCAR bands.

8.5 Conclusion

As a simple and highly reproducible molecular technique, SCAR markers have been widely used for the authentication of medicinal materials from adulterants. In this chapter, SCAR markers, generated from RAPD markers, were used to differentiate *P. ginseng* and *P. quinquefolius* from their congeneric species and common adulterants. Specific SCAR primers designed were able to amplify with *P. ginseng* and *P. quinquefolius* samples collected from different places and allowed differentiation among these two species with a fragment size difference of 30 bp. By conversing RAPD markers to SCAR markers, PCR assays can be improved in their sensitivity and specificity, and the result obtained is also simple to be analysed.

References

Asghari, M., Naghavi, M. R., Hosseinzadeh, A. H., Ranjbar, M., & Poorebrahim, M. (2015). Sequence characterized amplified region marker as a tool for selection of high-artemisinin containing species of Artemisia. *Res Pharm Sci, 10*(5), 453–459.

Barreneche, T., Bodenes, C., Lexer, C., Trontin, J. F., Fluch, S., Streiff, R., C. Plomion, G. Roussel, H. Steinkellner, K. Burg, J. M. Favre, J. Glössl, & Kremer, A. (1998). A genetic linkage map of *Quercus robur* L. (pedunculate oak) based on RAPD, SCAR, microsatellite, minisatellite, isozyme and 5S rDNA markers. *Theor Appl Genet,* 97(7), 1090–1103. doi:10.1007/s001220050996

Chao, W., Tang, C., Zhang, J., Yu, L., & Honda, Y. (2018). Development of a stable SCAR marker for rapid identification of *Ganoderma lucidum* Hunong 5 cultivar using DNA pooling method and inter-simple sequence repeat markers. *J Integr Agric, 17*(1), 130–138. doi:10.1016/S2095-3119(17)61825-2

Chaudhary, A. A., Yadav, D., Jamil, H. S. S., & Asil, M. (2013). Real time sequence characterized amplified region (RT-SCAR) marker: Development and its application for authentication and quantification of *Catharanthus roseus* L. Don. *J Med Plant Res,* 7(17), 1154–1160. doi:10.5897/JMPR12.615

Cho, K. H., Kwack, Y., Park, S. J., Kim, S. H., Lee, H. C., Chung, K. H., & Jun, J. H. (2020). Sequence-characterized amplified region markers and multiplex-polymerase chain reaction assays for kiwifruit cultivar identification. *Hortic Environ Biotechnol, 61*(2), 395–406. doi:10.1007/s13580-020-00227-9

Fu, J., Mei, Z., Tania, M., Yang, L., Cheng, J., & Khan, M. A. (2015). Development of RAPD-SCAR markers for different *Ganoderma* species authentication by improved RAPD amplification and molecular cloning. *Genet Mol Res, 14*(2), 5667–5676. doi:10.4238/2015.May.25.19

Fu, J., Yang, L., Khan, M. A., & Mei, Z. (2013). Genetic characterization and authentication of *Lonicera japonica* Thunb. by using improved RAPD analysis. *Mol Bio Rep, 40*(10), 5993–5999. doi:10.1007/s11033-013-2703-3

Gallego, F. J., Calles, B., & Benito, C. (1998). Molecular markers linked to the aluminium tolerance gene *alt1* in rye. *Theor Appl Genet,* 97, 1104–1109. doi:10.1007/s001220050997

Giovannelli, J. L., Farnham M. W., & Wang, M. (2002). Development of sequence characterised amplified region markers linked to downy mildew resistance in broccoli. *J Am Soc Hortic Sci, 127*(4), 597–601. doi:10.21273/JASHS.127.4.597

Huaracha, E., Xu, M., & Korban, S. S. (2004). Narrowing down the region of the Vf locus for scab resistance in apple using AFLP-derived SCARs. TAG. Theoretical and applied genetics. *Theor Appl Genet, 108*(2), 274–279. doi:10.1007/s00122-003-1435-5

Khan, M. A., Cheng, J. L., Mei, Z. Q., Wei, C. L., & Fu, J. J. (2016). Development of two novel specific SCAR markers by cloning improved RAPD fragments from the medicinal mushroom *Ganoderma lucidium* (Leysser: Fr) Karst. *Genet Mol Res, 15*(3), 15038536. doi:10.4238/gmr.15038536

Kim, W. J., Moon, B. C., Yang, S., Han, K. S., Choi, G., & Lee, A. Y. (2016). Rapid authentication of the herbal medicine plant species *Aralia continentalis* Kitag. and *Angelica biserrata* C.Q. Yuan and R.H. Shan using ITS2 sequences and multiplex-SCAR markers. *Molecules, 21*(3), 270. doi:10.3390/molecules21030270

Kim, W. J., Yang, S., Choi, G., Park, I., Noh, P., Seo, C. S., & Moon, B. C. (2019). Development of conventional PCR and real-time PCR assays to discriminate the origins of Chinese pepper oil and herbal materials from *Zanthoxylum*. *J Sci Food Agric, 99*(4), 2021–2029. doi:10.1002/jsfa.9458

Kumar, N. S., & Gurusubramanian, G. (2011). Random amplified polymorphic DNA (RAPD) markers and its applications. *Sci Vis, 11*, 116–124.

Lahogue, F., This, P., & Bouquet, A. (1998). Identification of a codominant SCAR marker linked to the seedlessness character in grapevine. *Theor Appl Genet, 97*, 950–959. Doi:10.1007/s001220050976

Laia, M. L., Alfenas, A. C., Brommonschenkel, S. H., Oda, S., José de Mello, E., Silva, I. M. A., J. F. Gonçalves, & Ferreira, M. S. (2015). Identification of a sequence characterized amplified region (SCAR) marker linked to the *Puccinia psidii* resistance Ggne 1 (Ppr1) in *Eucalyptus grandis*. *Afr J Microbiol Res, 10*(18), 1957–1964. doi:10.5897/AJAR2013.8016

Lam, K. Y., Chan, G. K., Xin, G. Z., Xu, H., Ku, C. F., Chen, J. P., Ping Yao, Huang-Quan Lin, Tina T X Dong, Tsim, K. W. (2015). Authentication of *Cordyceps sinensis* by DNA analyses: Comparison of ITS sequence analysis and RAPD-derived molecular markers. *Molecules, 20*(12), 22454–22462. doi:10.3390/molecules201219861

Lee, Y. M., Ji, Y., Kang, Y. M., Kim, W. J., Choi, G., & Moon, B. C. (2016). Molecular authentication of Pinelliae Tuber and its common adulterants using RAPD-derived multiplex sequence characterized amplified region (multiplex-SCAR) markers. *Int J Clin Exp Med, 9*, 40–50.

Mandolino, G., Carboni, A., Forapani, S., Faeti, V., & Ranalli, P. (1999). Identification of DNA markers linked to the male sex in dioecious hemp (*Cannabis sativa* L.). *Theor Appl Genet, 98*, 86–92. doi:10.1007/s001220051043

Mohan, M., Sathyanarayanan, P. V., Kumar, A., Srivastava, M. N., & Nair, S. (1997). Molecular mapping of a resistance-specific PCR-based marker linked to a gall midge resistance gene (*Gm4t*) in rice. *Theor Appl Genet, 95*(5), 777–782. doi:10.1007/s001220050625

Mohan, M., Nair, S., Bhagwat, A., Krishna, T. G., Yano, M., Bhatia, C. R., & Takuji, S. (1997). Genome mapping, molecular markers and marker-assisted selection in crop plants. *Mol Breed, 3*(2), 87–103. doi:10.1023/A:1009651919792

Moon, B. C., Kim, W. J., Park, I., Sung, G. H., & Noh, P. (2018). Establishment of a PCR assay for the detection and discrimination of authentic cordyceps and adulterant species in food and herbal medicines. *Molecules, 23*(8), 1932. doi:10.3390/molecules23081932

Nair, S., Kumar, A., Srivastava, M. N., & Mohan, M. (1996). PCR-based DNA marker linked to gall midge resistance gene, *Gm4t*, has potential for marker-aided selection in rice. *Theor Appl Genet, 92*(6), 660–665. doi:10.1007/BF00226086

Noh, P., Kim, W. J., Yang, S., Park, I., & Moon, B. C. (2018). Authentication of the herbal medicine Angelicae Dahuricae Radix using an ITS sequence-based multiplex SCAR assay. *Molecules, 23*(9), 2134. doi:10.3390/molecules 23092134.

Ohmori, T., Murata, M., & Motoyoshi, F. (1996). Molecular characterization of RAPD and SCAR markers linked to the *Tm-1* locus in tomato. *Theor Appl Genet, 92*(2), 151–156. doi:10.1007/BF00223369.

Paran, I., & Michelmore, R. W. (1993). Development of reliable PCR-based markers linked to downy mildew resistance genes in lettuce. *Theor Appl Genet, 85*, 985–993. doi:10.1007/BF00215038

Rameau, C., Dénoue, D., Fraval, F., Haurogné, K., Josserand, J., Laucou, V., S. Batge, & Murfet, I. C. (1998). Genetic mapping in pea. 2. Identification of RAPD and SCAR markers linked to genes affecting plant architecture. *Theor Appl Genet,* 97, 916–928. doi:10.1007/s001220050972

Semsang, N., Chundet, R., & Phanchisri, B. (2013). Development of a SCAR marker for discrimination of a Thai Jasmine Rice (*Oryza sativa* L. cv. KDML105) mutant, BKOS6, and associated with purple color trait in Thai Jasmine Rice-related varieties. *Am J Plant Sci, 4*(9), 1774–1783. doi:10.4236/ajps.2013.49218

Scovel, G., Ben-Meir, H., Ovadis, M., Itzhaki, H., & Vainstein, A. (1998). RAPD and RFLP markers tightly linked to the locus controlling carnation (*Dianthus caryophyllus*) flower type. *Theor Appl Genet, 96*(1), 117–122. doi:10.1007/s001220050717

Srivastava, R. K., Mishra, S. K., Singh, A. K., & Mohapatra, T. (2012). Development of a coupling-phase SCAR marker linked to the powdery mildew resistance gene 'er1' in pea (*Pisum sativum* L.). *Euphytica, 186*(3), 855–866. doi:10.1007/s10681-012-0650-z

Venter, E., & Botha, A. M. (2000). Development of markers linked to *Diuraphis noxia* resistance in wheat using a novel PCR-RFLP approach. *Theor Appl Genet, 100*, 965–970. doi:10.1007/s001220051377

William, M. N. V., Pande, N., Nair, S., Mohan, M., & Bennett, J. (1991). Restriction fragment length polymorphism analysis of polymerase chain reaction products amplified from mapped loci of rice (*Oryza sativa* L.) genomic DNA. *Theor Appl Genet,* 82(4), 489–498. doi:10.1007/BF00588604.

Williams, J. G. K., Kubelik, A. R., Livak, K. J., Rafalski, J. A., & Tingey, S. V. (1990). DNA polymorphisms amplified by arbitrary primers are useful as genetic markers. *Nucleic Acids Res, 18*(22), 6531–6535. doi:10.1093/nar/18.22.6531

Williamson, V. M., Ho, J. Y., Wu, F. F., Miler, N., & Kaloshian, I. (1994). A PCR-based marker tightly linked to the nematode resistance gene, *Mi*, in tomato. *Theor Appl Genet,* 87(7), 757–763. doi:10.1007/BF00221126

Yang, H., & Korban, S. S. (1996). Screening apples for OPD20/600 using sequence-specific primers. *Theor Appl Genet,* 92, 263–266. doi:10.1007/BF00223383

Yang, L., Khan, M. A., Mei, Z., Yang, M., Zhang, T., Wei, C., Yang, W., Zhu, L., Long, Y., Fu, J. J. (2014). Development of RAPD-SCAR markers for *Lonicera japonica* Thunb. (Caprifolicaceae) variety authentication by improved RAPD and DNA cloning. *Rev Biol Trop, 62*(4), 1649–1657. DOI:10.15517/rbt.v62i4.13493

Zhang, C., Mei, Z., Cheng, J., He, Y., Khan, M. A., Luo, P., Imani, S., Fu, J. (2015). Development of SCAR markers based on improved RAPD amplification fragments and molecular cloning for authentication of herbal medicines *Angelica sinensis*, *Angelica acutiloba* and *Levisticum officinale*. *Nat Prod Commun, 10*(10), 1743–1747. doi:10.1177/1934578X1501001027

Chapter 9

Authentication of Medicinal Materials by Multiplex Polymerase Chain Reaction

Zheng-Fei Lu

9.1 Introduction

Medicinal materials are widely used in traditional medicine, dietary supplements, spices and food for their therapeutic properties, flavour or scent (Chevallier, 1996; Duke, 2002; Jackson & Snowdon, 1990). To ensure the efficacy and safety of medicinal materials, fit-for-purpose identification methods are required in the quality assurance process to authenticate raw materials at the species level and verify the parts used (Ekor, 2014; Smillie & Khan, 2010). Traditionally, morphological and chemical analytical approaches are used for the authentication of medicinal materials (Applequist, 2006; Lazarowych & Pekos, 1998; Reich & Schibli, 2007; Upton, David, Gafner & Glasl, 2019). However, they face challenges in providing information to confirm the taxonomic identity of medicinal materials at the species level. First, medicinal materials in commerce are often traded in the form of slices or powders, or even extracts. For morphological approaches including macroscopic and microscopic identification (Techen, Crockett, Khan & Scheffler, 2004), they are either not the ideal method for differentiating species-specific morphological features or identifying samples that suffered from losing morphological features at various degrees. Second, medicinal materials in commerce are harvested from different geographic locations, undergo different processing, and are stored under different conditions. Those factors cause fluctuations in their phytochemical profiles, presenting difficulties in setting up acceptance criteria for chemical authentication methods. In contrast, genomic information, which can be retrieved from different forms of medicinal materials, is not subject to changes from environmental conditions, and has been used to trace the origin of medicinal materials (Böhme, Calo-Mata, Barros-Velázquez & Ortea, 2019; Heubl, 2010; Kumar, Gupta, Misra, Modi & Pandey, 2009; Lo & Shaw, 2018; Sucher & Carles, 2008). Therefore, molecular analytical methods are often required to assist traditional morphological and chemical authentication techniques (Techen *et al.*, 2004).

Among the different molecular analytical methods, species-specific polymerase chain reaction (PCR), designed to be specific to the target species, has become a popular choice for authenticating species in quality control of medicinal materials (Wallinger *et al.*, 2012). However, if the presence or absence of multiple targets need to be confirmed, additional reaction runs are required for each target, resulting in higher cost and time when performing the assay. In these circumstances, multiplex PCR could be used to improve the test efficiency. Compared to classical singleplex PCR that uses one pair of species-specific primers to amplify target DNA one at a time, multiplex PCR uses multiple sets of primers to generate a series of amplicons in one reaction system, with the same expense in terms of time and labour. Once successfully developed and validated, multiplex PCR can be applied in quality control processes to simultaneously verify the presence and absence of multiple species. Because of its reproducible, reliable and economical features, multiplex PCR is not only a quality control friendly option to aid compliance with regulations on medicinal material identification, but also reduces the risk of economically motived adulterations.

This chapter focuses on the topics related to the application of multiplex PCR in the authentication of medicinal materials. First, the unique advantages of multiplex PCR are listed. Then, various types of multiplex PCR used are introduced, followed by a summary of typical workflows and an example protocol to address multiplex PCR assay development and application. Next, published examples are highlighted to demonstrate how multiplex PCR could be used to achieve various goals in the authentication of medicinal materials. Finally, limitations and possible solutions regarding multiplex PCR are discussed.

9.2 Multiplex PCR as Fit-for-Purpose Methods for Authentication of Medicinal Materials

9.2.1 Precise Species Identification to Ensure Purported Health Benefits

Different species in the same genus may serve distinct medicinal purposes in traditional medicine (Zhao *et al.*, 2006). Given the complex phylogenetic relationship between plant species, conventional singleplex PCR, which only delivers binary results, may not be the ultimate choice for precise species identification. Multiplex PCR, which offers molecular diagnostic information from multiple genomic locations, is a cost-effective tool for the identification of medicinal materials and discrimination of closely related species.

9.2.2 Cost-Effective Tool to Detect Adulterants in Mixtures

As stated before, most medicinal materials in trade are not individual plants but presented in the form of slices, powders or even extracts, which may not constitute materials from a single origin. In other words, medicinal materials labelled as parts originating from a single species may be substituted or partially substituted by material from other species for economic gain. Therefore, confirming the absence of other species is as equally important as verifying the presence of target species in the medicinal materials. To fulfil this task, multiple specific targets need to be tested in the process of authentication, and multiplex PCR is a good choice to simultaneously identify the claimed species and to detect known adulterants in mixtures.

9.2.3 Built-in Internal Control to Investigate False Negative Findings

In PCR, inhibitors carried over from DNA extraction may interfere with the PCR process, leading to reduced sensitivity or even false negatives (Tan & Yiap, 2009). To identify a false negative result caused by PCR inhibitors, exogenous DNA is often added to the PCR reaction and amplified by a separate set of primers as amplification control. For medicinal materials, secondary metabolites, such as polyphenols and polysaccharides, are natural sources of PCR inhibitors and may not be completely removed in the DNA extraction process, resulting in false negative results (Do & Adams, 1991; Fang, Hammar & Grumet, 1992; Porebski, Bailey & Baum, 1997; Weishing, Nybom, Wolff & Meyer, 1995). In multiplex PCR, when a common amplicon is expected from all targeted species or the adulterant is present but not the claimed species, the amplified fragment provides an internal control for the other unamplified targets, revealing information to help address false negative findings.

9.3 Types of Multiplex PCR Used in the Authentication of Medicinal Materials

9.3.1 Multiplex End-Point PCR — Fragment Size Multiplexing

Agarose gel electrophoresis is the most widely used technique for analysing PCR products. In fact, as summarised in Table 9.1, the majority of the published multiplex PCR assays were developed to be visualised by agarose gel electrophoresis as end-point PCR.

In theory, an unlimited number of target amplicons can be detected and differentiated by fragment size multiplexing, as long as they can be resolved by agarose gel electrophoresis. However, in reality, the DNA quality of medicinal materials presents challenges. In the first place, genomic DNA extracted from commercial products are usually degraded at a certain level (Lu *et al.*, 2018). Consequently, a higher amplification failure rate is expected for large amplicons in multiplex PCR. In other words, to maintain the assay's universal applicability to authenticate commercial products, amplicons of multiplex PCR need to be designed that will yield as short a PCR product length as possible (<1,000 bp for crudes, less than 200 bp for highly processed materials). Moreover, for fragments in low molecular weight, although the decrease in fragment length comes with an increase in migration distance, the size measurement of PCR fragments may not be accurate due to the decrease in sharpness of bands in the agarose gel, not to mention that primer dimers may also show up in the same region to add another layer of complexity for the interpretation of diagnostic bands.

Table 9.1 Multiplex End-Point PCR in the Authentication of Medicinal Materials

Species in test scope	Target region	Design	Readout	Type of medicinal material	Application	Reference
Cimicifuga heracleifolia *C. dahurica* *C. foetida* *C. simplex*	ITS	ARMS-PCR	AGE	Root, whole plant	Species discrimination	(Jigden, *et al*., 2010c)
Panax ginseng *P. japonicus* *P. quinquefolius* *P. notoginseng* *P. vietnamensis*	*trnK* and 18S rRNA	ARMS-PCR	AGE	Voucher specimen, crude drug materials	Species discrimination	(Zhu, Fushimi, Cai & Komatsu, 2004)
P. ginseng *P. quinquefolius*	Unknown	ARMS-PCR	AGE	Commercial products	Species discrimination	(Cui, Tang & Huang, 2006)
Panax ginseng, other *Panax* spp.	ITS	ARMS-PCR	AGE	Voucher specimen	Species discrimination	(Park, Kim, In & Yang, 2006)
Rheum officinale *R. palmate* *R. tanguticum* *R. undulatum*	SCAR markers	RAPD-derived SCAR markers	AGE	Voucher specimen	Species discrimination	(Moon *et al*., 2009)
Angelica decursiva *Peucedanum decursivum* *P. praeruptorum* *Anthricus sylvestris*	SCAR marker and ITS	RAPD-derived SCAR markers; species-specific PCR	AGE	Voucher specimen	Species discrimination	(Choo *et al*., 2009)

Panax ginseng cultivar 'Chunpoong'	nad7 intron 4	ARMS-PCR, internal posCtrl	AGE	Voucher specimen	Cultivars discrimination	(Wang, Sun, Kwon, Jin & Yang, 2009)
Cynanchum wilfordii *C. auriculatum* *Polygonum multiflorum*	SCAR markers	RAPD-derived SCAR markers	AGE	Voucher specimen	Species discrimination	(Moon *et al.*, 2010)
Ligusticum tenuissimum *L. jeholense* *Ligusticum* sp.	ITS	Species-specific PCR	AGE	Died roots	Species discrimination	(Jigden, *et al.*, 2010a)
Schizonepeta tenuifolia *Agastache rugosa* *Elsholtzia ciliata*	*trnL-trnF*	ARMS-PCR, internal posCtrl	AGE	Voucher specimen, commercial products	Species discrimination	(Jigden, *et al.*, 2010b)
Anemarrhena asphodeloides *Belamcanda chinensis* *Paeonia albiflora* *Peucedanum japonicum*	*trnL-trnF*	ARMS-PCR, internal posCtrl	AGE	Voucher specimen	Species discrimination	(Jigden, Wang, Samdan & Yang, 2010)
Panax ginseng cultivar 'Chunpoong'	*Cox2*	ARMS-PCR, internal posCtrl	AGE	Voucher specimens	Cultivars discrimination	(Wang, Sun, Kwon, Jin & Yang, 2010)
Lentinula edodes (23 strains)	SCAR markers	RAPD-derived SCAR markers	AGE	Voucher specimen	Strain discrimination	(Wu *et al.*, 2010)
Acorus gramineus *A. calamus* *A. tatarinowii* *A. gramineus var. pusilus*	SCAR markers	RAPD-derived SCAR markers	AGE	Voucher specimen	Species discrimination	(Moon *et al.*, 2011)

(*Continued*)

Table 9.1 (*Continued*)

Species in test scope	Target region	Design	Readout	Type of medicinal material	Application	Reference
<u>*P. ginseng*</u> *P. quinquefolius*	rDNA ETS	ARMS-PCR, no control	AGE	Voucher specimen, commercial products	Species discrimination, adulterant detection in mixture	(Wang *et al.*, 2011)
<u>*Dendrobium tosaense*, *D. nobile*</u> *D. linawianum* *D. hercoglossum* *D. moniliforme* *D. huoshanense* 14 other *Dendrobium* spp.	ITS	Species-specific PCR	AGE	Voucher specimen	Species discrimination	(Chiang *et al.*, 2012)
Hypericum perforatum, *H. androsaemum* *H. athoum* *H. ascyron*	ITS	Species-specific PCR	CE	Voucher specimen, tablet, capsule	Species discrimination	(Howard *et al.*, 2012)
<u>*Schisandra chinensis*</u> *S. repanda* *Kadsura japonica*	*rbcL*, ITS	ARMS-PCR	AGE	Voucher specimens	Species discrimination	(Kim, Jang, Kim, Kim & Kim, 2012)

Epimedium koreanum *Caulophyllum robustum* *Thalictrum aquilegifolium* *Astilbe chinensis*	ITS	Species-specific PCR	AGE	Standard samples, commercial products	Species discrimination	(Kim, Subramaniyam, Kim, Kwon & Yang, 2012)
Citrus reticulata *C. unshiu* *C. japonica* *C. maxima* *C. trifoliata*	ITS	ARMS-PCR, internal posCtrl	AGE	Leaf	Species discrimination	(Wang *et al.*, 2012)
Rheum palmatum *R. tanguticum* *R. officinale* *R. franzenbachii* *R. undulatum* *R. rhaponticum* *R. crispus* *R. dentatus*	*matK*	ARMS-PCR, internal posCtrl	AGE	Voucher specimen	Species discrimination	(Xu *et al.*, 2013)
Schisandra chinensis *S. sphenanthera* *S. repanda* *Kadsura japonica*	SCAR markers	RAPD-derived SCAR markers	AGE	Voucher specimen	Species discrimination	(Lee, Moon, Ji, Seo & Kim, 2013)

(*Continued*)

Table 9.1 (*Continued*)

Species in test scope	Target region	Design	Readout	Type of medicinal material	Application	Reference
<u>*Crocus sativus*</u> *Carthamus* spp.	SCAR marker and ITS	RAPD-derived SCAR markers; species-specific PCR	AGE	Voucher specimen	Species discrimination, adulterant detection in mixture	(Babaei, Talebi & Bahar, 2014)
Aucklandia lappa *Inula helenium* *Vladimiria souliei* *Aristolochia debilis* *A. contorta*	ITS	Species-specific PCR	AGE	Voucher specimen	Species discrimination, adulterant detection in mixture	(Doh, Lee, Ju & Oh, 2014)
Dracocephalum moldavica *Melissa officinalis* *Nepeta cataria*	*rbcL*	ARMS-PCR, internal posCtrl	AGE	Voucher specimen, commercial products	Species discrimination, adulterant detection in mixture	(Horn *et al.*, 2014)
Eleutherococcus gracilistylus *E. senticosus* *E. sessiliflorus* *E. sieboldianus*	ITS	Species-specific PCR	AGE	Standard, commercial products	Species discrimination	(Kim *et al.*, 2014)
<u>*Akebia quinate*</u> *A. trifoliata* *A. manshuriensis* *Clematis armandii*	SCAR markers	RAPD-derived SCAR markers	AGE	Voucher specimen	Species discrimination	(Moon, Ji, Lee, Kang & Kim, 2015)

<u>*Panax ginseng*</u> *P. quinquefolius*	26S-18S, ITS2 and *psbA-trnH*	Species-specific PCR	AGE	Voucher specimen, decoctions	Species discrimination, multi-herb decoctions	(Lo, Li & Shaw, 2015)
Manolia denudate *M. biondii* *M. liliiflora* *M. kobus*	*ndhF*	ARMS-PCR, internal posCtrl	AGE	Standard, commercial products	Species discrimination	(Kim *et al.*, 2015)
<u>*Salvia miltiorrhiza*</u> *S. przewalskii* *S. yunnanensis* *S. sinica* *S. digitaloides*	ITS	Species-specific PCR & ARMS-PCR	AGE	Voucher specimen	Species discrimination	(Zhang, Wang, Wang & Wang, 2015)
<u>*Patrinia villosa*</u> <u>*P. scabiosifolia*</u> *P. rupestris* *P. saniculifolia*	SCAR markers	RAPD-derived SCAR markers	AGE	Voucher specimen	Species discrimination	(Moon *et al.*, 2016)
Terminalia bellirica *T. chebula* *T. catappa* *Phyllanthus emblica*	ITS	ARMS-PCR, no control	AGE	Voucher specimen, crude drug materials	Species discrimination, adulterant detection in mixture	(Intharuksa *et al.*, 2016)

(*Continued*)

Table 9.1 (*Continued*)

Species in test scope	Target region	Design	Readout	Type of medicinal material	Application	Reference
Poaceae family *Coix lacryma-jobi* *Zea mays* *Oryza sativa* subsp. *japonica* *Hordeum vulgare* *Triticum aestivum*	*rpoC2*	Species-specific PCR	AGE	Seed, commercial flour-mixed products	Species discrimination, adulterant detection in mixture, commercial product testing	(Moon, Kim & Jang, 2016)
Cymbopogon citratus, *C. nardus*	*trnL-trnF*	ARMS-PCR, internal posCtrl	AGE	Leaf or stalk	Species discrimination	(Ng *et al.*, 2016)
<u>*Convolvulus prostratus*,</u> *Evolvulus alsinoides*	ITS	Species-specific PCR	AGE	Voucher specimen, material heat dried from voucher specimen	Species discrimination, adulterant detection in mixture	(Sharma & Shrivastava, 2016)
Boerhavia diffusa *B. errecta* *Trianthema* spp.	SCAR markers	RAPD-derived SCAR markers	AGE	Voucher specimen	Species discrimination	(Vinay, 2016)
<u>*Aralia continentalis*</u> <u>*Angelica biserrate*</u> *Levisticum officinale* *Heracleum moellendorffii*	ITS1	Species-specific PCR	AGE	Voucher specimen, commercial products	Species discrimination, adulterant detection in mixture	(Kim *et al.*, 2016)

<u>*Sarcandra glabra,*</u> *Chloranthus spicatus* *C. serratus* *C. henryi*	*trnL-trnF*	ARMS-PCR, internal posCtrl	AGE, qPCR SYBR Green singleplex	Leaf, commercial products	Species discrimination, adulterant detection in mixture	(Wei, Chen, Huang, Liu & Liang, 2016)
<u>*Pinellia ternate*</u> *P. tripartite* *P. pedatisecta* *Typhonium flagelliforme*	SCAR markers	RAPD-derived SCAR markers	AGE	Voucher specimen	Species discrimination	(Lee *et al.*, 2016)
<u>*Adenophora stricta*</u> *A. triphylla* *Codonopsis lanceolata* *C. pilosula* *Glehnia littoralis*	ITS	Species-specific PCR	AGE	Voucher specimen, processed commercial products	Species discrimination, commercial product testing	(Moon *et al.*, 2017)
Panax ginseng cultivar 'G-1'	45S rDNA	ARMS-PCR, internal posCtrl	AGE	Voucher specimen	Cultivars discrimination	(Yang *et al.*, 2017)
<u>*Triticum durum*</u> *Triticum aestivum*	ITS	Species-specific PCR	AGE	Seed, commercial bakery products	Species discrimination, adulterant detection in mixture, commercial product testing	(Arlorio *et al.*, 2003)
Aristolochia pothieri *A. pierrei* *A. tagala* *A. ringens* *A. kerrii*	ITS2	Species-specific PCR	AGE	Voucher specimen, commercial crude drug	Species discrimination	(Dechbumroong, Aumnouypol, Denduangboripant & Sukrong, 2018)

(*Continued*)

Table 9.1 (*Continued*)

Species in test scope	Target region	Design	Readout	Type of medicinal material	Application	Reference
A. littoralis *A. grandiflora* *A. gigantea* *A. tentaculate* *A. anguicida* *Gymnopetalum integrifolium* *Raphistemma pulchellum* *Jasminum* sp. *J. sambac* *J. adenophyllum*						
<u>*Dendrobium devonianum*</u> *D. aphyllum,* *D. strongylanthum* *D. officinale* *D. nobile* *D. chrysotoxum* *D. huoshanense* *D. fimbriatum*	*trnL-trnF*	Species-specific PCR	AGE	Voucher specimen, commercial products	Species discrimination, adulterant detection in mixture, commercial product testing	(Jiang *et al.*, 2018)

<u>*Angelica dahurica*</u> <u>*A. dahurica* var.</u> *formosana*, *A. anomala*, *A. japonica*	ITS	Species-specific PCR	AGE	Voucher specimen, commercial products	Species discrimination, adulterant detection in mixture	(Noh, Kim, Yang, Park & Moon, 2018)
Dendrocalamus asper *D. copelandii* *D. latiflorus* *D. hamiltonii* *Dendrocalamus* sp.	SCAR markers	RAPD-derived SCAR markers	AGE	Voucher specimen	Species discrimination	(Rangsiruji, Binchai & Pringsulaka, 2018)
Lycium chinense *L. barbarum*	*psbA-trnH*	ARMS-PCR, internal posCtrl	AGE	Voucher specimen, commercial products	Species discrimination	(Wetters, Horn & Nick, 2018)
<u>*Angelica gigas*</u> *A. sinensis* *A. acutiloba*	ITS, *trnC-petN*	Species-specific PCR	AGE	Standard samples, commercial products	Species discrimination, adulterant detection in mixture	(Kim, Park, Lee & Kim, 2018)
Allium ochotense *A. microdictyon*	ITS	ARMS-PCR (Tetra), internal posCtrl	AGE	Voucher specimen	Species discrimination	(Kim *et al.*, 2018)
Gynostemma pentaphyllum *G. longipes* *G. burmanicum* *G. pubescens*	*ycf3*, *accD*, *petD*, *psbB*	Species-specific PCR	AGE	Fresh and dried samples	Species discrimination, adulterant detection in mixture	(Abid *et al.*, 2019)

(*Continued*)

Table 9.1 (*Continued*)

Species in test scope	Target region	Design	Readout	Type of medicinal material	Application	Reference
<u>*Rubus coreanus*</u> *R. chingi,* *R. crataegifolius* *R. occidentalis*	*Rpl16, trnG-trnS*	Species-specific PCR	AGE	Voucher specimen, commercial products	Species discrimination, adulterant detection in mixture	(Mohanan *et al.*, 2019)
<u>*Chrysanthemum indicum*</u> *C. morifolium* *C. boreale* *Aster spathulifolius*	*rpoC2*	ARMS-PCR, internal posCtrl	AGE	Fresh and dried samples	Species discrimination	(Abid *et al.*, 2020)
Cymbidium goeringii cultivars	SSR	SSR genotypes	CE	Leaf, root	Cultivar discrimination	(Lee *et al.*, 2020)
<u>*Dimocarpus longan,*</u> *Litchi chinensis,* *Nephelium lappaceum*	ITS	Species-specific PCR, cross-reactivity tested	AGE	Voucher specimen, commercial products	Species discrimination, adulterant detection in mixture	(Kim *et al.*, 2020)
<u>*Viscum coloratum,*</u> *Taxillus sutchuenensis var. duclouxii,* *Korthalsella japonica,* *Loranthus tanakae*	*matK*	Species-specific PCR, sensitivity in mixed samples	AGE, qPCR SYBR Green singleplex	Voucher specimen, commercial products	Species discrimination, adulterant detection in mixture	(Kim *et al.*, 2020)

ARMS-PCR: amplification refractory mutation system PCR; AGE: agarose gel electrophoresis; CE: capillary electrophoresis; ETS: external transcribed spacer; SCAR: sequence characterised amplification region; SSR: simple sequence repeat.

Note: For species in test scope column, the underlined scientific name represents the target species.

To overcome the limitation of agarose gel electrophoresis in the differentiation of amplicons that differ only by a few bp in length, polyacrylamide (PAA) gels or capillary electrophoresis can be used (Henegariu, Heerema, Dlouhy, Vance & Vogt, 1997; Lindstedt, Vardund, Aas & Kapperud, 2004; Yokoyama, Kishida, Uchimura & Ichinohe, 2006). Using St John's Wort (*Hypericum perforatum L.*) as an example, Howard and collaborators developed the 'PlantID' assay, which replaced traditional agarose gel electrophoresis by high-resolution capillary electrophoresis when evaluating multiplex PCR products (Howard *et al.*, 2012). In the same study, the authors also discussed the assay's potential to cover a broader range of species with a lower false-positive rate by using up to five types of fluorescent labels and requiring multiple peaks from different regions for individual species identification.

9.3.2 Multiplex Real-Time PCR

For multiplex end-point PCR, PCR products have to be visualised by electrophoresis for result interpretation. This additional step can be avoided by performing multiplex real-time PCR, which monitors cycle-to-cycle amplification by the change in florescent intensity (Logan, Logan, Edwards & Saunders, 2009). In contrast to multiplex end-point PCR, multiplex real-time PCR not only completes data generation and collection in a closed-tube system, which eliminates the need for post-amplification manipulation (i.e. reducing opportunities for contamination), but also shows high accuracy, sensitivity and the possibility of reporting quantitative measurements, although the main applications of multiplex PCR in the authentication of medicinal materials are still qualitative (Gachon, Mingam & Charrier, 2004; Kaltenboeck & Wang, 2005; Longo, Berninger & Hartley, 1990).

The detection chemistries used in monitoring amplification can be divided into two types: non-specific amplification product detection using DNA-intercalating dyes, such as SYBR® Green and EvaGreen®, or specific amplification product detection using fluorophore-labelled sequence-specific probes, such as TaqMan probes (Navarro, Serrano-Heras, Castaño & Solera, 2015). The selection of detection chemistry depends on the purpose of the assay and their applications are discussed in separate sections. Table 9.2 reviews and summarises previous publications on multiplex real-time PCR for the authentication of medicinal materials based on detection chemistries, types of medicinal materials and applications.

9.3.3 DNA-Intercalating Dyes — High-Resolution Melting Profile Multiplexing

There is a wide variety of commercially available DNA-intercalating fluorescent dyes. Among them, SYBR® Green is the most commonly used dye, followed by EvaGreen®, which offers additional advantages compared with SYBR® Green, such as being less inhibitory to PCR and less toxic (Mao, Leung & Xin, 2007). Compared with target-specific probe chemistry, these are much less expensive and more flexible choices for real-time PCR method development, because they only require primers to get the specific template region amplified. However, their non-selective binding affinity to all double-strand DNA, including primer dimers, compromises the specificity of the assay. To obtain target-specific readout, a melting curve analysis is necessary after the amplification stage to ensure a single amplicon is obtained. Due to this reason, DNA-intercalating dyes are less desirable for multiplex assays, where multiple amplicons are expected after amplification.

Table 9.2 Multiplex Real-Time PCR in the Authentication of Medicinal Materials

Species in test scope	Target region	Design	Readout	Type of medicinal material	Application	Reference
Cynanchum wilfordii *Cynanchum auriculatum*	*trnL-trnF*	Allele-specific probe	Fluorophore colour	Leaf, root, commercial products	Species discrimination	(Ryuk, Lee, Ju & Ko, 2014)
Salvia officinalis *Salvia fruticosa* *Matricaria chamomilla* *Sideritis scardica* *Origanum vulgare* *Oregano onites* *Achillea millefolium* *Melissa officinalis* *Rosmarinus officinalis*	ITS2	Species-specific PCR	DNA-intercalating dye +HRM	Standard	Species discrimination	(Xanthopoulou *et al.*, 2016)
Cannabis sativa *Merremia tuberosa* *Ipomoea purpurea* *Datura stramonium*	*UF3GT, adc1, waxy, THC*	Species-specific PCR	DNA-intercalating dye +HRM	Seed, other plant parts	Species discrimination	(Elkins, Perez & Quinn, 2017)

(*Continued*)

Table 9.2 (*Continued*)

Species in test scope	Target region	Design	Readout	Type of medicinal material	Application	Reference
Juglans regia *Quercus robur* *Matricaria recutita* *Salvia miltiorrhiza* *Aristolochia clematitis*	ITS	Species-specific PCR +target-specific probe	Fluorophore colour	Voucher specimen, commercial herbal mix	Species discrimination	(Doganay-Knapp, Orland, König & Knöss, 2018)
Various species originating from 29 different families	ITS2, *psbA-trnH*, *rbcL*, *(trnL c,d)*, *(trnL g,h)*	Universal primer mix	DNA-intercalating dye +HRM	Leaf, seed	Species, sub-species, and cultivars discrimination	(Ballin, Onaindia, Jawad, Fernandez-Carazo & Maquet, 2019)
Petroselinum crispum *Apium graveolens*	ITS2	Species-specific PCR+target-specific probe	Fluorophore colour	Leaf	Species discrimination	(Quan *et al.*, 2020)

HRM: high-resolution melting.

Note: For species in the test scope column, the underlined scientific name represents the target species.

However, successful examples still could be found. To differentiate fluorescence emitted from multiple distinctive amplification products after multiplex amplification, high-resolution melting (HRM) analysis is often required. Because of the unique base composition of PCR amplicons, a well-designed HRM analysis can produce unique melting profiles that are specific to each target, which further serve evidence for species identification (Ballin *et al.*, 2019; Xanthopoulou *et al.*, 2016). However, analysing results from multiplex PCR based on DNA-intercalating dyes is still challenging, especially when primer dimers or contaminating products are present; it is also prone to overlooking the characteristic melting peaks from targets that are in low abundance. This explains the fact that many multiplex quantitative polymerase chain reaction (qPCR)-HRM assays developed today are focused on medicinal materials with a single origin but not on mixtures. For further information, the principles and application of HRM are discussed in Chapter 16 of this book.

9.3.4 Probes — Fluorophore Colour Multiplexing

Although many types of fluorophore-labelled probes are used in real-time PCR to detect targets in a sequence-specific manner, hydrolysis probes, such as TaqMan probes, are the most popular choice (Holland, Abramson, Watson & Gelfand, 1991; Navarro *et al.*, 2015). The TaqMan probe contains a fluorescent dye on the 5′ end and is quenched by the quencher on the 3′ end. During amplification, Taq DNA polymerase synthesises new strands using the unlabelled primers and the template. When the polymerase encounters the TaqMan probe that specifically binds to template, its endogenous 5′ nuclease activity hydrolyses the probe, separating the fluorophore from the quencher and emitting a signal.

Therefore, by using different probes that are labelled by a unique fluorescence colour, simultaneous detection of multiple targets or species in mixed form can be easily achieved.

For instance, celery (*Apium graveolens*) leaf flakes, which share many morphological characteristics and exhibit similar phytochemical profiles with parsley (*Petroselinum crispum*), are traded at a lower price. To properly authenticate parsley leaf materials and also detect economically motivated adulteration such as celery leaf, Quan and collaborators developed a probe-based multiplex qPCR assay to prevent parsley material misidentification (Quan *et al*., 2020). In their design, parsley, celery and internal amplification control (IAC) DNA were amplified by species-specific primers. During amplification, three probes (labelled with FAM, HEC and Cy3) that target variable regions in these amplicons were hydrolysed to emit fluorescence signals at different wavelengths. To demonstrate the assay's value in the authentication of parsley, it was further validated to reliably detect 1% (w/w) of celery in parsley leaf materials. The list of target species that can be differentiated depends on the emission spectrum characteristics of fluorophores. Because the emission wavelengths of individual fluorophores need to be separated, the maximal number of targets that can be differentiated per reaction ranges from four to six (Marras, 2006). To authenticate mixed medicinal products, Doganay-Knapp and collaborators developed a 5-plex qPCR assay to simultaneously trace *Juglans regia*, *Quercus robur*, *Matricaria recutita*, *Salvia miltiorrhiza* and *Aristolochia clematitis* (Doganay-Knapp *et al*., 2018). The assay was able to successfully detect all components in a set of defined mixture with highly variable quantities of each medicinal materials and demonstrated superior sensitivity than similar multiplex end-point PCR assays evaluated in the same study.

9.4 Workflow to Develop Multiplex PCR Assays for the Authentication of Medicinal Materials

The same primer design and optimisation principles apply regardless of whether traditional end-point PCR or real-time PCR is chosen. For real-time PCR, there are additional factors to consider in design, such as the design of fluorophore-labelled probes based on projected amplicons and assessing the uniqueness of amplicon melting profiles. The basic steps to develop and optimise multiplex PCR assays for the authentication of medicinal materials are summarised in Figure 9.1.

9.4.1 Definition of Targets

To develop multiplex PCR for species identification and discrimination, the scope of the multiplex PCR targets, including the target species, close species and common adulterants, should be defined first.

9.4.2 Design of Primers

9.4.2.1 *Homologous Sequence-Based Primer Design*

DNA barcode sequences, such as the internal transcribed spacer (ITS) from ribosomal RNA in nuclear genome, ribulose bisphosphate carboxylase large chain (*rbcL*) from chloroplast, cyclooxygenase 2 (*cox2*) from mitochondria, are the frequent choices for target-specific primer design (CBOL Plant Working Group, 2009; Chen *et al.*, 2010). To start the homologous sequence-based primer design, barcode sequences from every species or target in the test

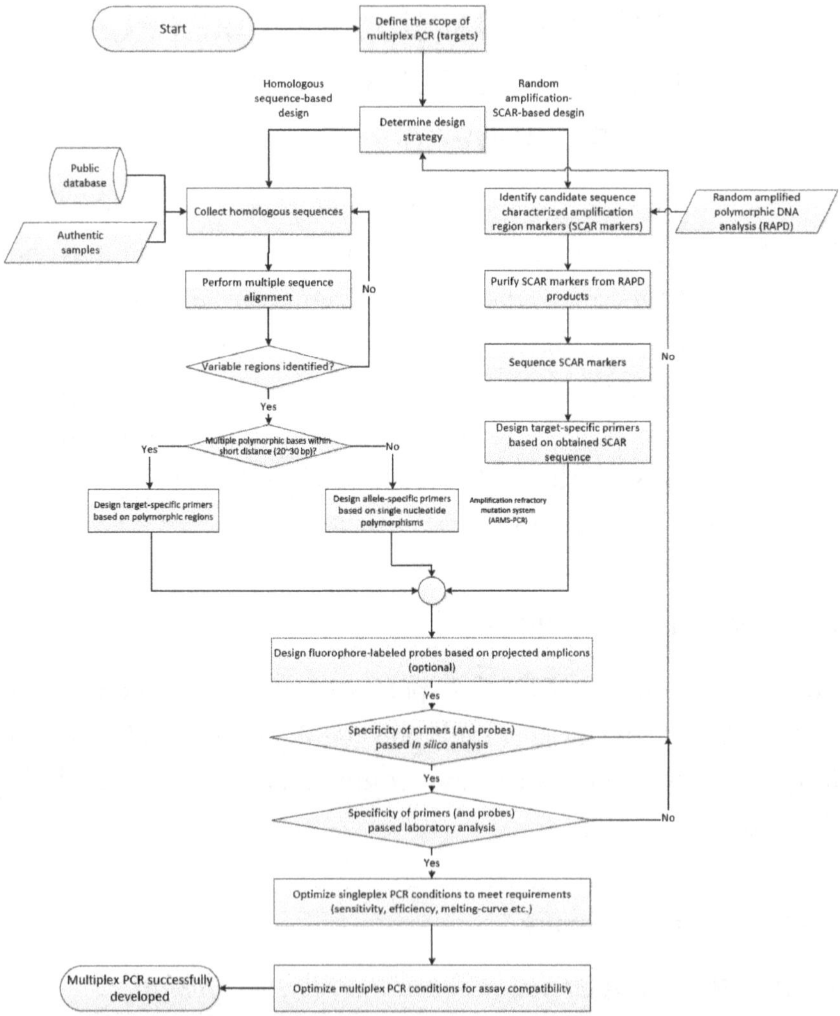

Fig. 9.1 Schematic representation of various steps in the development of a multiplex PCR assay for authentication.

scope are collected either from the public database or samples certified to be authentic. Then, multiple sequence alignment is performed to identify intraspecies conserved regions and interspecies variable regions. Depending on the phylogenetic relationship between individual species in the pre-defined test scope, different levels of variations may be observed in the aligned sequences. For phylogenetically distant species, species-specific primers may be placed at sites that contain multiple polymorphic bases, insertions or deletions, so specific amplification in target species can be achieved through the differences in primer hybridisation efficiency and polymerase elongation efficiency between target and non-target species (Cha & Thilly, 1993). In contrast, for closely related species, the differences between homologues sequences are often at a single nucleotide polymorphism (SNP) level.

9.4.2.2 *Random Amplification Sequence Characterised Amplification Region Marker-Based Primer Design*

In addition to designing multiplex PCR primers based on differences between homologous sequences, random amplified polymorphic DNA (RAPD) analysis result can serve as another starting point, even under circumstances where sequence information is not available (Welsh & McClelland, 1990; Williams, Kubelik, Livak, Rafalski & Tingey, 1990). In this approach, RAPD analysis is first performed using a group of short oligonucleotides of 10 bp long (such as Operon primers) on all species in the test scope to generate distinctive amplification profiles. Since the RAPD amplification profile is sensitive to test conditions, to reliably distinguish different species, representative polymorphism bands for each species are identified from RAPD amplification products (Paran & Michelmore, 1993). Then, candidate amplicons are purified from agarose gel, sequenced and sometimes queried in GenBank using the Basic Local Alignment Search Tool (BLAST) program to select and convert the unique sequences to sequence characterised amplification region (SCAR) markers. Next, SCAR primers are designed by either extending the original RAPD primer towards the centre of the SCAR marker with an additional six to ten bases, or nesting the primer binding site to completely exclude the RAPD primer sequences. Provided that the SCAR primers are longer in length, species-specific amplicons can be generated consistently in PCR reactions for identification purpose (Hernández, Martín & Dorado, 1999).

9.4.3 Screening of Candidate Primers, Optimisation and Pooling

Ideally, prior to laboratory analysis, the specificity and properties of all candidate primers should be evaluated by *in silico* analysis. The former could be surveyed and verified by BLAST searches in public databases, whereas the properties, such as melting temperature, GC content and secondary structures, could be calculated by various oligo analyser tools that available online.

To ensure the PCR primers are indeed discriminative among species, singleplex PCR should be performed to further evaluate the individual primer set's specificity, sensitivity and efficiency. Particularly, primers should be tested against all target species in the scope of multiplex PCR, sometimes even expanding the test subjects to other species used (Kim *et al.*, 2020). Based on experimental observation, the best primer pair for each species are identified.

Finally, these selected primers are pooled together in a single reaction for compatibility optimisation. Specific attention must be paid to (1) prevent the dominance of a small subset of PCR reaction, resulting in early consumption of reagents, and (2) minimise the interaction between different primers, to prevent the occurrence of undesired amplification artefacts (Sint, Raso & Traugott, 2012). At this stage, thermocycling conditions are unified, and parameters such as the primer ratio, dNTP, $MgCl_2$ and DNA polymerase concentration are adjusted, so that balanced amplification of each target can be achieved (Markoulatos, Siafakas & Moncany,

2002). To reduce non-specific interactions between primers, multiplex PCR design software and web applications are also available (Holleley & Geerts, 2009; Rachlin, Ding, Cantor & Kasif, 2005; Shen *et al.*, 2010). Although the development of multiplex PCR represents an investment, it is still the method of choice for medicinal materials that require repetitive identification testing, and the initial investments can be easily justified by the advantages that multiplex PCR brings.

9.5 Multiplex PCR for *P. ginseng* Identification and Its Adulteration Detection

To illustrate the principles of designing multiplex PCR assays and demonstrate the procedure of performing multiplex PCR for the authentication of medicinal materials, a brief multiplex end-point Amplification Refractory Mutation System PCR (ARMS-PCR) protocol for *P. ginseng* identification and its adulteration detection is illustrated as an example.

9.5.1 Design of ARMS-PCR for *P. ginseng* Identification

To differentiate *P. ginseng* from its adulterants in genus *Panax*, the chloroplast *trnL-trnF* intergenic spacers of common *Panax* spp. were downloaded from GenBank, aligned and assessed for variations that are unique to *P. ginseng*. As shown in Figure 9.2A, the *P. ginseng* consensus sequence exhibits Thymine (T) at the boxed SNP position, while *P. quinquefolius*, *P. notoginseng* and *P. japonicus* exhibit adenine (A). Four primers are designed around the SNP position to give PCR fragments of different lengths for *P. ginseng* and other species: the outer primer pair amplifies a large 181 bp internal control fragment from all genomic DNA in *Panax* spp., whereas the inner primers amplify two smaller diagnostic

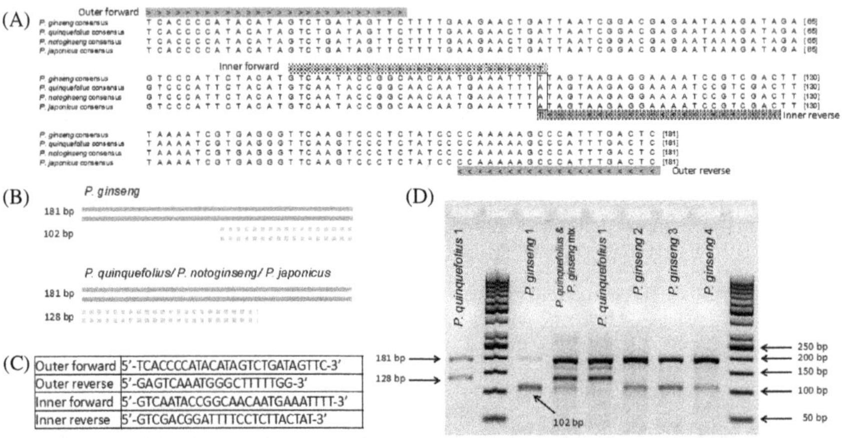

Fig. 9.2 (A) Alignment of *Panax* spp. *trnL-trnF* intergenic spacer sequences and multiplex primer locations. The outer primer set is indicated by arrows with grey background. The inner primer set is designed based on the SNP site (open square box). To better illustrate the design, the last bases of inner primers are shown. Reverse inner primer is shown as complement to the displayed sequences. (B) A schematic diagram of PCR products expected from multiplex PCR assay. A 181 bp outer fragment and a 102 bp inner fragment are expected from *P. ginseng*; a 181 bp outer fragment and a 102 bp inner fragment are expected from other *Panax* spp. (C) Primer sequences used in multiplex PCR. (D) *Panax* spp. PCR products visualised in 2% agarose gel.

fragments representing two allelic states in *P. ginseng* and other species. When *P. ginseng* DNA is present, a perfect match is formed between the *P. ginseng* specific inner forward primer and DNA template from *P. ginseng*, resulting in a 102 bp fragment. On the other hand, the inner reverse primer could pair with the outer forward primer to generate a 128 bp fragment only when a perfect match is formed between the 3′ terminus of inner reverse primer and template DNA from other ginseng species (Figure 9.2B).

9.5.2 Genomic DNA Extraction from Ginseng Roots

1. Grind ginseng root materials into fine powder using the 1600 MiniG from SPEX SamplePrep.

2. Extract genomic DNA using the DNeasy *mericon* Food Kit from Qiagen, according to the manufacturer's standard protocol, with input powder weighing between 50 and 100 mg.
3. At the end of extraction, elute genomic DNA in 150 μL of the elution buffer provided in the kit.
4. Quantify the eluted DNA using Qubit 3.0 Fluorometer from Thermo Fisher Scientific.

9.5.3 Multiplex PCR

1. Dilute all genomic DNA to 1.0 ng/μL in nuclease-free water. If the concentration of extracted DNA is lower than 1.0 ng/μL, no dilution is needed.
2. Set up a 20 μL PCR system, containing 10 μL AmpliTaq Gold™ 360 Master Mix, 2 μL primer mix (2.5 μM each primer in Figure 9.2C), 2 μL genomic DNA (1.0 ng/μL or lower) and 6 μL nuclease-free water.
3. Use the following thermal profile for amplification: (1) an initial step of 3 min at 95°C and (2) 28 cycles of 30 s at 95°C, 30 s at 58°C and 30 s at 72°C; and (3) a final extension of 72°C for 5 min. DNA isolation control and negative control are included. *Note: For ARMS-PCR, Taq DNA polymerase lacks 3′ to 5′ exonuclease activity and is required.*

9.5.4 Visualisation of PCR Product

1. Separate PCR products with a 50 bp DNA size marker on a 2% pre-stained agarose gel at 120 V for 30 min.
2. Visualise the PCR product on an ultraviolet (UV) transilluminator.
3. *P. ginseng* exhibits two major bands, one slightly above the 100

bp marker, the other slightly below the 200 bp marker. Other ginseng in *Panax* spp. also exhibit two major bands on agarose gel. However, the lower band is in the middle between the 100 and 150 bp markers. A sample containing *P. ginseng* and other adulterants would exhibit three bands, one slightly above 100 bp marker, one in the middle between the 100 and the 150 bp marker and a third band slightly below the 200 bp marker (Figure 9.2D).

9.6 Application of Multiplex PCR in the Authentication of Medicinal Materials

9.6.1 Close Species Discrimination

Indeed, the majority of the multiplex PCR methods developed for medicinal materials aim to differentiate target species from close species and various adulterants. In terms of close species discrimination, the multiplex PCR assay developed for *Dendrobium* spp. identification serves as a noteworthy example. *Dendrobium caulis* (Shihu) is a valuable medicine derived from the stems of several closely related species in the genus *Dendrobium*. However, the biological activities and pharmacological actions of different Dendrobii species vary (Lam *et al.*, 2015). Therefore, precise identification and discrimination of Dendrobii at the species level is critical for ensuring the efficacy and safety of medicinal materials in the genus *Dendrobium*. In a study by Jiang and collaborators, an octaplex PCR assay was developed to generate PCR products of different sizes for eight *Dendrobium* spp. (Jiang *et al.*, 2018). The authors concluded that the assay could be used as a cost-effective method for the routine terminal market control of mainstream, closely related *Dendrobium* spp.

9.6.2 Adulteration Detection

Once a candidate multiplex PCR method demonstrated its specificity in discriminating target species and its close species, its capability in detecting economically motivated adulterants in mixtures was also frequently evaluated as the next step. Saffron (*Crocus sativus*), known as the world's most expensive spice by weight, has long been subject to adulteration from cheaper medicinal materials, such as safflower stamens (*Carthamus* spp.) (Gresta, Lombardo, Siracusa & Ruberto, 2008). To simultaneously identify saffron and detect safflower, which is the most common and cheapest substitute, Babaei and collaborators combined the saffron SCAR marker and ITS-specific primer in a single reaction system and developed a multiplex PCR assay that is able to produce a 613 bp ITS region amplicon from safflower adulterants in saffron samples (Babaei *et al.*, 2014). Additional examples for adulteration detection in mixtures are summarised in Tables 9.1 and 9.2.

9.6.3 Multi-Component Medicinal Materials Verification

Medicinal materials may present in the form of multi-component mixture. In fact, in traditional Chinese medicine (TCM) and ayurvedic medicine, the majority of medicinal products are used as multi-component mixtures. Analysing such mixed preparations containing many compounds from different species by chemical analytical methods presents challenges. To verify the presence of each ingredient in complex mixtures in a specific and sensitive manner, multiplex PCR becomes an indispensable tool. For example, Triphala is one of the most important formulations used in Ayurvedic medicine and Thai folk medicine. It consists of fruit powder from *Terminalia chebula* var. *chebula*, *T. bellirica* and *Phyllanthus emblica* (Nariya, Shukla, Jain, & Ravishankar, 2009). Although authentication of Triphala powder is difficult by morphological and chemical analytical methods, Intharuksa and collaborators developed a multiplex ARMS-PCR assay to detect all ingredients in several commercial Triphala formulations (Intharuksa *et al.*, 2016).

9.6.4 Cultivar Identification

To identify medicinal materials at the species level, multiplex PCR could also be applied to further identify cultivars of the same species. For example, among the *P. ginseng* cultivars, because of its superior quality and high yield, 'Chunpoong' is a high market value cultivar (Kwon, Chung, Kim, Lee & Choi, 1998). To discriminate 'Chunpoong' from other cultivars, several multiplex ARMS-PCR assay were designed based on SNPs located in the mitochondrial NADH dehydrogenase subunit (*nad7*) intron 4 region or cytochrome oxidase subunit 2 (*cox2*) intron II region (Wang *et al.*, 2009; 2010). These assays were demonstrated as time-saving and effective tools to facilitate the selection and breeding of *P. ginseng* cultivars.

9.7 Limitations

9.7.1 Unknown Targets Remain Unidentified

PCR-based authentication methods require the amplification of specific DNA loci with pre-designed oligonucleotide primers. As a result, the identity assessment can only be performed against a defined species list. If the medicinal materials contain adulterants that are unknown to the method developer or not considered in the multiplex PCR design stage, two types of outcomes are expected:

(1) no cross-activity between multiplex primers and unknown adulterants, so the adulterants will likely remain unidentified; and (2) multiplex primers amplify fragments from unknown adulterants, resulting in a new amplification profile. In this case, the amplification profile cannot be assigned to any species in the pre-defined scope. From a quality control standpoint, none of the outcomes are desired. The first outcome can be addressed from two angles. In the first place, a comprehensive literature review on the target material is necessary at the method development stage; other untargeted genomic methods, such as DNA barcoding, also need to be performed on a regular basis to survey medicinal materials, so that the risk of adulteration from not well-documented medicinal materials can be further reduced. For the second outcome, to investigate the potential new amplification profile, purifying and sequencing the additional amplicons from gel electrophoresis may also provide valuable information for decision-making.

9.7.2 Uneven Detection Limit

Another issue for multiplex PCR is the uneven detection limit for each target. Even when each primer is tested to specifically identify its target species in singleplex mode, because different targets compete with each other for resources, there is no guarantee that when they are combined in multiplex mode, the amplification efficiency of each pair is balanced. Among the multiple targets, certain targets may have a lower amplification efficiency, which translates to a higher detection limit, compared to other ingredients in the same scope. As a result, certain target species may be dropped out due to either the target species being represented at a lower percentage in the mixture or the extracted DNA having a low concentration. This often happens to longer amplicons in multiplex systems and has been reported in multiple studies (Doganay-Knapp *et al.*, 2018; Moon *et al.*, 2015). Therefore, to achieve a balanced amplification for each target, extensive efforts must be made to optimise the composition of the PCR buffer, the relative ratio of primer pairs, cycling conditions and the amount of DNA polymerase (Markoulatos *et al.*, 2002). Sometimes, the concentration of each primer set needs to be limited to overcome the early depletion of resources, or certain amplicons need to be redesigned to improve their amplification efficiency in the multiplex PCR system.

9.7.3 Limit on the Number of Analytes per Multiplex Assay

The limit on the number of analyte measurements per assay is another challenge that multiplex PCR faces when authenticating medicinal materials. For multiplex end-point PCR, the generated amplicons need to exhibit appropriate size differences to allow the unambiguous differentiation of fragments in electrophoresis. In theory, amplicons ranging between less than 100 bp and several kb can be resolved in agarose gel. However, considering the nonlinear relationship between DNA fragment size and migration distance, separating two DNA fragments of 1,000 bp and 1,050 bp in agarose gel is not as easy as separating fragments of 100 bp and 150 bp. Furthermore, given the level of DNA degradation in medicinal materials, all amplicons should be preferably less than 250 bp in length, which dramatically limits the number of analytes that can be resolved. To better differentiate amplicons of short length, capillary electrophoresis, which provides higher resolution than agarose gel electrophoresis, may be an option (Howard *et al.*, 2012). However, this additional step complicates the procedure and incurs higher cost and longer testing time, offsetting the benefits of choosing multiplex PCR in the first place. Similarly, in real-time PCR, the number of multiplexing is also constrained by the fluorophore emission spectra and available detection channels provided in the qPCR system. Usually no more than six unique fluorophores can be evaluated in a single reaction, including fluorophores reserved for the reference dye and IAC. To monitor more than six targets in multiplex real-time PCR, an amplitude modulation strategy, which combines colour and signal intensity measurements at the plateau phase has been proposed (Rajagopal *et al.*, 2019). However, successful application of this strategy in the authentication of medicinal materials has yet to be demonstrated.

9.8 Conclusion

Using a single assay to identify multiple components in medicinal materials is a long-term desire for traditional medicine, dietary supplement and spice industries. Multiplex PCR, combining the easy-to-use feature of regular PCR assays and targeting multiple objects to extract additional information that otherwise may require several parallel singleplex reactions, can be integrated into current quality control systems with minimal cost. Therefore, multiplex PCR is a promising tool to improve the efficiency of the authentication of medicinal materials in routine quality control practice without driving up the required cost and time.

Acknowledgement

I thank Dr. Tiffany Chua, Dr. Yanjun Zhang, Silva Babajanian, Peter Chang and Gary Swanson from Herbalife Nutrition for their valuable comments.

References

Abid, S., Kaliraj, L., Arif, M. H., Hurh, J., Ahn, J. C., Yang, D. C., & Jung, S. K. (2020). Molecular and morphological discrimination of Chrysanthemum indicum using allele-specific PCR and T-shaped trichome. *Mol Biol Rep, 47*(10), 7699–7708. doi:10.1007/s11033-020-05844-2

Abid, S., Mohanan, P., Kaliraj, L., Park, J. K., Ahn, J. C., & Yang, D. C. (2019). Development of species-specific chloroplast markers for the authentication of Gynostemma pentaphyllum and their distribution in the Korean peninsula. *Fitoterapia, 138*(1186), 104295. doi:10.1016/j.fitote.2019.104295

Applequist, W. (2006). *The Identification of Medicinal Plants: A Handbook of the Morphology of Botanicals in Commerce*. St. Louis: Missouri Botanical Garden Press.

Arlorio, M., Coïsson, J., Cereti, E., Travaglia, F., Capasso, M., & Martelli, A. (2003). Polymerase chain reaction (PCR) of puroindoline b and ribosomal/puroindoline b multiplex PCR for the detection of common wheat (Triticum aestivum) in Italian pasta. *Eur Food Res Technol, 216*(3), 253–258. doi:10.1007/s00217-002-0634-7

Babaei, S., Talebi, M., & Bahar, M. (2014). Developing an SCAR and ITS reliable multiplex PCR-based assay for safflower adulterant detection in saffron samples. *Food Control, 35*(1), 323–328. doi:10.1016/j.foodcont.2013.07.019

Ballin, N. Z., Onaindia, J. O., Jawad, H., Fernandez-Carazo, R., & Maquet, A. (2019). High-resolution melting of multiple barcode amplicons for plant species authentication. *Food Control, 105*, 141–150. doi:10.1016/j.foodcont.2019.05.022

Böhme, K., Calo-Mata, P., Barros-Velázquez, J., & Ortea, I. (2019). Review of recent DNA-based methods for main food-authentication topics. *J Agric Food Chem, 67*(14), 3854–3864. doi:10.1021/acs.jafc.8b07016

CBOL Plant Working Group. (2009). A DNA barcode for land plants. *PNAS, 106*(31), 12794–12797. doi:10.1073/pnas.0905845106

Cha, R. S., & Thilly, W. G. (1993). Specificity, efficiency, and fidelity of PCR. *PCR Methods Appl, 3*(3), S18–S29. doi:10.1101/gr.3.3.s18

Chen, S., Yao, H., Han, J., Liu, C., Song, J., Shi, L., Zhu, Y., Ma, X., Gao, T., Pang, X., Luo, K., Li, Y., Li, X., Jia, X., Lin, Y., Leon, C. (2010). Validation of the ITS2 region as a novel DNA barcode for identifying medicinal plant species. *PLoS One, 5*(1), e8613. doi:10.1371/journal.pone.0008613

Chevallier, A. (1996). *The Encyclopedia of Medicinal Plants*. New York: DK Publishing.

Chiang, C. H., Yu, T. A., Lo, S. F., Kuo, C. L., Peng, W. H., & Tsay, H. S. (2012). Molecular authentication of Dendrobium species by multiplex polymerase chain reaction and amplification refractory mutation system analysis. *J Am Soc Hortic Sci, 137*(6), 438–444. doi:10.21273/JASHS.137.6.438

Choo, B. K., Moon, B. C., Ji, Y., Kim, B. B., Choi, G., Yoon, T., & Kim, H. K. (2009). Development of SCAR markers for the discrimination of three species of medicinal plants, Angelica decursiva (Peucedanum decursivum), Peucedanum praeruptorum and Anthricus sylvestris, based on the internal transcribed spacer (ITS) sequence and random amplified polymorphic DNA (RAPD). *Biol Pharm Bull, 32*(1), 24–30. doi:10.1248/bpb.32.24

Cui, G. H., Tang, X. J., & Huang, L. Q. (2006). Application of multiplex allele-specific PCR for authentication of Panax ginseng and P. quinquefolius. *Zhongguo Zhong Yao Za Zhi, 31*(23), 1940–1943.

Dechbumroong, P., Aumnouypol, S., Denduangboripant, J., & Sukrong, S. (2018). DNA barcoding of Aristolochia plants and development of species-specific multiplex PCR to aid HPTLC in ascertainment of Aristolochia herbal materials. *PLoS One, 13*(8), e0202625. doi:10.1371/journal.pone.0202625

Do, N., & Adams, R. (1991). A simple technique for removing plant polysaccharide contaminants from DNA. *BioTechniques, 10*(2), 162, 164, 166.

Doganay-Knapp, K., Orland, A., König, G. M., & Knöss, W. (2018). The potential of three different PCR-related approaches for the authentication of mixtures of herbal substances and finished herbal medicinal products. *Phytomedicine, 43*, 60–67. doi:10.1016/j.phymed.2018.03.062.

Doh, E. J., Lee, G., Ju, Y. S., & Oh, S. E. (2014). Identification 4 kinds of Muxiang using multiplex PCR. *Korean J Herbology, 29*(3), 19–26. doi:10.6116/kjh.2014.29.3.19

Doh, E.J & Oh, SE. (2012) Multiplex PCR method to discriminate artemisia iwayomogi from other artemisia plants. In Sucher, N., Hennell, J., Carles, M. (Eds.) *Plant DNA Fingerprinting and Barcoding. Methods in Molecular Biology (Methods and Protocols), vol 862*. Humana Press. https://doi.org/10.1007/978-1-61779-609-8_12

Duke, J. A. (2002). *Handbook of Medicinal Herbs*. Florida, Boca Raton: CRC Press.

Ekor, M. (2014). The growing use of herbal medicines: Issues relating to adverse reactions and challenges in monitoring safety. *Front Pharmacol, 4*, 177–177. doi:10.3389/fphar.2013.00177

Elkins, K. M., Perez, A. C., & Quinn, A. A. (2017). Simultaneous identification of four 'legal high' plant species in a multiplex PCR high-resolution melt assay. *J Forensic Sci, 62*(3), 593–601. doi:10.1111/1556-4029.13321.

Fang, G., Hammar, S., & Grumet, R. (1992). A quick and inexpensive method for removing polysaccharides from plant genomic DNA. *BioTechniques, 13*(1), 52–54, 56.

Gachon, C., Mingam, A., & Charrier, B. (2004). Real-time PCR: What relevance to plant studies? *J Exp Bot, 55*(402), 1445–1454. doi:10.1093/jxb/erh181

Gresta, F., Lombardo, G., Siracusa, L., & Ruberto, G. (2008). Saffron, an alternative crop for sustainable agricultural systems: A review. *Agron Sustain Dev 28*(1), 95–112. doi:10.1051/agro:2007030

Henegariu, O., Heerema, N., Dlouhy, S., Vance, G., & Vogt, P. (1997). Multiplex PCR: Critical parameters and step-by-step protocol. *BioTechniques, 23*(3), 504–511. doi:10.2144/97233rr01

Hernández, P., Martín, A., & Dorado, G. (1999). Development of SCARs by direct sequencing of RAPD products: A practical tool for the introgression and marker-assisted selection of wheat. *Mol Breed, 5*(3), 245–253. doi:10.1023/A:1009637928471

Heubl, G. (2010). New aspects of DNA-based authentication of Chinese medicinal plants by molecular biological techniques. *Planta Med, 76*(17), 1963–1974. doi:10.1055/s-0030-1250519

Holland, P. M., Abramson, R. D., Watson, R., & Gelfand, D. H. (1991). Detection of specific polymerase chain reaction product by utilizing the 5′–3′ exonuclease activity of Thermus aquaticus DNA polymerase. *PNAS, 88*(16), 7276–7280. doi:10.1073/pnas.88.16.7276

Holleley, C. E., & Geerts, P. G. (2009). Multiplex Manager 1.0: A cross-platform computer program that plans and optimizes multiplex PCR. *BioTechniques, 46*(7), 511–517. doi:10.2144/000113156

Horn, T., Völker, J., Rühle, M., Häser, A., Jürges, G., & Nick, P. (2014). Genetic authentication by RFLP versus ARMS? The case of Moldavian dragonhead (Dracocephalum moldavica L.). *Eur Food Res Technol, 238*(1), 93–104.

Howard, C., Socratous, E., Williams, S., Graham, E., Fowler, M. R., Scott, N. W., Bremner, P. D., & Slater, A. (2012). PlantID — DNA-based identification of multiple medicinal plants in complex mixtures. *Chin Med, 7*(1), 18. doi:10.1186/1749-8546-7-18

Intharuksa, A., Ando, H., Miyake, K., Sirisa-Ard, P., Mikage, M., & Sasaki, Y. (2016). Molecular analysis of Terminalia spp. distributed in Thailand and authentication of crude drugs from Terminalia plants. *Biol Pharm Bull, 39*(4), 492–501. doi:10.1248/bpb.b15-00673

Jackson, B. P., & Snowdon, D. W. (1990). *Atlas of Microscopy of Medicinal Plants, Culinary Herbs and Spices*. London: Belhaven Press.

Jiang, C., Luo, Y., Yuan, Y., Dong, X., Zhao, Y., & Huang, L. (2018). Conventional octaplex PCR for the simultaneous identification of eight mainstream closely related Dendrobium species. *Ind Crops Prod, 112*, 569–576. doi:10.1016/j.indcrop.2017.12.048

Jigden, B., Wang, H., Kim, M. K., Kim, Y. J., In, J. G., & Yang, D. C. (2010a). Authentication of the oriental medicinal plant Ligusticum tenuissimum (Nakai) Kitagawa (Korean Go-Bon) by multiplex PCR. *Planta Med, 76*(06), 648–651. doi:10.1055/s-0029-1240632

Jigden, B., Wang, H., Kim, Y. J., Samdan, N., In, J. G., & Yang, D. C. (2010b). Molecular identification of oriental medicinal plant Schizonepeta tenuifolia bunge (Hyung-Gae) by multiplex PCR. *Plant Biotechnol Rep, 4*(3), 223–228. doi:10.1007/s11816-010-0142-3

Jigden, B., Wang, H., Kim, Y. J., Noh, J. H., Gotov, C., Lee, J. I., & Yang, D. C. (2010c). Development of a multiplex polymerase chain reaction method for simultaneous detection of four Cimicifuga Species. *Crop Sci, 50*(5), 1961–1966. doi:10.2135/cropsci2009.07.0412

Jigden, B., Wang, H., Samdan, N., & Yang, D. C. (2010). Molecular identification of oriental medicinal plant Anemarrhena asphodeloides Bunge ('Jimo') by multiplex PCR. *Mol Biol Rep, 37*(2), 955–960. doi:10.1007/s11033-009-9747-4

Joshi K., & Chavan P. (2012). Development of sequence characterized amplified region from random amplified polymorphic DNA amplicons. In Sucher N., Hennell J., Carles M. (Eds.) *Plant DNA Fingerprinting and Barcoding. Methods in Molecular Biology (Methods and Protocols), vol 862*. Totowa NJ: Humana Press. https://doi.org/10.1007/978-1-61779-609-8_10

Kaltenboeck, B., & Wang, C. (2005). Advances in real-time PCR: Application to clinical laboratory diagnostics. *Adv Clin Chem, 40*, 219–259. doi:10.1016/s0065-2423(05)40006-2

Kim, J. S., Jang, H. W., Kim, J. S., Kim, H. J., & Kim, J. H. (2012). Molecular identification of Schisandra chinensis and its allied species using multiplex PCR based on SNPs. *Genes Genomics, 34*(3), 283–290. doi:10.1007/s13258-011-0201-3

Kim, M. K., Jang, G. H., Yang, D. C., Lee, S., Lee, H. N., & Jin, C. G. (2014). Molecular authentication of Acanthopanacis cortex by multiplex-PCR analysis tools. *Korean J Plant Res, 27*(6), 680–686.

Kim, M. K., Noh, J. H., Yan, D. C., Lee, S., Lee, H. N., & Jin, C. G. (2015). Molecular authentication of Magnoliae flos using robust SNP marker base on trnL-F and ndhF region. *Korean J Plant Res, 28*(3), 341–349.

Kim, M. K., Subramaniyam, S., Kim, Y. J., Kwon, W. S., & Yang, D. C. (2012). Authentication of Epimedii Herba and adulterant plants by Multiplex PCR. *Korean J Med Crop Sci, 2012*(5), 321–322.

Kim, W. J., Moon, B. C., Yang, S., Han, K. S., Choi, G., & Lee, A. Y. (2016). Rapid authentication of the herbal medicine plant species Aralia continentalis Kitag. and Angelica biserrata CQ Yuan and RH Shan using ITS2 sequences and multiplex-SCAR markers. *Molecules, 21*(3), 270. doi:10.3390/molecules21030270

Kim, W. J., Yang, S., Choi, G., Park, I., Noh, P., Kim, M. J., & Moon, B. C. (2020a). Accurate and rapid identification of Longan arillus and Litchi semen by a multiplex PCR assay. *Plants, 9*(8), 948. doi:10.3390/plants9080948

Kim, W. J., Yang, S., Choi, G., Park, I., Noh, P., Lee, A. Y., Kim, H. S., & Moon, B. C. (2020b). Establishment of conventional PCR and real-time PCR assays for accurate, rapid and quantitative authentication of four mistletoe species. *Phytochemistry, 176*, 112400. doi:10.1016/j.phytochem.2020.112400.

Kim, Y. B., Ramekar, R. V., Choi, S. J., Choi, B. G., Kim, S. W., Moon, Y. K., Noh, H. S., Lee, J. K., Hong, J. S., Park, N. I., Choi, I. Y., Choi, S. K., & Park, K. C. (2018). Molecular identification of Allium ochotense and Allium microdictyon using multiplex-PCR based on single nucleotide polymorphisms. *Hortic Environ Biotechnol, 59*(6), 865–873. doi:10.1007/s13580-018-0069-0

Kim, Y. S., Park, H. J., Lee, D. H., & Kim, H. K. (2018). Development of multiplex polymerase chain reaction assay for identification of Angelica species. *Korean J Med Crop Sci, 26*(1), 26–31.

Kumar, P., Gupta, V., Misra, A., Modi, D., & Pandey, B. (2009). Potential of molecular markers in plant biotechnology. *Plant Omics, 2*(4), 141–162.

Kwon, W. S., Chung, C. M., Kim, Y. T., Lee, M. G., & Choi, K. T. (1998). Breeding process and characteristics of KG101, a superior line of Panax ginseng CA Meyer. *J Ginseng Res, 22*(1), 11–17.

Lam, Y., Ng, T. B., Yao, R. M., Shi, J., Xu, K., Sze, S. C. W., & Zhang, K. Y. (2015). Evaluation of chemical constituents and important mechanism of pharmacological biology in dendrobium plants. *Evid Based Complement Alternat Med, 2015*, 841752. doi:10.1155/2015/841752

Lazarowych, N. J., & Pekos, P. (1998). Use of fingerprinting and marker compounds for identification and standardization of botanical drugs: Strategies for applying pharmaceutical HPLC analysis to herbal products. *Drug Inf J, 32*(2), 497–512. doi:10.1177/009286159803200222

Lee, H. J., Park, H. R., Lee, A. J., Nam, D. E., Lee, D. G., Do, Y., & Chung, K. W. (2020). Genetic authentication of cultivars with flower-variant types using SSR markers in spring orchid, Cymbidium goeringii. *Hortic Environ Biotechnol, 61*(3), 1–14. doi:10.1007/s13580-020-00243-9

Lee, O. R., Kim, M. K., & Yang D. C. (2012) Authentication of medicinal plants by SNP-based multiplex PCR. In Sucher, N., Hennell, J., Carles, M. (Eds.) *Plant DNA Fingerprinting and Barcoding. Methods in Molecular Biology (Methods and Protocols), vol 862*. Totowa NJ: Humana Press.

Lee, Y. M., Ji, Y., Kang, Y. M., Kim, W. J., Choi, G., & Moon, B. C. (2016). Molecular authentication of Pinelliae Tuber and its common adulterants using RAPD-derived multiplex sequence characterized amplified region (multiplex-SCAR) markers. *Int J Clin Exp Med, 9*(1), 40–50.

Lee, Y. M., Moon, B. C., Ji, Y., Seo, H. S., & Kim, H. K. (2013). Development of RAPD-derived SCAR markers and multiplex-PCR for authentication of the Schisandrae Fructus. *Korean J Med Crop Sci, 21*(3), 165–173. doi:10.7783/KJMCS.2013.21.3.165

Lindstedt, B.-A., Vardund, T., Aas, L., & Kapperud, G. (2004). Multiple-locus variable-number tandem-repeats analysis of Salmonella enterica subsp. enterica serovar Typhimurium using PCR multiplexing and multicolor capillary electrophoresis. *J Microbiol Methods, 59*(2), 163–172. doi:10.1016/j.mimet.2004.06.014

Lo, Y. T., Li, M., & Shaw, P. C. (2015). Identification of constituent herbs in ginseng decoctions by DNA markers. *Chin Med, 10*(1), 1. doi:10.1186/s13020-015-0029-x

Lo, Y. T., & Shaw, P. C. (2018). DNA-based techniques for authentication of processed food and food supplements. *Food Chem, 240*, 767–774. doi:10.1016/j.foodchem.2017.08.022

Logan, J., Logan, J. M., Edwards, K. J., & Saunders, N. A. (2009). *Real-time PCR: Current Technology and Applications*. Norfolk, UK: Horizon Scientific Press.

Longo, M. C., Berninger, M. S., & Hartley, J. L. (1990). Use of uracil DNA glycosylase to control carry-over contamination in polymerase chain reactions. *Gene, 93*(1), 125–128. doi:10.1016/0378-1119(90)90145-H

Lu, Z., Rubinsky, M., Babajanian, S., Zhang, Y., Chang, P., & Swanson, G. (2018). Visualization of DNA in highly processed botanical materials. *Food Chem, 245*, 1042–1051. doi:10.1016/j.foodchem.2017.11.067

Mao, F., Leung, W. Y., & Xin, X. (2007). Characterization of EvaGreen and the implication of its physicochemical properties for qPCR applications. *BMC Biotechnol, 7*(1), 76. doi:10.1186/1472-6750-7-76

Markoulatos, P., Siafakas, N., & Moncany, M. (2002). Multiplex polymerase chain reaction: A practical approach. *J Clin Lab Anal, 16*(1), 47–51. doi:10.1002/jcla.2058.

Marras, S. A. E. (2006). Selection of fluorophore and quencher pairs for fluorescent nucleic acid hybridization probes. In Didenke, V. V. (Ed.) *Fluorescent Energy Transfer Nucleic Acid Probes: Designs and Protocols* (pp. 3–16). Totowa, NJ: Humana Press.

Mohanan, P., Hurh, J., Kim, S. O., Na, J. R., Kim, Y. J., Lee, H. A., Kim, M. K., &, Yang, D. C. (2019). Chloroplast DNA-derived markers for the authentication of oriental medicinal Rubus species and mistaken identity of bokbunja in the local markets of Korea. *Plant Biotechnol Rep, 13*(22), 305–314. doi:10.1007/s11816-019-00540-5

Moon, B. C., Ji, Y. U., Lee, Y. M., Chun, J. M., Lee, A., Choo, B. K., & Kim, H. K. (2011). Development of SCAR markers for the authentication of Acori rhizoma based on the analysis of RAPD and multiplex-PCR. *Korean J Med Crop Sci, 19*(3), 162–169. doi:10.7783/KJMCS.2011.19.3.162

Moon, B. C., Lee, Y. M., Chun, J. M., Lee, A., Yoon, T. S., Cheon, M. S., Choo, B. K., & Kim, H. K. (2009). Development of SCAR markers for the discrimination of Rhei Radix et Rhizoma and Rhei undulatai Rhizoma based on the RAPD. *Korean J Herbology, 24*(4), 115–120.

Moon, B. C., Choo, B. K., Cheon, M. S., Yoon, T., Ji, Y., Kim, B. B., Lee, A-Young, Kim, H. K. (2010). Rapid molecular authentication of three medicinal plant species, Cynanchum wilfordii, Cynanchum auriculatum, and Polygonum multiflorum (Fallopia multiflorum), by the development of RAPD-derived SCAR markers and multiplex-PCR. *Plant Biotechnol Rep, 4*(1), 1–7. doi:10.1007/s11816-009-0114-7

Moon, B. C., Ji, Y., Lee, Y. M., Kang, Y. M., & Kim, H. K. (2015). Authentication of Akebia quinata D ECNE from its common adulterant medicinal plant species based on the RAPD-derived SCAR markers and multiplex-PCR. *Genes Genomics, 37*(1), 23–32.

Moon, B. C., Kim, W. J., Han, K. S., Yang, S., Kang, Y., Park, I., & Piao, R. (2017). Differentiating authentic Adenophorae Radix from its adulterants in commercially-processed samples using multiplexed ITS sequence-based SCAR markers. *Appl Sci, 7*(7), 660. doi:10.3390/app7070660

Moon, B. C., Lee, Y. M., Kim, W. J., Ji, Y., Kang, Y. M., & Choi, G. (2016). Development of molecular markers for authentication of the medicinal plant species Patrinia by random amplified polymorphic DNA (RAPD) analysis and multiplex-PCR. *Hortic Environ Biotechnol, 57*(2), 182–190. doi:10.1007/s13580-016-0064-2

Moon, S. C., Kim, J. H., & Jang, C. S. (2016). Development of multiplex PCR for species-specific identification of the Poaceae family based on chloroplast gene, rpoC2. *Appl Biol Chem, 59*(2), 201–207. doi:10.1007/s13765-016-0155-x

Nariya, M., Shukla, V., Jain, S., & Ravishankar, B. (2009). Comparison of enteroprotective efficacy of triphala formulations (Indian Herbal Drug) on methotrexate-induced small intestinal damage in rats. *Phytother Res, 23*(8), 1092–1098. doi:10.1002/ptr.2744

Navarro, E., Serrano-Heras, G., Castaño, M., & Solera, J. (2015). Real-time PCR detection chemistry. *Clin Chim Acta, 439*, 231–250. doi:10.1016/j.cca.2014.10.017.

Ng, W. L., Yeap, S. K., Bakar, N. A., Nurfatin, W., Jaafar, W., & Tan, S. (2016). Multiplex PCR assays for species discrimination of Cymbopogon citratus (DC.) Stapf and C. nardus (L.) Rendle, two common 'Serai' (lemon grass) species in Peninsular Malaysia. *Sains Malays, 45*(3), 323–327. doi:10.17576/jsm-2016-4503-01

Noh, P., Kim, W. J., Yang, S., Park, I., & Moon, B. C. (2018). Authentication of the herbal medicine Angelicae Dahuricae Radix using an ITS sequence-based multiplex SCAR assay. *Molecules, 23*(9), 2134. doi:10.3390/molecules23092134

Paran, I., & Michelmore, R. W. (1993). Development of reliable PCR-based markers linked to downy mildew resistance genes in lettuce. *Theor Appl Genet, 85*(8), 985–993. doi:10.1007/BF00215038

Park, M. J., Kim, M. K., In, J. G., & Yang, D. C. (2006). Molecular identification of Korean ginseng by amplification refractory mutation system-PCR. *Food Res Int, 39*(5), 568–574. doi:10.1016/j.foodres.2005.11.004

Porebski, S., Bailey, L. G., & Baum, B. R. (1997). Modification of a CTAB DNA extraction protocol for plants containing high polysaccharide and polyphenol components. *Plant Mol Biol Rep, 15*(1), 8–15. doi:10.1007/BF02772108

Quan, Z., Yang, Z., Chua, T., Li, L., Zhang, Y., Babajanian, S., Chua, T., Chang, P., Swanson, G., Lu, Z. (2020). Development and validation of a probe-based qPCR method to prevent parsley leaf material misidentification. *Fitoterapia, 146*, 104666. doi:10.1016/j.fitote.2020.104666

Rachlin, J., Ding, C., Cantor, C., & Kasif, S. (2005). MuPlex: Multi-objective multiplex PCR assay design. *Nucleic Acids Res, 33*(Suppl. 2), W544–W547.

Rajagopal, A., Yurk, D., Shin, C., Menge, K., Jacky, L., Fraser, S., Thomas A. Tombrello, Tsongalis, G. J. (2019). Significant expansion of real-time PCR multiplexing with traditional chemistries using amplitude modulation. *Sci Rep, 9*, 1053. doi:10.1038/s41598-018-37732-y

Rangsiruji, A., Binchai, S., & Pringsulaka, O. (2018). Species identification of economic bamboos in the genus Dendrocalamus using SCAR and multiplex PCR. *Songklanakarin J Sci Technol, 40*(3), 640–647. doi:10.14456/sjst-psu.2018.86

Reich, E., & Schibli, A. (2007). *High-Performance Thin-Layer Chromatography for the Analysis of Medicinal Plants*. New York: Thieme.

Ryuk, J. A., Lee, H. W., Ju, Y. S., & Ko, B. S. (2014). Monitoring and identification of Cynanchum wilfordii and Cynanchum auriculatum by using molecular markers and real-time polymerase chain reaction. *J Korean Soc Appl Biol Chem, 57*(2), 245–251. doi:10.1007/s13765-013-4248-5

Sharma, S., & Shrivastava, N. (2016). Internal transcribed spacer guided multiplex PCR for species identification of Convolvulus prostratus and Evolvulus alsinoides. *Acta Pharm Sin B, 6*(3), 253–258.

Shen, Z., Qu, W., Wang, W., Lu, Y., Wu, Y., Li, Z., Hang, X., Wang, X., Zhao, D., Zhang, C. (2010). MPprimer: A program for reliable multiplex PCR primer design. *BMC Bioinform, 11*, 143. doi:10.1186/1471-2105-11-143

Sint, D., Raso, L., & Traugott, M. (2012). Advances in multiplex PCR: Balancing primer efficiencies and improving detection success. *Methods Ecol Evol, 3*(5), 898–905. doi:10.1111/j.2041-210X.2012.00215.x

Smillie, T., & Khan, I. (2010). A comprehensive approach to identifying and authenticating botanical products. *Clin Pharmacol Ther, 87*(2), 175–186. doi:10.1038/clpt.2009.287

Sucher, N. J., & Carles, M. C. (2008). Genome-based approaches to the authentication of medicinal plants. *Planta Med, 74*(6), 603–623. doi:10.1055/s-2008-1074517

Tan, S. C., & Yiap, B. C. (2009). DNA, RNA, and protein extraction: The past and the present. *J Biomed Biotechnol, 2009*, 574398.

Techen, N., Crockett, S., Khan, I., & Scheffler, B. (2004). Authentication of medicinal plants using molecular biology techniques to compliment conventional methods. *Curr Med Chem, 11*(11), 1391–1401. doi:10.2174/0929867043365206

Upton, R., David, B., Gafner, S., & Glasl, S. (2019). Botanical ingredient identification and quality assessment: Strengths and limitations of analytical techniques. *Phytochem Rev, 19*(21) 1–21. doi:10.1007/s11101-019-09625-z

Vinay, K. (2016). Development of PCR based SCAR markers for rapid authentication of Boerhavia errecta, B. diffusa and their adulterant Trianthema species. *Res J Biotechnol, 11*, 3.

Wallinger, C., Juen, A., Staudacher, K., Schallhart, N., Mitterrutzner, E., Steiner, E. M., Thalinger, B., & Traugott, M. (2012). Rapid plant identification using species-and group-specific primers targeting chloroplast DNA. *PLoS One, 7*(1), e29473. doi:10.1371/journal.pone.0029473

Wang, H., Kim, M. K., Kim, Y. J., Lee, H. N., Jin, H., Chen, J., & Yang, D. C. (2012). Molecular authentication of the oriental medicines Pericarpium Citri Reticulatae and Citri Unshius Pericarpium using SNP markers. *Gene, 494*(1), 92–95. doi:10.1016/j.gene.2011.11.026

Wang, H., Kim, M. K., Kwon, W. S., Jin, H., Liang, Z., & Yang, D. C. (2011). Molecular authentication of Panax ginseng and ginseng products using robust SNP markers in ribosomal external transcribed spacer region. *J Pharm Biomed Anal, 55*(5), 972–976. doi:10.1016/j.jpba.2011.03.037.

Wang, H., Sun, H., Kwon, W. S., Jin, H., & Yang, D. C. (2009). Molecular identification of the Korean ginseng cultivar 'Chunpoong' using the mitochondrial nad7 intron 4 region. *Mitochondrial DNA, 20*(2–3), 41–45. doi:10.1080/19401730902856738

Wang, H., Sun, H., Kwon, W. S., Jin, H., & Yang, D. C. (2010). A PCR-based SNP marker for specific authentication of Korean ginseng (Panax ginseng) cultivar 'Chunpoong'. *Mol Biol Rep 37*(2), 1053–1057. doi:10.1007/s11033-009-9827-5

Wei, Y., Chen, Y., Huang, Y., Liu, J., & Liang, Y. (2016). Molecular authentication and quantitative analysis of Sarcandra glabra and adulterated chloranthus products using SNP markers. *Mitochondrial DNA A DNA Mapp Seq Anal, 27*(5), 3618–3625. doi:10.3109/19401736.2015.1079826

Weising, K., Nybom, H., Wolff, K., & Meyer, W. (1995). DNA Isolation and Purification. In *DNA Fingerprinting in Plants and Fungi* (pp. 44–50). Boca Raton: CRC Press. 44–59.

Welsh, J., & McClelland, M. (1990). Fingerprinting genomes using PCR with arbitrary primers. *Nucleic Acids Res, 18*(24), 7213–7218. doi:10.1093/nar/18.24.7213

Wetters, S., Horn, T., & Nick, P. (2018). Goji Who? Morphological and DNA based authentication of a 'Superfood'. *Front Plant Sci, 9*, 1859. doi:10.3389/fpls.2018.01859

Williams, J. G., Kubelik, A. R., Livak, K. J., Rafalski, J. A., & Tingey, S. V. (1990). DNA polymorphisms amplified by arbitrary primers are useful as genetic markers. *Nucleic Acids Res, 18*(22), 6531–6535. doi:10.1093/nar/18.22.6531

Wu, X., Li, H., Zhao, W., Fu, L., Peng, H., He, L., Cheng, J., Wei, H., & Wu, Q. (2010). SCAR makers and multiplex PCR-based rapid molecular typing of Lentinula edodes strains. *Curr Microbiol, 61*(5), 381–389. doi:10.1007/s00284-010-9623-4

Xanthopoulou, A., Ganopoulos, I., Kalivas, A., Osathanunkul, M., Chatzopoulou, P., Tsaftaris, A., & Madesis, P. (2016). Multiplex HRM analysis as a tool for rapid molecular authentication of nine herbal teas. *Food Control, 60*, 113–116. doi:10.1016/j.foodcont.2015.07.021

Xu, G., Wang, X., Liu, C., Li, W., Wei, S., Liu, Y., Cheng, X., & Liu, J. (2013). Authentication of official Da-huang by sequencing and multiplex allele-specific PCR of a short maturase K gene. *Genome, 56*(2), 109–113. doi:10.1139/gen-2012-0182

Yang, D. U., Kim, M. K., Mohanan, P., Mathiyalagan, R., Seo, K. H., Kwon, W. S., & Yang, D. C. (2017). Development of a single-nucleotide-polymorphism marker for specific authentication of Korean ginseng (Panax ginseng Meyer) new cultivar 'G-1'. *J Ginseng Res, 41*(1), 31–35. doi:10.1016/j.jgr.2015.12.007

Yokoyama, E., Kishida, K., Uchimura, M., & Ichinohe, S. (2006). Comparison between agarose gel electrophoresis and capillary electrophoresis for variable numbers of tandem repeat typing of Mycobacterium tuberculosis. *J Microbiol Methods, 65*(3), 425–431. doi:10.1016/j.mimet.2005.08.014

Zhang, T., Wang, J., Wang, D., & Wang, H. (2015). Development of an authentication system for genuine radix Salviae Miltiorrhizae (Salvia miltiorrhiza) using SNP markers. *Planta Med Lett, 2*(1), e65–e68. doi:10.1055/S-0035-1558205

Zhao, Z., Hu, Y., Liang, Z., Yuen, J. P. S., Jiang, Z., & Leung, K. S. Y. (2006). Authentication is fundamental for standardization of Chinese medicines. *Planta Med, 72*(10), 865–874. doi:10.1055/s-2006-947209

Zhu, S., Fushimi, H., Cai, S., & Komatsu, K. (2004). Species identification from ginseng drugs by multiplex amplification refractory mutation system (MARMS). *Planta Med, 70*(02), 189–192. doi:10.1055/s-2004-815502

Part IV
DNA Sequencing-based Techniques for Molecular Authentication

Chapter 10

Identification of Medicinal Materials Using Forensically Informative Nucleotide Sequencing

Ming Li

10.1 Introduction

Molecular authentication of medicinal materials has been employed worldwide since the 1990's. Thanks to the advancement in molecular technology, a number of molecular technologies have been used to identify a wide range of medicinal materials in the last three decades. In early 2000, DNA barcodes have been proposed for the identification of organisms (Hebert, Cywinska, Ball & deWaard, 2003). They have been continuously demonstrated as useful loci for molecular authentication in the last two decades. These carefully selected loci consist sufficient nucleotide polymorphisms and are useful to differentiate the genuine medicinal materials from the adulterants, in particular, those derived from phylogenetically closely related species. Meanwhile, whole genome sequencing has become more accessible in recent years. Genome-wide polymorphism provides comprehensive information to differentiate genuine medicinal species from the adulterants (Chen, Wu, & Zhang, 2020).

Among these technologies, DNA sequencing of specific loci, DNA barcodes and the whole genomes retrieve the most reliable information of polymorphic sites for identification. With the help of phylogenetic analysis, the species of genuine medicinal materials, substitutes, adulterant and commodities can be readily identified. Forensically informative nucleotide sequencing (FINS) is an identification technique that combines DNA sequencing and phylogenetic analysis. It was first used to identify the animal origin of biological specimen (Bartlett & Davidson, 1992), and subsequently applied in other food products, forensic investigations and wildlife protection (Lago, Herrero, Vieites & Espiñeira, 2011; Thakur *et al.*, 2013; Sahajpal & Goyal, 2009; Singh *et al.*, 2020). For medicinal materials, animal- and plant-based alternative medicines provide accessible healthcare all over the world. They are important treatments for the well-being of developing regions in particular. In the market, adulteration is commonly due to accidental substitution of materials with similar organoleptic characters; intentional substitution of less expensive materials; and confusion caused by the use of local substitutes and inconsistent local names. Different from conventional authentication methods (morphology and chemistry), which are sensitive to growing stages, environmental factors, and post-harvest processing, FINS is a definitive method to identify the biological origin of the medicinal materials.

Taking traditional Chinese medicine (TCM) as an example, more than 800 species are recorded in the *Pharmacopoeia of the People's Republic of China* for medicinal use (State Pharmacopoeia Commission of People's Republic of China, 2010). Some of them are economically important and ecologically valuable (e.g., Dendrobii Caulis), and some are highly toxic (e.g., Aristolochiae Fructus and Radix Tripterygii Wilfordii). The authenticity of their biological origins is thus crucial to ensure the safety, efficacy and fair use of these medicines. FINS showed successful applications for the identification of Chinese medicinal materials in some early studies (reviewed in Li, Zhang, But & Shaw, 2011b). It has been continuously employed for the identification in the last decades. Some of the studies are summarised in Table 10.1.

10.2 Major Steps in FINS

FINS identification requires the DNA sequences of a defined loci of the examined specimen, which are compared with reference sequences using a phylogenetic analysis (Bartlett & Davidson, 1992). A general workflow for FINS identification is illustrated in Figure 10.1. Four major steps are involved:

(1) Sample preparation and DNA isolation
(2) Loci selection and DNA amplification
(3) DNA sequencing and sequence database analysis
(4) Phylogenetic analysis and identification

10.2.1 Sample Preparation and DNA Isolation

There are two types of samples: target samples and reference samples. Target samples refer to those which need to be identified by FINS. Most commonly, these samples include raw plant and animal parts, commodities, food products and processed ingredients. Reference samples refer to the materials derived from the species for comparison in phylogenetic analysis. They should include the species used for the medicinal materials and their closely related species. Species used as suspected adulterants and their closely related species should also be included as reference samples. The

Table 10.1 Studies of Identification of Medicinal Materials Using FINS

Sample materials	DNA loci	Major findings	References
Shihu samples and *Dendrobium* species	ITS	Four inspected samples of 'Fengdou' were identified	Ding, Wang, Xu, Xu, & Zhou, 2002
Rhinoceros horns, Rhinoceros species and other mammals	*Cyt b*	Two samples were of white rhinoceros, and four samples were of dark rhinoceros	Hsieh *et al.*, 2003
Snake blood and meat, and 90 snake species	*Cyt b*	Six unknown samples were identified as *Python molurus* and *P. reticulates*	Wong, Wang, But & Shaw, 2004
Chinese sika deer and *Cervus nippon* subspecies	Mitochondrial control region	Two suspected samples were derived from wild population of *C. nippon kopschi*	Wu, Wan, Fang, & Zhang, 2005
Fresh samples of Dangshen	5S rDNA spacer	Two samples of Hong Dangshen were identified as *Codonopsis pilosula* var. *modesta*	Zhang *et al.*, 2007
Snake venom	16S rDNA	One snake venom was identified as derived from *Naja atra*	Chen,Zhao, & Han, 2008
Shihu samples and *Dendrobium* species	*psbA-trnH*	Identification of various 'Fengdou' *Dendrobium* species and 20 Shihu samples	Shao *et al.*, 2009
Madouling samples, *Aristolochia*, *Cardiocrinum* and *Lilium* species	*psbA-trnH*, *trnL-trnF*	Two out of four Madouling samples from Taiwan and Yunnan were substituted by *C. giganteum* var. *yunnanense*	Li *et al.*, 2010b
Cordyceps samples and related *Cordyceps* species	*EF-1α*, ITS, *nrLSU*, *rpb1*	Three Cordyceps samples were genuine derived from *C. sinensis*, five samples were *C. gunni* from China and one sample was *C. gunni* from Tasmania	Chan *et al.*, 2011

Ephedrae Herba (*Ephedra sinica*, *E. intermedia* and *E. equisetina*) and its adulterants	ITS2	13 authentic samples of Ephedrae Herba and 14 samples of adulterants were successfully differentiated	Pang, Song, Xu & Yao, 2012
Zijingpi (*Kasura longipedunculata*) and its adulterants	ITS	Eight out of eight inspected samples of Zijingpi were identified as its adulterant *Schisandra sphenanthera*	Chen *et al.*, 2012
Rhei Rhizoma (*Rheum palmatum*, *R. tanguticum* and *R. officinale*) and their adulterants	*matK*	47 authentic Rhei Rhizoma samples and 15 samples of adulterants were successfully differentiated; three inspected samples were identified as genuine	Zhang *et al.*, 2013
Cynomorii Herba (*Cynomorium songaricum*) and its adulterants	ITS2	11 authentic *C. songaricum* samples and 20 adulterants were successfully differentiated	Hou *et al.*, 2013
Pyrrosiae Foliumas (*Pyrrosia sheareri*, *P. lingua*, and *P. petiolosa*)	*psbA-trnH*	26 authentic samples of *P. sheareri*, 31 of *P. lingua*, 41 of *P. petiolosa*, and eight adulterant *P. assimilis* were successfully differentiated	Zhang *et al.*, 2014
Radix Astragali (*Astragalus membranaceus and A. mongholicus*) 'Huang Qi'	*COI*, ITS, *matK*, *rbcL*, *psbA-trnH*	40 authentic samples of Radix Astragali and 37 adulterants were successfully differentiated	Zheng *et al.*, 2014
Anoectochilus roxburghi	*matK*, *psbA-trnH*, and ITS2	Eight authentic samples of A. *roxburghi* and seven adulterants were successfully differentiated; ITS2 was the best candidate for differentiation	Lv *et al.*, 2015

(Continued)

Table 10.1 (*Continued*)

Sample materials	DNA loci	Major findings	References
Gentiana robusta	ITS, *matK*, *rbcL*, *psbA-trnH*, *atpB-rbcL*, *trnL-trnF*, etc.	12 authentic samples of *G. robusta* and 12 adulterants were successfully differentiated	Xiong, Zhao, Ni, Gaawe, & Mi 2015
Zaocys (*Z. dhumnades*)	*COI*	11 authentic samples of *Z. dhumnades* and 40 counterfeits were successfully differentiated; five out of 10 commercial samples were identified as genuine	Cao *et al.*, 2014
Notopterygium seeds (*N. incisum* and *N. franchetii*)	ITS2	24 out of 27 inspected samples were identified as genuine	Zhang *et al.*, 2016
Buffalo horns (*Bubalus bubalis*)	*COI*	20 authentic samples of *B. bubalis* and 73 adulterants of four species were successfully differentiated; 34 out of 62 commercial samples were identified as genuine	Liu, Gao, & Zhou, 2017
Pulsatilla chinensis 'Baitouweng'	ITS2	25 authentic samples of *P. chinensus*, 32 relatives of 12 *Pulsatilla* species, and 48 adulterants of 10 species were successfully differentiated; two out of 30 commercial samples of 'Baitouweng' were identified as genuine	Shi *et al.*, 2017
Marsdenia tenacissima	ITS2	58 samples of *M. tenacissima* and its adulterants were successfully differentiated; an adulterant was found in 62 commercial samples	Yu *et al.*, 2018

Fructus Arctii (*Arctium lappa*)	ITS2	Authentic samples of *A. lappa* were successfully differentiated from five counterfeit species	Xing *et al.*, 2018
Cordyceps sinensis	ITS and *COI*	116 *fungi* samples and 146 hosts samples of *C. sinensis* and six adulterants were successfully differentiated; among 29 commercial samples of six products, four products were identified as genuine	Su, Li, Yang, Ding, & Xiang, 2019
Ligustici Rhizoma et Radix (*Ligusticum sinense* and *L. jeholense*) 'Gao-ben'	ITS2	43 authentic samples of Ligustici Rhizoma et Radix and six potential substitutes were successfully differentiated; six out of 25 commercial samples were identified as genuine	Liu, Gao, & Zhou, 2019
Pueraria montana var. *lobata* and *P. montana* var. *thomsonii*	ITS2	27 authentic samples of the 2 *P. montana* varieties were successfully differentiated; 28 out of 30 commercial raw material samples, five out of 10 food products, and 10 out of 12 medicinal products Yufeng Ningxin were identified as genuine	Zhang *et al.*, 2020
Fritillariae cirrhosae bulbus	Whole plastid genome, ITS, *psbA-trnH*, *rbcL*, *psbM-psdD*, *matK* etc.	32 authentic samples of five original species of Fritillariae cirrhosae bulbus, three adulterants and one outgroup were successfully differentiated	Chen *et al.*, 2020

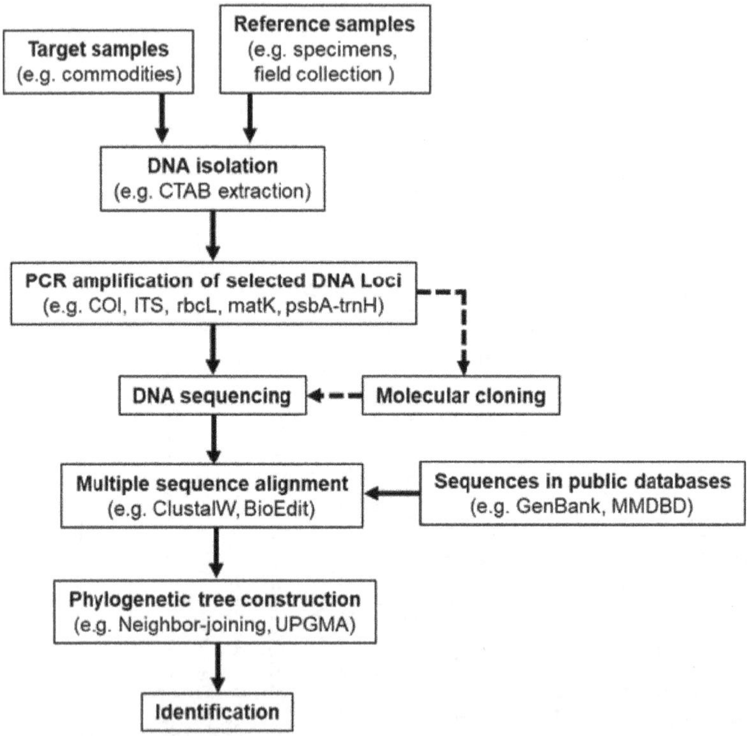

Fig. 10.1 Schematic diagram of performing FINS.

reference samples should be obtained from a reliable source and must be identified correctly. These materials could be fresh or preserved specimens. It is worth noticing that a sufficient amount of relatively intact DNA from the sample is required for FINS. Materials derived from low-DNA-content region or highly processed samples, such as the highly processed Chinese medicinal materials Asini Corii Colla (Ejiao) derived from the donkey skin extract (Lv, Zhou, You, Ye & Zhang, 2009), affect DNA isolation and amplification, and hence the success of FINS for identification. These materials may have very short DNA fragments with less than 200 bp or be short as 50 bp (Lo, Li & Shaw, 2015; Lv *et al.*, 2009; Teletchea, Maudet & Hanni, 2005). The short DNA fragments do not only bring challenges for primer design, DNA amplification and sequencing, but also for the location of enough informative nucleotide polymorphism for FINS.

DNA can be isolated from the samples by DNA extraction and DNA release (Hajibabaei *et al.*, 2005). DNA extraction is an invasive method that disrupts the tissue and cells and extracts the DNA through physical and chemical treatments. One of the most commonly used DNA extraction methods is cetyl trimethylammonium bromide (CTAB) and phenol/chloroform extraction (Kang, Cho, Yoon & Eun, 1998), with details given in Section 10.3.1.2. Disruption of samples may not always be possible, in particular, when the reference sample is derived from voucher specimens. DNA may be released from the sample into the solution without destruction. The amount and purity of the isolated DNA are critical for the subsequent steps of FINS. There are many commercially available DNA purification kits for removing the impurity and concentrating the DNA. The DNA extracts should be frozen for long-term storage and kept away from chemicals such as ethyl acetate or formaldehyde, which may damage the DNA (Prendini, Hanner & DeSalle, 2002).

10.2.2 Loci Selection and DNA Amplification

The selection of a DNA loci for amplification is the most crucial factor for FINS identification. The identification power or resolution relies on the number of informative polymorphic sites in the DNA loci between the target and reference samples. The variability of different DNA loci depends on their evolutionary rates. Slowly evolving loci contain less polymorphic sites. They are more conserved and are used to differentiate at the genus and family levels. Rapidly evolving loci contain more polymorphic sites that enable the differentiation at the species level. A superfast evolving locus may be too varied, such that it is difficult to identify the informative polymorphic sites between the authentic species and the related species. Ideal DNA loci for FINS identification should show high interspecific variation but low intraspecific variation. These loci should process sufficient interspecific nucleotide polymorphism for the differentiation of the authentic species and its closely related species in phylogenetic analysis. Sometimes, a combination of different DNA loci is needed for such a purpose.

There is no single universal DNA locus that is suitable for FINS identification of all species. The evolutionary rate of a locus varies among animals, plants and fungi. Take mitochondrial cytochrome c oxidase subunit 1 (*COI*) as an example; it shows sufficient interspecific variations in animals in general and thus is suitable to differentiate animal species (Hebert *et al*., 2003). It, however, is too conserved in plant species because of its low mutational rate in plants (Cho, Mower, Qiu & Palmer, 2004; Santamaria *et al*., 2009). Having the knowledge of the variability of different DNA loci is helpful to facilitate the selection of DNA loci for FINS identification. Since early 2000, DNA barcodes have been used to identify organisms. The most commonly used barcode for animals is *COI*; for fungi is the internal transcribed spacer (ITS); for plants are the chloroplast large subunit of the ribulose-bisphosphate carboxylase gene (*rbcL*), maturase K coding region (*matK*), *psbA-trnH* intergenic spacer (*psbA-trnH*) and ITS (CBOL Plant Working Group, 2009; Hebert *et al*., 2003; Kress, Wurdack, Zimmer, Weigt & Janzen, 2005).

Thanks to the international endeavours for developing DNA barcodes worldwide in the last two decades, DNA barcodes have become very popular for molecular identification of medicinal materials (Li, Cao, But & Shaw, 2011a; Li *et al*., 2012b; Lou *et al*., 2010; Techen, Parveen, Pan & Khan, 2014; Wong *et al*., 2018).

They are the primary target for FINS identification. The value of FINS depends on the choice of these DNA loci (Yu *et al.*, 2012). Other loci might be required to achieve higher resolution for discriminating closely related species. In most cases, fresh or properly preserved samples have no problem in retrieving enough quality DNA. However, some medicinal materials are processed or improperly stored, so the quality and quantity of the DNA may be low. Shorter DNA loci are preferred in these samples. ITS2 has been demonstrated as a good DNA locus because of its small size (200–300 bp) and high variation among closely related species (Chen *et al.*, 2010). It, however, has the problems of multiple copies and a secondary structure (Alvarez & Wendel, 2003; Baldwin *et al.*, 1995), and molecular cloning is sometimes needed to alleviate the problems. Fungal contamination of the samples is another challenge for using ITS2 in FINS. Specific primers may be designed to minimise the false positive results in amplification due to fungal contamination. The primers commonly used for the amplification of the DNA loci by polymerase chain reaction (PCR) are listed in Table 10.2. Details of the PCR are discussed in Section 10.3.1.3.

10.2.3 DNA Sequencing and Sequence Database Analysis

Reading the sequence of a locus obtains the maximum genetic information for identification. Owing to the advancement in molecular technology in these years, DNA sequencing is much more accessible and affordable. Massively, parallel sequencing and real-time single-molecule sequencing are available for more accurate high-throughput sequencing (reviewed in Shendure *et al.*, 2017). For molecular identification of medicinal materials, although next-generation sequencing has been used most recently (Chen *et al.*, 2020),

Table 10.2 Common Primers Used for PCR Amplification

DNA locus	Primer (5′ to 3′)	Reference
12S rDNA	Forward: CAA ACT GGG ATT AGA TAC CCC ACT AT Reverse: GAG GGT GAC GGG CGG TGT GT	Girish *et al.*, 2004
16S rDNA	Forward: CGC CTG TTT ATC AAA AAC AT Reverse: CTC CGG TTT GAA CTC AGA TC	Mitchell, Cockburn & Seawright, 1993
18S rDNA	Forward: CAA CCT GGT TGA TCC TGC CAG T Reverse: CTG ATC CTT CTG CAC CTT CAC CTA C	Sogin, 1990
COI	Forward: GGT CAA CAA ATC ATA AAG ATA TTG G Reverse: TAA ACT TCA GGG TGA CCA AAA AAT CA	Hebert *et al.*, 2003
Cyt b	Forward: TAC CAT GAG GAC AAA TAT CAT TCT G Reverse: CCT CCT AGT TTG TTA GGG ATT GAT CG	Verma & Singh, 2003
ITS	Forward: TCC TCC GCT TAT TGA TAT GC Reverse: CCT TAT CAT TTA GAG GAA GGA G	Kress *et al.*, 2005
ITS1	Forward: CAC ACC GCC CGT CGC TCC TAC CGA Reverse: TTG CGT TCA AAG ACT CGA TG	White, Burms, Lee & Taylor, 1990
ITS2	Forward: AAC CAT CGA GTC TTT GAA CGC A Reverse: ACT CGC CGT TAC TAG GGG AA	White *et al.*, 1990
matK	Forward: CGT ACA GTA CTT TTG TGT TTA CGA G Reverse: ACC CAG TCC ATC TGG AAA TCT TGG TTC	CBOL Plant Working Group, 2009
rbcL	Forward: ATG TCA CCA CAA ACA GAG ACT AAA GC Reverse: GTA AAA TCA AGT CCA CCR CG	CBOL Plant Working Group, 2009
psbA-trnH	Forward: GTT ATG CAT GAA CGT AAT GCT C Reverse: CGC GCA TGG TGG ATT CAC AAT CC	Kress *et al.*, 2005
trnL-trnF	Forward: CGA AAT CGG TAG ACG CTA CG Reverse: ATT TGA ACT GGT GAC ACG AG	Taberlet, Gielly, Pautou & Bouvet, 1991

Sanger DNA sequencing remains the most used. Although direct sequencing of amplified loci is possible, molecular cloning is sometimes required. For instances, some DNA loci, such as ITS and the 5S rRNA gene spacer, have non-homogenous multiple copies or secondary structures (Alvarez & Wendel, 2003; Baldwin *et al.*, 1995); there may be interference of the poly-A/T sequence in some loci, such as *psbA-trnH* (Zhu *et al.*, 2010); multiple amplicons with a similar size can be generated by non-specific amplification or fungal contamination; small-size amplicons (e.g., <100 bp) may not be sequenced properly. These issues affect the results of direct sequencing, and molecular cloning should be performed before sequencing to ensure the sequencing results are readable.

FINS identification relies on the comparison of DNA sequences among the target sequence and reference samples. Similar to the studies in taxonomy or phylogeny, the authenticity, quality and reliability of the DNA sequences are important (Nilsson *et al.*, 2006; Vilgalys, 2003). Benefitting from the ongoing research on DNA barcoding and phylogenetic studies, millions of DNA sequences can be downloaded from public databases such as NCBI GenBank (https://www.ncbi.nlm.nih.gov/genbank/). The Medicinal Materials DNA Barcoding Database (https://rdccm.cuhk.edu.hk/mherbsdb/) focuses on medicinal materials that contain over 65,000 DNA sequences of 2,200 medicinal species (Lou *et al.*, 2010; Wong *et al.*, 2018). The availability of a large amount of reference sequences in these databases makes rough identification possible. However, the quality and authenticity of public DNA sequences could be the concerns. It might be necessary to generate reference DNA sequences, in particular, for those closely related species, for confirmation.

10.2.4 Phylogenetic Analysis and Identification

DNA sequences of the samples are subjected to multiple sequence alignment to compute the homologous sites and site polymorphism (reviewed in Chowdhury & Garai, 2017). A number of multiple sequence alignment tools are available, and they have different strengths and weaknesses (Essoussi, Boujenfa & Limam, 2008; Pais, Ruy, Oliveira & Coimbra, 2014; Pervez *et al.*, 2014). Based on the sequence alignment, a phylogenetic tree is constructed to infer the evolutionary relationships among the species using the methods such as neighbour-joining, maximum parsimony and maximum likelihood (Kapli, Yang & Telford, 2020). The commonly used programs for the tree construction include MEGA and PAUP (Bhargava & Sharma, 2013; Schmitt & Barker, 2009).

Different from the molecular identification methods based entirely on the comparison of polymorphic sites (Li *et al.*, 2012a; 2014), FINS relies on the discrimination power of the DNA loci in phylogenetic analysis. A phylogram consisting the target samples and reference samples is constructed for the identification of the biological origin of the samples (Bartlett & Davidson, 1992). FINS users focus on the topology instead of the evolutionary history among the species in the phylogenetic tree. DNA distance-matrix methods, such as the Unweighted Pair-group Mean Analysis (UPGMA) tree and the neighbour-joining tree, are constructed based on the genetic distance shown in multiple sequence alignments. These cladograms reveal the similarities among the target samples and the reference samples. It was suggested that the DNA distance-based tree construction methods are preferred for FINS identification (Forrest & Carnegie, 1994). Other phylogram construction methods, such as Maximum Parsimony, were also used in FINS identification (Rajpoot, Kumar, Bahuguna & Kumar, 2016; Yu *et al.*, 2012).

10.3 Case Study of FINS on Baihuasheshecao

According to Appendix III in the *Pharmacopoeia* of the People's Republic of China (2005), Baihuasheshecao (Herba Hedyotidis) is the entire plant of *Oldenlandia diffusa* (Willd.) Roxb., which is regarded as a synonymous of *Hedyotis diffusa* Willd, in the family Rubiaceae (Ko, 1999). Traditionally, Baihuasheshecao can clear 'heat', remove toxic materials and promote diuresis to eliminate 'wetness-evil'. It is used to treat cough, sore throats, intestinal carbuncle, snake bites, oedema, dysentery, enterocolitis, 'damp-heat', jaundice and tumours. In the market, there are several common adulterants derived from related *Hedyotis* species, including *H. corymbosa* (Linn.) Lam., *H. tenelliflora* Bl. and *H. pinifolia* Wall. ex G. Don. They have different functions and medicinal values (Wang & Ye, 2003), and thus should be differentiated.

10.3.1 Materials and Methods

10.3.1.1 *Sample Collection and Preparation*

Equipment

- Glass bottle container

Reagent

- Silica gel

Procedures

1. Collection of target samples: seven commodity samples labelled as Baihuasheshecao from the markets in Hong Kong and mainland China (Table 10.3).
2. Collection of reference samples: 21 authentic *Hedyotis* species from Hong Kong, including seven field samples and 14 herbarium specimens (Table 10.3).
3. Dry and store the samples in glass bottles with silica gel.

10.3.1.2 *DNA Extraction (Kang et al., 1998)*

Equipment

- Fine scissors
- NanoDrop™ Micro-UV/Vis Spectrophotometer
- Plastic rods

Table 10.3 Authentic Samples of the *Hedyotis* Species and the Baihuasheshecao Commodity Samples Used in this Study

Sample	Code	Source
Baihuasheshecao	Hed2, Hed3, Hed4	Commodity purchased from Hong Kong
Baihuasheshecao	Hed12, Hed14. Hed15, Hed16	Commodity purchased from mainland China
H. corymbosa	Hed7, Hed8	Collected in the field in Hong Kong
H. diffusa	Hed9, Hed10, Hed11	Collected in the field in Hong Kong
H. hedyotidea	Hhed	Collected in the field in Hong Kong
H. acutangula	Hacu	Collected in the field in Hong Kong
H. aurricularia	Haur1, Haur2	Specimen from the Hong Kong Herbarium
H. biflora	Hbif2	Specimen from the Hong Kong Herbarium
H. bracteosa	Hbr1, Hbr2	Specimen from the Hong Kong Herbarium
H. consanguinea	Hcon1	Specimen from the Hong Kong Herbarium
H. costata	Hctt3	Specimen from the Hong Kong Herbarium
H. effuse	Hef2	Specimen from the Hong Kong Herbarium
H. pinifolia	Hpin1	Specimen from the Hong Kong Herbarium
H. tenelliflora	Hten 1	Specimen from the Hong Kong Herbarium
H. verticillata	Hve1, Hve2	Specimen from the Hong Kong Herbarium
H. yangchunensis	Hya1, Hya2	Specimen from the Hong Kong Herbarium

Reagents

- Extraction buffer (2% Cetyltrimethylammonium-bromide, 20 mM EDTA·Na2·2H2O, 1.4 M NaCl and 100 mM Tris, pH 8)
- CTAB solution
- Chloroform:isoamyl alcohol (24:1) with 5% phenol
- Isopropanol
- Proteinase K (Armersham Pharmacia Biotech)

Procedures

1. Wash 0.01–0.1 g field samples and 0.05–0.5 g herbarium specimens or commodity samples with 75% ethanol and distilled water to remove dust and minimise fungal contamination.
2. Place the samples in a 1.5-mL Eppendorf tube containing 400 μL extraction buffer and 50 μg proteinase K.
3. Cut each sample into small pieces using fine scissors and incubate at 37°C for 30 min.
4. Ground the sample into powder in the Eppendorf tube using a sterile plastic rod and incubate at 37°C for another 30 min.
5. Add an 400 μL CTAB solution and mix with the sample by inversion.
6. Add an equal volume of chloroform: isoamyl alcohol (24:1) with 5% phenol, gently invert the Eppendorf tube for several times.
7. Centrifuge the mixture at 10,000 ×g at room temperature for 10 min.
8. Transfer the supernatant into a new Eppendorf tube and mix with 2/3 volume of isopropanol, followed by incubation at room temperature for 10 min.
9. Centrifuge the mixture at 10,000 ×g at room temperature for 5 min.
10. Discard the supernatant and wash the remaining DNA pellet by 70% ethanol twice followed by air-drying.

11. Resuspend the DNA pellet in 40–60 μL distilled water, and determine the DNA concentration by a spectrophotometer, as described in Chapter 3.
12. Store the DNA extract at −20°C for future use.

10.3.1.3 *DNA Amplification and Purification*

Equipment

- Benchtop centrifuge
- Thermal cycler

Reagent

- GoTaq® G2 Flexi DNA Polymerase kit (Promega, Madison, WI)

Procedures

1. Prepare the reaction mixture of 1–2 μL total DNA, 0.2 μL Taq polymerase, 2.5 μL 10× PCR buffer, 0.5 μL 10 mM forward primer of the ITS region (5′-CAC ACC GCC CGT CGC TCC TAC CGA-3′), 0.5 μL 10 mM reverse primer (5′-ACT CGC CGT TAC TAG GGG AA-3′), 1 μL 2.5 mM dNTPs, 2 μL 25 mM $MgCl_2$ and 17.3 μL distilled water into a 200-μL Eppendorf tube.
2. Perform PCR using a thermocycler with the following profile:
    1. 95°C for 2 min
    2. 95°C for 40 s
    3. 56°C for 30 s
    4. 72°C for 1 min
    5. Repeat Steps 2–4 for an additional 30 cycles
    6. 72°C for 5 min
    7. 14°C until the end

3. Analyse the quality of PCR products by agarose gel electrophoresis as described in Chapter 3.
4. Purify the PCR products as described in Chapter 3.
5. Keep the purified PCR products at –20°C for storage.

10.3.1.4 *Molecular Cloning*

Equipment

- Rotary shaking incubator

Reagents

- pGEM®-T Easy Vector System (Promega)
- *Escherichia coli* competent cells
- Luria-Bertani (LB) medium
- Ampicillin
- Mini Plus Plasmid DNA Extraction System (Viogene-Biotek Corp, New Taipei City)

Procedures

1. Prepare *E. coli* competent cells as described in Chapter 3.
2. Ligate the purified PCR product to the DNA vector using the pGEM®–T Easy Vector System and transfer the *E. coli* competent cells with the plasmid as described in Chapter 3. Use ampicillin as the antibiotic.
3. Grow the cells on the LB plates overnight and pick white colonies for cell cultivation.
4. Place each colony in a sterile culture tube containing 1.8 mL LB medium and 50 μg/mL ampicillin.
5. Place the cell culture tubes in a shaker to shake at 250 rpm at 37°C for 16 h.
6. Pour the cell culture into a sterile Eppendorf tube and centrifuge at 10,000 ×g for 10 s.

7. Completely resuspend the cell pellet in 250 μL MX1 buffer of the Mini-Plus Plasmid DNA Extraction System by vortex.
8. Add 250 μL MX2 buffer with gentle inversion, and incubate at room temperature for 5 min.
9. Add 350 μL MX3 buffer and then gently mix immediately. Centrifuge at 10,000 × g for 10 min.
10. Transfer the supernatant into the Mini-MTM column, followed by centrifugation at 10,000 × g for 1 min.
11. Wash the column by washing buffers, followed by drying.
12. Place the column into a new Eppendorf tube and add 40 μL warm distilled water to the membrane, followed by standing at room temperature for 5 min.
13. Centrifuge at 10,000 ×g for 3 min to elute the purified plasmids, which are then stored at –20°C before use.

    Remark: Work should be carried out under sterile conditions to avoid contamination. Molecular cloning is an optional step for FINS. It takes an additional three days, but a better DNA sequencing result may be obtained.

10.3.1.5 *DNA Sequencing*

Equipment

- ABI PRISM 3100 Genetic Analyzer (Thermo Fisher Scientific, Waltham, MA)
- Thermal cycler

Reagents

- BigDye® Terminator v3.1 Cycle Sequencing Kit (Thermo Fisher Scientific)

- Sodium acetate (3 M, pH 5.2)
- Hi-diformamide (Applied Biosystems)

Procedures

1. The cycle sequencing reaction mixture consists of 5–20 ng of purified PCR product or plasmid, 2 μL Big Dye reaction mix, 1 μL 2× sequencing buffer, 1 μL of 2 μM sequencing primers, and sterile distilled water, adding up to a final volume of 10 μL.
2. For direct sequencing of PCR products, the PCR primers are used as the sequencing primers. For sequencing the plasmids, universal primers T7-promoter (5′-TAA TAC GAC TCA CTA TAG GG-3′) and Sp6-promoter (5′-ATT TAG GTG ACA CTA TAG AAT-3′) are used.
3. Put the reaction mixture in a thermocycler using the following cycle sequencing profile:
   1. 95°C for 1 min
   2. 95°C for 10 s
   3. 50°C for 5 s
   4. 60°C for 5 min
   5. Repeat Steps 2–4 for an additional 24 cycles
   6. 14°C until the end
4. Add 1 μL of 3 M sodium acetate (pH 5.2) and 25 μL of 95% ethanol to each cycle sequencing product and then place at −20°C for 10 min.
5. Centrifuge the mixture at 10,000 ×g for 30 min. Discard the supernatant.
6. Add 200 μL of 75% ethanol and mix by vortex. Centrifuge at 10,000 ×g for another 5 min and remove the supernatant as much as possible.

7. Air-dry the pellet and dissolve in 12 μL Hi-Di Formamide.
8. Load the solution into a 96-well sequencing plate and denature at 95°C for 2 min followed by chilling on ice immediately.
9. Detect the DNA sequence using the ABI Prism 3100 Genetic Analyzer.

10.3.1.6 *Multiple Sequence Alignment*

Programs

- ClustalW2 (European Bioinformatics Institute)
- Biological Sequence Alignment Editor (BioEdit, Ibis Biosciences, Carlsbad, CA)

Procedures

1. Align ITS sequences of the 21 authentic *Hedyotis* reference samples and the seven commodity samples together with an ITS sequence (GenBank accession no.: AY438319), which was identified as *H. corymbosa* (Li *et al.*, 2010a), using ClustalW2 and edit the alignment using the BioEdit Sequence Alignment Editor (Hall, 1999).
2. Procedures of multiple sequence alignment have been described in Chapter 4.
3. The multiple sequence alignment is shown in Figure 10.2.
4. Compute the percentage similarity among the sequences.

10.3.2 Results

The intraspecific similarities of *H. diffusa* and *H. corymbosa* are 99.5% and 99.3%, respectively, showing that this region was very

```
                            ....|....| ....|....| ....|....| ....|....| ....|....| ....|....| ....|....| ....|....|
                                    5         15         25         35         45         55         65         75
H_diffusa_Hed9              GAGGAAGGAG AAGTCGTAAC AAGGTTTCCG TAGGTGAACC TGCGGAAGGA TCATTGTCGA ATCCTGCAAA CCACCGCGAA
H_diffusa_Hed10             ---------G AAGTCGTAAC AAGGTTTCCG TAGGTGAACC TGCGGAAGGA TCATTGTCGA ATCCTGCAAA CCACCGCGAA
H_diffusa_Hed11             ---------G AAGTCGTAAC AAGGTTTCCG TAGGTGAACC TGCGGAAGGA TCATTGTCGA ATCCTGCAAA CCACCGCGAA
Baihuasheshecao_Hed12       ---------G AAGTCGTAAC AAGGTTTCCG TAGGTGAACC TGCGGAAGGA TCATTGTCGA ATCCTGCAAA CCACCGCGAA
Baihuasheshecao_Hed14       ---------G AAGTCGTAAC AAGGTTTCCG TAGGTGAACC TGCGGAAGGA TCATTGTCGA ATCCTGCAAA CCACCGCGAA
Baihuasheshecao_Hed15       ---------G AAGTCGTAAC AAGGTTTCCG TAGGTGAACC TGCGGAAGGA TCATTGTCGA ATCCTGCAAA CCACCGCGAA
H_corymbosa_Hed7            ---------- ---------- ---------- ---------- ---------- ---TTGTCGA ATCCTGCAAA CGACCGCGAA
H_coymbosa_Hed8             GAGGAAGGAG AAGTCGTAAC AAGGTTTCCG TAGGTGAACC TGCGGAAGGA TCATTGTCGA ATCCTGCAAA CGACCGCGAA
Baihuasheshecao_Hed2        GAGGAAGGAG AAGTCGTAAC AAGGTTTCCG TAGGTGAACC TGCGGAAGGA TCATTGTCGA ATCCTGCAAA CGACCGCGAA
Baihuasheshecao_Hed3        GAGGAAGGAG AAGTCGTAAC AAGGTTTCCG TAGGTGAACC TGCGGAAGGA TCATTGTCGA ATCCTGCAAA CGACCGCGAA
Baihuasheshecao_Hed4        GAGGAAGGAG AAGTCGTAAC AAGGTTTCCG TAGGTGAACC TGCGGAAGGA TCATTGTCGA ATCCTGCAAA CGACCGCGAA
AY438319                    ---------- ---------- ---------- ---------C TGCGGAAGGA TCATTGTCGA ATCCTGCAAA CGATCGCGAA
H_tenelliflora_Hten1        GAGGAAGGAG AAGTCGTAAC AAGGTTTCCG TAGGTGAACC TGCGGAAGGA TCATTGTCGA ATCCTGCAAA CCACCGCGAA
Baihuasheshecao_Hed16       ---------- -------AAC AAGGTTTCCG TAGGTGAACC TGCGGAAGGA TCATTGTCGA ATCCTGCAAA CCACCGTGAA
H_pinifolia_Hpin1           GAGGAAGGAG AAGTCGTAAC AAGGTTTCCG TAGGTGAACC TGCGGAAGGA TCATTGTCGA ATCCTGCAAA CCACCGCGAA
H_aurricularia_Haur1        GAGGAAGGAG AAGTCGTAAC AAGGTTTCCG TAGGTGAACC TGCGGAAGGA TCATTGTCGA ATCCTGCAAA CCACCGCGAA
H_aurricularia_Haur2        GAGGAAGGAG AAGTCGTAAC AAGGTTTCCG TAGGTGAACC TGCGGAAGGA TCATTGTCGA ATCCTGCAAA CCACCGCGAA
H_hedyotidea_Hhed           ---------G AAGTCGTAAC AAGGTTTCCG TAGGTGAACC TGCGGAAGGA TCATTGTCGA ATCCTGCAAA CCACCGCGAA
H_costata_Hctt3             GAGGAAGGAG AAGTCGTAAC AAGGTTTCCG TAGGTGAACC TGCGGAAGGA TCATTGTCGA ATCCTGCAAA CCACCGCGAA
H_verticillata_Hve1         GAGGAAGGAG AAGTCGTAAC AAGGTTTCCG TAGGTGAACC TGCGGAAGGA TCATTGTCGA ATCCTGCAAA CCACCGCGAA
H_verticillata_Hve2         GAGGAAGGAG AAGTCGTAAC AAGGTTTCCG TAGGTGAACC TGCGGAAGGA TCATTGTCGA ATCCTGCAAA CCACCGCGAA
H_biflora_Hbif2             GAGGAAGGAG AAGTCGTAAC AAGGTTTCCG TAGGTGAACC TGCGGAAGGA TCATTGTCGA ATCCTGCAAA CCACCGTGAA
H_effusa_Hef2               GAGGAAGGAG AAGTCGTAAC AAGGTTTCCG TAGGTGAACC TGCGGAAGGA TCATTGTCGA TGCCCTAAGA CCACCGCGAA
H_consanguinea_Hcon1        GAGGAAGGAG AAGTCGTAAC AAGGTTTCCG TAGGTGAACC TGCGGAAGGA TCATTGTCGA ATCCTGCGAA CCACCGCGAA
H_acutangula_Hacu           ---------G AAGTCGTAAC AAGGTTTCCG TAGGTGAACC TGCGGAAGGA TCATTGTCGA ATCCTGGGAT CCACTGCGAA
H_bracteosa_Hbr2            GAGGAAGGAG AAGTCGTAAC AAGGTTTCCG TAGGTGAACC TGCGGAAGGA TCATTGTCGA ATCTTGCAAA CCACCGCGAA
H_bracteosa_Hbr1            GAGGAAGGAG AAGTCGTAAC AAGGTTTCCG TAGGTGAACC TGCGGAAGGA TCATTGTCGA ATCCTGCGAA CCACCGTGAA
H_yangchunensis_Hya1        GAGGAAGGAG AAGTCGTAAC AAGGTTTCCG TAGGTGAACC TGCGGAAGGA TCATTGTCGA ATCCTGCGAA CCACCGCGAA
H_yangchunensis_Hya2        GAGGAAGGAG AAGTCGTAAC AAGGTTTCCG TAGGTGAACC TGCGGAAGGA TCATTGTCGA ATCCTGCGAA CCACCGCGAA


                            ....|....| ....|....| ....|....| ....|....| ....|....| ....|....| ....|....| ....|....|
                                   85         95        105        115        125        135        145        155
H_diffusa_Hed9              CACGT-T--T TAAAAACCAG CGGGCTGCGG GCGGACAGCC GTCTGCCAGC A--CCCGCGC CCAAC-AAAC TTCCGGCGCG
H_diffusa_Hed10             CACGT-T--T TAAAAACCAG CGGGCTGCGG GCGGACAGCC GTCTGCCAGC A--CCCGCGC CCAAC-AAAC TTCCGGCGCG
H_diffusa_Hed11             CACGT-T--T TAAAAACCAG CGGGCTGCGG GCGGACAGCC GTCTGCCAGC A--CCCGCGC CCAAC-AAAC TTCCGGCGCG
Baihuasheshecao_Hed12       CACGT-T--T TAAAAACCAG CGGGCTGCGG GCGGACAGCC GTCTGCCAGC A--CCCGCGC CCAAC-AAAC TTCCGGCGCG
Baihuasheshecao_Hed14       CACGT-T--T TAAAAACCAG CGGGCTGCGG GCGGACAGCC GTCTGCCAGC A--CCCGCGC CGAAC-AAAC TTCCGGCGCG
Baihuasheshecao_Hed15       CACGT-T--T TAAAAACCAG CGGGCTGCGG GCGGACAGCC GTCTGCCAGC A--CCCGCGC CCAAC-AAAC TTCCGGCGCG
H_corymbosa_Hed7            CACGTTT--T TATAAACCCG CGGGGCACGG ACGGACTCCC GTCTGGCCGT TGCCCCGCAC CCAACAAAAC TTCCGGCGCG
H_coymbosa_Hed8             CACGTTT--T TATAAACCCG CGGGGCACGG ACGGACTCCC GTCTGGCCGT TGCCCCGCAC CCAACAAAAC TTCCGGCGCG
Baihuasheshecao_Hed2        CACGTTT--T TATAAACCCG CGGGGCACGG ACGGACTCCC GTCTGGCCGT TGCCCCGCAC CCAACAAAAC TTCCGGCGCG
Baihuasheshecao_Hed3        CACGTTT--T TATAAACCCG CGGGGCACGG ACGGACTCCC GTCTGGCCGT TGCCCCGCAC CCAACAAAAC TTCCGGCGCG
Baihuasheshecao_Hed4        CACGTTT--T TATAAACCCG CGGGGCACGG ACGGACTCCC GTCTGGCCGT TGCCCCGCAC CCAACAAAAC TTCCGGCGCG
AY438319                    CACGTTT--T TATAAACCCG CGGGGCACGG ACGGACTCCC GTCTGGCCGT TGCCCCGCAC CCAACAAAAC TTCCGGCGCG
H_tenelliflora_Hten1        CACGT-T--T AAAAACCTG- CGGGCTGCGG TCGGACTACC GTCTGCCGGC G--CCCGCAC CTAAC-AAAC TTCCGGCGCG
Baihuasheshecao_Hed16       CACGT-T--T AAAAACCCG- CGGGCTGCGG GCGGACTGCC GTCCGCCGGC G--CCCGCAC CTAAC-AAAC TTCCGGCGCG
H_pinifolia_Hpin1           CACGTAT--T CACAAACTAG CGGGTTGCGG GCGGACCGAG TTCGCCTGCT C--CCCGCAC CAAAC-GAAC TTCCGGCGCG
H_aurricularia_Haur1        CACGT-T--T TGAAAACC-G CGGGCCGTCG GCGCGCTCAG GTTTGCCGGC A--ACCGCAC CAAACTTAAC TTCCGGCGCG
H_aurricularia_Haur2        CACGT-T--T TGGAAACC-G CGGGCCGTCG GCGCGCTCAG GTTTGCCGGC A--ACCGCAC CAAGCTTAAC TTCCGGCGCG
H_hedyotidea_Hhed           CACGT-T--T CGAAAAACAG CGGGCCGTCG GCGCGCTCCG GTTCGCCGGC G--CCCGCAC CTAACAAAAC TCCCGGCGCG
H_costata_Hctt3             CACGT-T--T CAAAAAACTG CGGGCCGTCG GCGCGCTCCG GTGTGCCGGC G--CCCGCAA CTAACTAAAC TTCCGGCGCG
H_verticillata_Hve1         CACGT-T--T TATAACCCGG CGGGCTGCGG GCGGACTAAC GTCTGCCGGC A--CCCGCAC CTAAC-AAAA TTCCGGCGCG
H_verticillata_Hve2         CACGT-T--T TATAACCCGG CGGGCTGCGG GCGGACTAAC GTCTGCCGGC A--CCCGCAC CTAAC-AAAA TTCCGGCGCG
H_biflora_Hbif2             CATGT----T TGTAAACTTG CGGGACGCGG GCTGACACCC GTCTGCCGGC T--CCCGCAC CTAACAAAAC TTCCGGCGCG
H_effusa_Hef2               CACGT-T--A AAAAAACTCT CGGGGAGACG AAGGGCTTAG TGTCTGGATT TTCCCCGGTC CCAACTTAAT TTCCGGCGCG
H_consanguinea_Hcon1        CACGTTTGAT AACAAAAGTT GGGGGTGCGG CTGGGCTAAG TTTGGCTGCC C-TCCCGAAC TTAAAAAAAC TTCCGGCGCG
H_acutangula_Hacu           CACGTTTGAT AACAAAAATC GGGGGTGCGG CCGGGCCAAG CTCGACAGCC C-CCCCGAAC CTAACAAAAC TTCCGGCGCG
H_bracteosa_Hbr2            CACGTTTGAT AACAAAAATC GGGGGCGCAG TCGGGCCAAG CTTGGC-GGC C-CCCCGTGC CTAACAAAAC TTCCGGCGCG
H_bracteosa_Hbr1            CACGTTTGAT AACAAAAATC GGGGGCGCAG TCGGGCCAAG ATTGGC-TGC C-CCC-GTGC CTAACAAAAC TTCCGGCGCG
H_yangchunensis_Hya1        CACGTTTGAT AACAAAAATC GGGGACGCGG TCGTGCCAAG CTTGGCCTGC C-CCCCGTGC CTAACAAAAC TTCCGGCGCG
H_yangchunensis_Hya2        CACGTTTGAT AACAAAAATC GGGGACGCGG TCGTGCCAAG CTTGGCCTGC C-CCCCGTGC CTAACAAAAC TTCCGGCGCG
```

Fig. 10.2 Multiple sequence alignment of the complete sequence of the ITS region of the authentic *Hedyotis* samples and Baihuasheshecao commodities in this study. Details of the samples are given in Table 10.3.

```
                          ....|....| ....|....| ....|....| ....|....| ....|....| ....|....| ....|....| ....|....|
                                165        175        185        195        205        215        225        235
H_diffusa_Hed9            GAAAGCGCCA AGGACTACTC AAA-CGGATC GTCCGCGTCC CCCCTGCGGG TTCCGCGGGG CGGGCGCCGG TCTTCTGAAT
H_diffusa_Hed10           GAAAGCGCCA AGGACTACTC AAA-CGGATC GTCCGCGTCC CCC-TGCGGG TTCCGCGGGG CGGGCGCCGG TCTTCTGAAT
H_diffusa_Hed11           GAAAGCGCCA AGGACTACTC AAA-CGGATC GTCCGCGTCC CCC-TGCGGG TTCCGCGGGG CGGGCGCCGG TCTTCTGAAT
Baihuasheshecao_Hed12     GAAAGCGCCA AGGACTACTC AAA-CGGATC GTCCGCGTCC CCCCTGCGGG TTCCGCGGGG CGGGCGCCGG TCTTCTGAAT
Baihuasheshecao_Hed14     GAAAGCGCCA AGGACTACTC AAA-CGGATC GTCCGCGTCC CCC-TGCGGG TTCCGCGGGG CGGGCGCCGG TCTTCTGAAT
Baihuasheshecao_Hed15     GAAAGCGCCA AGGACTACTC AAA-CGGATC GTCCGCGTCC CCCCTGCGGG TTCCGCGGGG CGGGCGCCGG TCTTCTGAAT
H_corymbosa_Hed7          GAAAGCGCCA AGGACTACAC AAA-AGGATC GTCCGCATCC CCC-GGCGGT TTCCGTTGGG CGGGTGTGAC GTGTCTGAAT
H_coymbosa_Hed8           GAAAGCGCCA AGGACTACAC AAA-AGGATC GTCCGCATCC CCC-GGCGGT TTCCGTTGGG CGGGTGTGAC GTGTCTGAAT
Baihuasheshecao_Hed2      GAAAGCGCCA AGGACTACAC AAA-AGGATC GTCCGCATCC CCC-GGCGGT TTCCGTTGGG CGGGTGTGAC GTGTCTGAAT
Baihuasheshecao_Hed3      GAAAGCGCCA AGGACTACAC AAA-AGGATC GTCCGCATCC CCC-GGCGGT TTCCGTTGGG CGGGTGTGAC GTGTCTGAAT
Baihuasheshecao_Hed4      GAAAGCGCCA AGGACTACAC AAA-AGGATC GTCCGCATCC CCC-GGCGGT TTCCGTTGGG CGGGTGTGAC GTGTCTGAAT
AY438319                  GAAAGCGCCA AGGACTACAC AAA-AGGATC GTCCGCATCC CCC-GGCGGT TTCCGTTGGG CGGGTGTGAC GTGTCTGAAT
H_tenelliflora_Hten1      GTATGCGCCA AGGACTACTC AAAACGGATC GTCCGCATCC CCC-TACGGA TTCCGCAGGG CGGGTGCCGG TCGTCTGAAT
Baihuasheshecao_Hed16     GTATGCGCCA AGGACTACTC AAAACGGATC GTCCGCATCC CCC-TACGGA TTCCGCAGGG CGGGTGCCGG TCGTCTGAAT
H_pinifolia_Hpin1         GAATGCGCCA AGGACTACTC AAA-CGGATC GTCCGCGTCC CCC-TTCGGA TTCCGCAGGG CGGGCGCTGG TCGTCTGAAT
H_aurricularia_Haur1      GATTGCGCCA AGGACTACTA AAA-CGGATC GTCCGCGTCC CCC-TGCAAA TTCCGCAGGC GGGGCGCGGG GCGTCTGAAT
H_aurricularia_Haur2      GATTGCGCCA AGGACTACTA AAA-CGGATC GTCCGCGTCC CCC-TGCAAA TTCCGCAGGC GGGGCGCGGG GCGTCTGAAT
H_hedyotidea_Hhed         GAATGCGCCA AGGATTACTA AAA-CGGATC GTCCGTGTCC CCC-GGCGGA TTCCGCAGGC GGGGCGCGGG GCGTCTGAAT
H_costata_Hctt3           GAATGCGCCA AGGACTACTA AAA-CGGATC GTCCGCGTCC CCC-TGCGGA TTCTGCGGGC GGGGCACGGT GCGTCTGAAT
H_verticillata_Hve1       GAACGCGCCA AGGACTACTC AAA-CGGATC GTCCGCATCC CCC-TGCGGA TTCCGCAGGG CGGGTGCCGG TCGTCTGAAT
H_verticillata_Hve2       GAACGCGCCA AGGACTACTC AAA-CGGATC GTCCGCATCC CCC-TGCGGA TTCCGCAGGG CGGGTGCCGG TCGTCTGAAT
H_biflora_Hbif2           GAATGCGCCA AGGACTACTC AAA-TGGAAC GTCCGCGTCC CCC-CACGGT TTCCGCGGGG TGGGCGCGGG TCTTCTGAAT
H_effusa_Hef2             GATAGCGCCA AGGACTACTT GAA-CGGATC GCCTGCACAC TCC-CACGGC TTCCGCGGTG CGGGTGCGGC GCGTCTGAAT
H_consanguinea_Hcon1      GAACGCGTCA AGGACTACTC GAA-CGGATC GTCCGCATCC TCC-CACGGC TTCCGCCGGG AGGGCGCGGC GCGTCTGAAA
H_acutangula_Hacu         GAACGCGTCA AGGACTACTC AAA-CGGATC GTCCGCATCC CCC-CACGGC TTCCGTCGGG AGGGTGCGGC GTGTCTGAAA
H_bracteosa_Hbr2          GAACGCGTCA AGGACTACTC GAA-CGGATC GTTCGCGTCC CAC-CACGGC TTCTGTCGGG AGGGCGCGGC GCGTCTGAAA
H_bracteosa_Hbr1          GAACGCGTCA AGGACTACTC GAA-CGGATC GTCCGCGTCC CAC-CACGGC TTCCGTC-GG AGGGCGTGGC GCGTCTGAAA
H_yangchunensis_Hya1      GAATGCGTCA AGGACTACTC AAA-CGGATC GTCCGCGTCC CCC-CACGGA TCCCGTCGGG ATGGCGCGGC GTGTCTGAAA
H_yangchunensis_Hya2      GAATGCGTCA AGGACTACTC AAA-CGGATC GTCCGCGTCC CCC-CACGGA TCCCGTCGGG AGGGCGCGGC GCGTCTGAAA
```

```
                          ....|....| ....|....| ....|....| ....|....| ....|....| ....|....| ....|....| ....|....|
                                245        255        265        275        285        295        305        315
H_diffusa_Hed9            CGTA--ACCA ATACGACTCT CGGCAACGGA TATCTAGGCT CTCGCATCGA TGAAGAACGT AGCGAAATGC GATACTTGGT
H_diffusa_Hed10           CGTA--ACCA ATACGACTCT CGGCAACGGA TATCTAGGCT CTCGCATCGA TGAAGAACGT AGCGAAATGC GATACTTGGT
H_diffusa_Hed11           CGTA--ACCA ATACGACTCT CGGCAACGGA TATCTAGGCT CTCGCATCGA TGAAGAACGT AGCGAAATGC GATACTTGGT
Baihuasheshecao_Hed12     CGTA--ACCA ATACGACTCT CGGCAACGGA TATCTAGGCT CTCGCATCGA TGAAGAACGT AGCGAAATGC GATACTTGGT
Baihuasheshecao_Hed14     CGTA--ACCA ATACGACTCT CGGCAACGGA TATCTAGGCT CTCGCATCGA TGAAGAACGT AGCGAAATGC GATACTTGGT
Baihuasheshecao_Hed15     CGTA--ACCA ATACGACTCT CGGCAACGGA TATCTAGGCT CTCGCATCGA TGAAGAACGT AGCGAAATGC GATACTTGGT
H_corymbosa_Hed7          CGTATAACCA ATACGACTCT CGGCAACGGA TATCTAGGCT CTCGCATCGA TGAAGAACGT AGCGAAATGC GATACTTGGT
H_coymbosa_Hed8           CGTATAACCA ATACGACTCT CGGCAACGGA TATCTAGGCT CTCGCATCGA TGAAGAACGT AGCGAAATGC GATACTTGGT
Baihuasheshecao_Hed2      CGTATAACCA ATACGACTCT CGGCAACGGA TATCTAGGCT CTCGCATCGA TGAAGAACGT AGCGAAATGC GATACTTGGT
Baihuasheshecao_Hed3      CGTATAACCA ATACGACTCT CGGCAACGGA TATCTAGGCT CTCGCATCGA TGAAGAACGT AGCGAAATGC GATACTTGGT
Baihuasheshecao_Hed4      CGTATAACCA ATACGACTCT CGGCAACGGA TATCTAGGCT CTCGCATCGA TGAAGAACGT AGCGAAATGC GATACTTGGT
AY438319                  CGTATAACCA ATACGACTCT CGGCAACGGA TATCTAGGCT CTCGCATCGA TGAAGAACGT AGCGAAATGC GATACTTGGT
H_tenelliflora_Hten1      CGTA--ACCA ATACGACTCT CGGCAACGGA TATCTAGGCT CTCGCATCGA TGAAGAACGT AGCGAAATGC GATACTTGGT
Baihuasheshecao_Hed16     CGTA--ACCA ATACGACTCT CGGCAACGGA TATCTAGGCT CTCGCATCGA TGAAGAACGT AGCGAAATGC GATACTTGGT
H_pinifolia_Hpin1         CGTA--ACCA ATACGACTCT CGGCAACGGA TATCTAGGCT CTCGCATCGA TGAAGAACGT AGCGAAATGC GATACTTGGT
H_aurricularia_Haur1      CGTA--ACCA ATACGACTCT CGGCAACGGA TATCTAGGCT CTCGCATCGA TGAAGAACGT AGCGAAATGC GATACTTGGT
H_aurricularia_Haur2      CGTA--ACCA ATACGACTCT CGGCAACGGA TATCTAGGCT CTCGCATCGA AGAAGAACGT AGCGAAATGC GATACTTGGT
H_hedyotidea_Hhed         CGTA--ACCA ATACGACTCT CGGCAACGGA TATCTAGGCT CTCGCATCGA TGAAGAACGT AGCGAAATGC GATACTTGGT
H_costata_Hctt3           CGTA--ACCA ATACGACTCT CGGCAACGGA TATCTAGGCT CTCGCATCGA TGAAGAACGT AGCGAAATGC GATACTTGGT
H_verticillata_Hve1       CGTA--ACCA ATACGACTCT CGGCAACGGA TATCTAGGCT CTCGCATCGA TGAAGAACGT AGCGAAATGC GATACTTGGT
H_verticillata_Hve2       CGTA--ACCA ATACGACTCT CGGCAACGGA TATCTAGGCT CTCGCATCGA TGGAGAACGT AGCGAAATGC GATACTTGGT
H_biflora_Hbif2           TGTA--ACCA ATACGACTCT CGGCAACGGA TATCTAGGCT CTCGCATCGA TGAAGAACGT AGCGAAATGC GATACTTGGT
H_effusa_Hef2             CGTATAACCA ATACGACTCT CGGCAACGGA TATCTAGGCT CTCGCATCGA TGAAGAACGT AGCGAAATGC GATACTTGGT
H_consanguinea_Hcon1      GATA--ACCA ATACGACTCT CGGCAACGGA TATCTAGGCT CTCGCATCGA TGAAGAACGT AGCGAAATGC GATACTTGGT
H_acutangula_Hacu         GATA--ACCA ATACGACTCT CGGCAACGGA TATCTAGGCT CTCGCATCGA TGAAGAACGT AGCGAAATGC GATACTTGGT
H_bracteosa_Hbr2          ATAA--ACCA ATACGACTCT CGGCAACGGA TATCTAGGCT CTCGCATCGA TGAAGAACGT AGCGAAATGC GATACATGGT
H_bracteosa_Hbr1          GATA--ACCA ATACGACTCT CGGCAACGGA TATCTAGGCT TTTGCATCGA TGAAGAACGT AGCGAAATGC GATACTTGGT
H_yangchunensis_Hya1      GATA--ACCA ATACGACTCT CGGCAACGGA TATCTAGGCT CTCGCATCGA TGAAGAACGT AGCGAAATGC GATACTTGGT
H_yangchunensis_Hya2      GATA--ACCA ATACGACTCT CGGCAACGGA TATCTAGGCT CTCGCATCGA TGAAGAACGT AGCGAAATGC GATACTTGGT
```

Fig. 10.2 (*Continued*)

```
                            ....|....| ....|....| ....|....| ....|....| ....|....| ....|....| ....|....| ....|....|
                                  325        335        345        355        365        375        385        395
H_diffusa_Hed9              GTGAATTGCA GAATCCCGTG AACCATCGAG TTTTTGAACG CAAGTTGCGC CCGAAGCCAT TAGGCCGAGG GCACGTCTGC
H_diffusa_Hed10             GTGAATTGCA GAATCCCGTG AACCATCGAG TTTTTGAACG CAAGTTGCGC CCGAAGCCAT TAGGCCGAGG GCACGTCTGC
H_diffusa_Hed11             GTGAATTGCA GAATCCCGTG AACCATCGAG TTTTTGAACG CAAGTTGCGC CCGAAGCCAT TAGGCCGAGG GCACGTCTGC
Baihuasheshecao_Hed12       GTGAATTGCA GAATCCCGTG AACCATCGAG TTTTTGAACG CAAGTTGCGC CCGAAGCCAT TAGGCCGAGG GCACGTCTGC
Baihuasheshecao_Hed14       GTGAATTGCA GAATCCCGTG AACCATCGAG TTTTTGAACG CAAGTTGCGC CCGAAGCCAT TAGGCCGAGG GCACGTCTGC
Baihuasheshecao_Hed15       GTGAATTGCA GAATCCCGTG AACCATCGAG TTTTTGAACG CAAGTTGCGC CCGAAGCCAT TAGGCCGAGG GCACGTCTGC
H_corymbosa_Hed7            GTGAATTGCA GAATCCCGTG AACCATCGAG TTTTTGAACG CAAGTTGCGC CCGAAGCCAT TTGGCTGAGG GCACGCCTGC
H_coymbosa_Hed8             GTGAATTGCA GAATCCCGTG AACCATCGAG TTTTTGAACG CAAGTTGCGC CCGAAGCCAT TTGGCTGAGG GCACGCCTGC
Baihuasheshecao_Hed2        GTGAATTGCA GAATCCCGTG AACCATCGAG TTTTTGAACG CAAGTTGCGC CCGAAGCCAT TTGGCTGAGG GCACGCCTGC
Baihuasheshecao_Hed3        GTGAATTGCA GAATCCCGTG AACCATCGAG TTTTTGAACG CAAGTTGCGC CCGAAGCCAT TTGGCTGAGG GCACGCCTGC
Baihuasheshecao_Hed4        GTGAATTGCA GAATCCCGTG AACCATCGAG TTTTTGAACG CAAGTTGCGC CCGAAGCCAT TTGGCTGAGG GCACGCCTGC
AY438319                    GTGAATTGCA GAATCCCGTG AACCATCGAG TTTTTGAACG CAAGTTGCGC CCGAAGCCAT TTGGCTGAGG GCACGCCTGC
H_tenelliflora_Hten1        GTGAATTGCA GAATCCCGTG AACCATCGAG TTTTTGAACG CAAGTTGCGC CCGAAGCCAT TAGGCTGAGG GCACGTCTGC
Baihuasheshecao_Hed16       GTGAATTGCA GAATCCCGTG AACCATCGAG TTTTTGAACG CAAGTTGCGC CCGAAGCCAT TAGGCTGAGG GCACGTCTGC
H_pinifolia_Hpin1           GTGAATTGCA GAATCCCGTG AACCATCGAG TTTTTGAACG CAAGTTGCGC CCGAAGCCAT TAGGCCGAGG GCACGTCTGC
H_aurricularia_Haur1        GTGAATTGCA GAATCCCGTG AACCATCGAG TTTTTGAACG CAAGTTGCGC CCGAAGCCAT TAGGCTGAGG GCACGTCTGC
H_aurricularia_Haur2        GTGAATTGCA GAATCCCGTG AACCATCGAG TTTTTGAACG CAAGTTGCGC CCGAAGCCAT TAGGCTGAGG GCACGTCTGC
H_hedyotidea_Hhed           GTGAATTGCA GAATCCCGTG AACCATCGAG TTTTTGAACG CAAGTTGCGC CCGAAGCCAT CAGGCTGAGG GCACGTCTGC
H_costata_Hctt3             GTGAATTGCA GAATCCCGTG AACCATCGAG TTTTTGAACG CAAGTTGCGC CCGAAGCCAT TAGGCTGAGG GCACGTCTGC
H_verticillata_Hve1         GTGAATTGCA GAATCCCGTG AACCATCGAG TTTTTGAACG CAAGTTGCGC CCGAAGCCAT TAGGCTGAGG GCACGTCTGC
H_verticillata_Hve2         GTGAATTGCA GAATCCCGTG AACCATCGAG TTTTTGAACG CAAGTTGCGC CCGAAGCCAT TAGGCTGAGG GCACGTCTGC
H_biflora_Hbif2             GTGAATTGCA GAATCCCGTG AACCATCGAG TTTTTGAACG CAAGCTGCGC CCGAAGCCAT TTGGCTGAGG ACACGTCTGC
H_effusa_Hef2               GTGAATTGCA GAATCCCGTG AACCATCGAG TTTTTGAACG CAAGTTGCGC CCGAAGCCAT TAGGCTGAGG GCACGTCTGC
H_consanguinea_Hcon1        GTGAATTGCA GAATCCCGTG AACCATCGAG TTTTTGAACG CAAGTTGCGC CCGAAGCCAT TAGGCCGAGG GCACGTCTGC
H_acutangula_Hacu           GTGAATTGCA GAATCCCGTG AACCATCGAG TTTTTGAACG CAAGTTGCGC CCGATGCCAT TAGGCCGAGG GCACGTCTGC
H_bracteosa_Hbr2            GTGAATTGCA GAATCCCGTG AACCATCGAG TTTTTGAACG CAAGTTGCGC CCAAAGCCAT TAGGCCGAGG GCACGTCTGC
H_bracteosa_Hbr1            GTGAATTGCA GAATCCCGTG AACCATCGAG TTTTTGAACG CAAGTTGCGC CCGAAGCCAT TAGGCCGAGG GCACGTCTGC
H_yangchunensis_Hya1        GTGAATTGCA GAATCCCGTG AACCATCGAG TTTTTGAACG CAAGTTGCGC CCAAAGCCAT TAGGCCGAGG GCACGTCTGC
H_yangchunensis_Hya2        GTGAATTGCA GAATCCCGTG AACCATCGAG TTTTTGAACG CAAGTTGCGC CCAAAGCCAT TAGGCCGAGG GCACGTCTGC

                            ....|....| ....|....| ....|....| ....|....| ....|....| ....|....| ....|....| ....|....|
                                  405        415        425        435        445        455        465        475
H_diffusa_Hed9              CTGGGCGTCA CGCAACGTCG CCACCCCC-- TC-GCCTCGC GCCTGCGCGT CGAGTCGGGC GGCGGAAGCT GGCCTCCCGT
H_diffusa_Hed10             CTGGGCGTCA CGCAACGTCG CCACCCCC-- TC-GCCTCGC GCCTGCGCGT CGAGTCGGGC GGCGGAAGCT GGCCTCCCGT
H_diffusa_Hed11             CTGGGCGTCA CGCAACGTCG CCACCCCC-- TC-GCCTCGC GCCTGCGCGT CGAGTCGGGC GGCGGAAGCT GGCCTTCCGT
Baihuasheshecao_Hed12       CTGGGCGTCA CGCAACGTCG CCACCCCC-- TC-GCCTCGC GCCTGCGCGT CGAGTCGGGC GGCGGAAGCT GGCCTCCCGT
Baihuasheshecao_Hed14       CTGGGCGTCA CGCAACGTCG CCACCCCC-- TC-GCCTCGC GCCTGCGCGT CGAGTCGGGC GGCGGAAGCT GGCCTCCCGT
Baihuasheshecao_Hed15       CTGGGCGTCA CGCAACGTCG CCACCCCC-- TC-GCCTCGC GCCTGCGCGT CGAGTCGGGC GGCGGAAGCT GGCCTCCCGT
H_corymbosa_Hed7            CTGGGCGTCA CGCATCGTCG CCACCCCCC- TC-------- -GCAATGCGA AGCGCGGGGT GACGGAAGTT GGCCTCCCGT
H_coymbosa_Hed8             CTGGGCGTCA CGCATCGTCG CCACCCCCC- TC-------- -GCAATGCGA AGCGCGGGGT GACGGAAGTT GGCCTCCCGT
Baihuasheshecao_Hed2        CTGGGCGTCA CGCATCGTCG CCACCCCCC- TC-------- -GCAATGCGA AGCGCGGGGT GACGGAAGTT GGCCTCCCGT
Baihuasheshecao_Hed3        CTGGGCGTCA CGCATCGTCG CCACCCCCC- TC-------- -GCAATGCGA AGCGCGGGGT GACGGAAGTT GGCCTCCCGT
Baihuasheshecao_Hed4        CTGGGCGTCA CGCATCGTCG CCACCCCCC- TC-------- -GCAATGCGA AGCGCGGGGT GACGGAAGTT GGCCTCCCGT
AY438319                    CTGGGCGTCA CGCATCGTCG CCACCCCCC- TC-------- -GCAATGCGA AGCGCGGGGT GACGGAAGTT GGCCTCCCGT
H_tenelliflora_Hten1        CTGGGCGTCA CGCACCGTCG CCACCCCCCC T-CACCGCGT GCTAACGCGT CGAGGCGGAT GGCGGATGTT GGCCTCCCGT
Baihuasheshecao_Hed16       CTGGGCGTCA CGCACCGTCG CCACCCCCCC T-CACCGCGT GCTAACGCGT CGAGGCGGAT GGCGGATGTT GGCCTCCCGT
H_pinifolia_Hpin1           CTGGGCGTCA CGCACCGTCG CCTCCCCCAC AACGTCGCGT GCCGACGCGT GTGGACGGGT GGCGGATGTT GGCCTCCCGT
H_aurricularia_Haur1        CTGGGCGTCA CGCATCGTCG CCACCCCCC- TC-ACCGCGC TCCGGCGCAT CGAGGCGGGT GACGGATGTT GGCCTCCCGT
H_aurricularia_Haur2        CTGGGCGTCA CGCATCGTCG CCACCCCCC- TC-ACCGCGC TCCGGCGCAT CGAGGCGGGT GACGGATGTT GGCCTCCCTT
H_hedyotidea_Hhed           CTGGGCGTCA CGCATCGTCG CCACCCCCA- TC-GCCGCGC TCCTGCGCCA CGAGGCGGGT GACGGATGTT GGCCTCCCGT
H_costata_Hctt3             CTGGGCGTCA CGCATCGTCG CCGCCCCCC- TC-ACCGCGC TCTGGCGCAG CGTGGCGGGT GACGGATGTT GGCCTCCCGT
H_verticillata_Hve1         CTGGGCGTCA CGCATCGTCG CCACCCCCCC T-CTTCGCGT GCTAACGAGT TTTGGCGGGC GGCGGATGTT GGCCTCCCGT
H_verticillata_Hve2         CTGGGCGTCA CGCATCGTCG CCACCCCCCC T-CATCGCGT GCTAACGTGT TTTGGCGGGC GGCGGATGTT GGCCTCCCGT
H_biflora_Hbif2             CTGGGCGTCA CGCATCGTCG CCACCCCCTC C---CTGTGC CTTTG-GCAT TGAGTCGGGT GACGGATGTT AGCCTCCCGT
H_effusa_Hef2               CTGGGCGTCA CGCATCGTCG CCACCTCCCC C-----TCTT TCTCCGATCG AGTATGGGGT GGCGGAAACT GGCCTCCCGT
H_consanguinea_Hcon1        CTGGGCGTCA CGCATCGTCG CCACCCCCC- -------TTT TCACACGCCC TGCGGTGGGT GACGGACATT GGCCCCCCGT
H_acutangula_Hacu           TTGGGCGTCA CGCATCGTCG CCACCCCCC- -------TC- GCACACGCT- TGCGGTGGGT GACGGACATT GGCCCCCCGT
H_bracteosa_Hbr2            CTGGGCGTCA CGCAACGTCG CCACCCCCCG -------TTC GCACACGCCA TGCGGTGGGT GACGGAAATT GGCCCCCCGT
H_bracteosa_Hbr1            CTGGGCGTCA CGCAACGTCG CCACCCCCC- -------TTC GCACACGCCA TGCGGTAGGT GACGGACATT GGCCCCCCGT
H_yangchunensis_Hya1        CTGGGCGTCA CGCATCGTCG CCACCCCCC- -------TTC GCACACGCCC TGCGGTGGGT GACGGACATT GGCCCCCCGT
H_yangchunensis_Hya2        CTGGGCGTCA CGCATCGTCG CCACCCCCC- -------TTC GCACACGCCC TGCGGTGGGT GACGGACATT GGCCCCCCGT
```

Fig. 10.2 (*Continued*)

```
                            ....|....| ....|....| ....|....| ....|....| ....|....| ....|....| ....|....| ....|....|
                                  485        495        505        515        525        535        545        555
H_diffusa_Hed9              GTCC-GCAG- GGCGCGGCCG GCCTAAATCC GAGTCCTCCG TTCGG-GACG TCACGACAAG TGGTGGTTGA AAACTTCAA-
H_diffusa_Hed10             GTCC-GCAG- GGCGCGGCCG GCCTAAATCC GAGTCCTCCG TTCGG-GACG TCACGACAAG TGGTGGTTGA AAACTTCAA-
H_diffusa_Hed11             GTCC-GCAG- GGCGCGGCCG GCCTAAATTC GAGTCCTCCG TTCGG-GACG TCACGACAAG TGGTGGTTGA AAACTTCAA-
Baihuasheshecao_Hed12       GTCC-GCAG- GGCGCGGCCG GCCTAAATCC GAGTCCTCCG TTCGG-GACG TCACGACAAG TGGTGGTTGA AAACTTCAA-
Baihuasheshecao_Hed14       GTCC-GCAG- GGCGCGGCCG GCCTAAATCC GAGTCCTCCG TTCGG-GACG TCACGACAAG TGGTGGTTGA AAACTTCAA-
Baihuasheshecao_Hed15       GTCC-GCAG- GGCGCGGCCG GCCTAAATCC GAGTCCTCCG TTCGG-GACG TCACGACAAG TGGTGGTTGA AAACTTCAA-
H_corymbosa_Hed7            GTCTCCTGGC AGCGCGGCCG GCCTAAATTC GAGTCCTCCG TTCGGAGACG TCACGACTAG TGGTGGTTGA AAACTTCAT-
H_coymbosa_Hed8             GTCTCCTGGC AGCGCGGCCG GCCTAAATTC GAGTCCTCCG TTCGGAGACG TCACGACTAG TGGTGGTTGA AAACTTCAT-
Baihuasheshecao_Hed2        GTCTCCTGGC AGCGCGGCCG GCCTAAATTC GAGTCCTCCG TTCGGAGACG TCACGACTAG TGGTGGTTGA AAACTTCAT-
Baihuasheshecao_Hed3        GTCTCCTGGC AGCGCGGCCG GCCTAAATTC GAGTCCTCCG TTCGGAGACG TCACGACTAG TGGTGGTTGA AAACTTCAT-
Baihuasheshecao_Hed4        GTCTCCTGGC AGCGCGGCCG GCCTAAATTC GAGTCCTCCG TTCGGAGACG TCACGACTAG TGGTGGTTGA AAACTTCAT-
AY438319                    GTCTCCTGGC AGCGCGGCCG GCCTAAATTC GAGTCCTCCG TTCGGAGACG TCACGACTAG TGGTGGTTGA AAACTTCAT-
H_tenelliflora_Hten1        GTCCACCCG- GGCGCGGCCG GCCTAAATCC GAGTCCCCCG TTCGG-GACG TCACGACAAG TGGTGGTTGA AAACTTCAA-
Baihuasheshecao_Hed16       GTCCACCCT- GGCGCGGCCG GCCTAAATCC GAGTCCCCCG TTCGG-GACG TCACGACAAG TGGTGGTTGA AAACTTCAA-
H_pinifolia_Hpin1           GTCC-TCCG- GGCGCGGCCG GCCCAAATAC GAGCACCCCG TTCGG-GACG TCGCGACAAG TGGTGGTTGA AAACCTCAA-
H_aurricularia_Haur1        GCCC-CCGC- GGCGCGGCCG GCCTAAATCC GAGTCCTCCG CTCGG-GACG TCACGACAAG TGGTGGTTGA AAACCTCAA-
H_aurricularia_Haur2        GCCC-CCGC- GGCGCGGCCG GCCTAAATCC GAGTCCTCCG CTCGG-GACG TCACGACAAG TGGTGGTTGA AAACCTCAA-
H_hedyotidea_Hhed           GCCC-CCGA- GGCGCGGCCG GCCTAAATCC GAGTCCTCCG TTCGG-GACG TCACGACAAG TGGTGGTTGA AAACCTCAA-
H_costata_Hctt3             GCCC-TC-T- GGCGCGGCCG GCCTAAATCA GAGTCCTCCG TTCGG-GACG TCACGACAAG TGGTGGTTGA AAACTTCAA-
H_verticillata_Hve1         GTCC-CTCG- GGCGCGGCCG GCCTAAATCC GAGTCCTCCG TTCGG-GACG TCACGACAAG TGGTGGTTGA AAACTTCAA-
H_verticillata_Hve2         GTCC-CTCG- GGCGCGGCCG GCCTAAATCC GAGTCCTCCG TTCGG-GACG TCACGACAAG TGGTGGTTGA AAACTTCAA-
H_biflora_Hbif2             GTCTCCTAC- GGCGCGGCTG GCCTAAATGC GAGTCCTCCG TTCGG-GACG TCACGACAAG TGGTGGTTGA AAATTTCAA-
H_effusa_Hef2               GCTCCTCCG- AGCGCGGCCG GCCTAAATAA GAGTCCTCCC CTCGG-GACG TCACGACTTG TGGTGGTTGA AATCCTCAA-
H_consanguinea_Hcon1        GTCT-CCAG- CACGCGGTCG GCCCAAAATT GAGTTCCCGA CTCGG-GACG TCACGGCGAG TGGTGGTTGA AACGCTCAA-
H_acutangula_Hacu           GTCT-CCAG- CACGCGGTCG GCCCAAAACA GAGTACCCGT CTCGG-GACG TCACGGCGAG TGGTGGTTGA AATGTTCAA-
H_bracteosa_Hbr2            GTCT-CCAG- CATGCGGTCG GCCCAAAACG GAGTCCCCGT CTCGG-GACG TCACGGCGAG TGGTGGTTGA AATGCTCAA-
H_bracteosa_Hbr1            GTCT-CCAG- CACGCGGTCG GCCTAAAACG GAGTCCCTGT CTCGG-GACG TCACGGCGAG TGGTGGTTGA AACGCCCAA-
H_yangchunensis_Hya1        GTCT-CCAG- CACGCGGTCG GCCCAAAATA GAGTCCCCGT CTCGG-GACG TCACGGCGAG TGGTGGTTGA AACGCTCAAA
H_yangchunensis_Hya2        GTCT-CCAG- CACGCGGTCG GCCCAAAATA GAGTCCCCGT CTCGG-GACG TCACGGCGAG TGGTGGTTGA AACGCTCAA-
```

```
                            ....|....| ....|....| ....|....| ....|....| ....|....| ....|....| ....|....| ....|....|
                                  565        575        585        595        605        615        625        635
H_diffusa_Hed9              CTCGATCGTA GCCGTGACCG AGAACGCATG GTAGGCCTCT --AAAGACCC TGGAGCCTCC --GGGCCCTC GACCATGACC
H_diffusa_Hed10             CTCGATCGTA GCCGTGACCG AGAACGCATT GTAGGCCTCT --AAAGACCC TGGAGCCTCC --GGGCCCTC GACCATGACC
H_diffusa_Hed11             CTCGATCGTA GCCGTGACCG AGAACGCATT GTAGGCCTCT --AAAGACCC TGGAGCCTCC --GGGCCCTC GACCATGACC
Baihuasheshecao_Hed12       CTCGATCGTA GCCGTGACCG AGAACGCATG GTAGGCCTCT --AAAGACCC TGGAGCCTCC --GGGCCCTC GACCATGACC
Baihuasheshecao_Hed14       CTCGATCGTA GCCGTGACCG AGAACGCATT GTAGGCCTCT --AAAGACCC TGGAGCCTCC --GGGCCCTC GACCATGACC
Baihuasheshecao_Hed15       CTCGATCGTA GCCGTGACCG AGAACGCATG GTAGGCCTCT --AAAGACCC TGGAGCCTCC --GGGCCCTC GACCATGACC
H_corymbosa_Hed7            CCCGATCGAA GCCGTGGCTC TTGCCGACGC GGGGCGTGCT C-AAAGACCC TAGAGCCTCT CGAGGCCCTC GACCATGACC
H_coymbosa_Hed8             CCCGATCGAA GCCGTGGCTC TTGCCGACGC GGGGCGTGCT C-AAAGACCC TAGAGCCTCT CGAGGCCCTC GACTATGACC
Baihuasheshecao_Hed2        CCCGATCGAA GCCGTGGCTC TTGCCGACGC GGGGCGTGCT C-AAAGACCC TAGAGCCTCT CGAGGCCCTC GACTATGACC
Baihuasheshecao_Hed3        CCCGATCGAA GCCGTGGCTC TTGCCGACGC GGGGCGTGCT C-AAAGACCC TAGAGCCTCT CGAGGCCCTC GACTATGACC
Baihuasheshecao_Hed4        CCCGATCGAA GCCGTGGCTC TTGCCGACGC GGGGCGTGCT C-AAAGACCC TAGAGCCTCT CGAGGCCCTC GACTATGACC
AY438319                    CCCGATCGAA GCCGTGGCTC TTGCCGACGC GGGGCGTGCT C-AAAGACCC TAGAGCCTCT CGAGGCCCTC GACCATGACC
H_tenelliflora_Hten1        CTCGATCGTA GCCGTGACCG AGACCGTGCG GGAGACCCC- --ACAGACCC TGGAGCCTCC --GGGCCCTC GACCATGACC
Baihuasheshecao_Hed16       CTCGATCGTA GCCGTGACCG AGACCGTGCG GGAGACCCC- --ATAGACCC TGGAGCCTCC --GGGCCCTC GACCATGACC
H_pinifolia_Hpin1           CTCGATCGTG GCCGCGACCG AGACCGCGCG GGATAACTC- --AGAGACCC TGGAGCCTCC --GGGCCCTC GACCATGACC
H_aurricularia_Haur1        CTCGATCGAA GCCGTGACCG AATCCGTTCG GCAGAGCTCA CGCAAGACCC CAGAGCCTTC --GGGCCATC GACCATGACC
H_aurricularia_Haur2        CTCGATCGAA GCCGTGACCG AATCCGTTCG GCAGAGCTCA CGCAAGACCC CAGAGCCTTC --GGGCCATC GACCATGACC
H_hedyotidea_Hhed           CTCGATCGAA GCCGTGGCCG AAACCGTGCG GCGGTGCTCA CGGAAGACCC AGGAGCCTTC --GGGCCCTC GACCATGACC
H_costata_Hctt3             CTCGATCGAA GCCGTGACTG AAACCGTGCG GCAGAGCTCG CGATAGACCC TGGAGCCTTC --GGGCCCTC GACCATGACC
H_verticillata_Hve1         CTCGATCGTA GCCGTGACCG ATACCGTGCG GATGAACCC- --ATAGGCCC TGGAGCCTTC --GGGCCCTC GACCATGACC
H_verticillata_Hve2         CTCGATCGTA GCCGTGACCG ATACCGTGCG GATGAACCC- --ATAGACCC CGGAGCCTTC --GGGCCCTC GACCATGACC
H_biflora_Hbif2             CTCGATCGAA GCCGTGATTG AGCCCGTGCC GGAGATCTCC ---AAGACCC TGGAGCCTTG --TGGCCCTC GACCATGACC
H_effusa_Hef2               CTCGATCGGC GTCGTGTCTA AGCCCGTCGC GGAGCGTTCT C-CGAGACCC AGGAGCCTTG --AGGCCCTC GACAATGACC
H_consanguinea_Hcon1        CTCGATCGAA GCCGCGACGC TACCGACGGC GGGGCAACT- ---AAGACCC CGGAGCCCTC --GGGCCCTC GACAATGACC
H_acutangula_Hacu           CTCGATCGAA GCCGCGATGC GACCGACGGT GGGGCG-TCT ---AAGACCC CGGAGCCCTA --GGGCCCTC GACAATGACC
H_bracteosa_Hbr2            CTCGATCGAA GCCGCGACGC GACCGACGGC AGGGCG-TCT ---AACACCC CAGAGCCCTC --GGGTCCTC GACAATGACC
H_bracteosa_Hbr1            CTCGATCGAA GCCGCGACGC GACCGACGGC GGGGCG-TCT ---AAGACCC CGGAGCCCTT --GGGCCCTC GACAATGACC
H_yangchunensis_Hya1        CTCGATCCAA GCTGCGACGC GACCGACGGC GGGGCG-TCT ---AAGACCC TGGACCCTTC --GGGCCCTC GACAATGACC
H_yangchunensis_Hya2        CTCGATCCAA GCTGCGACGC GACCGACGGC GGGGCG-TCT ---AAGACCC CGGAGCCTTC --GGGCCCTC GACAATGACC
```

Fig. 10.2 *(Continued)*

conserved intraspecifically. The interspecific similarities among the 14 species ranged from 76.1% to 94.5%, which indicate that this region was variable enough for the differentiation of the *Hedyotis* species included in this study. The similarities between *H. diffusa*, and each of the adulterant species ranged from 83.2% to 90.7%. The interspecific polymorphisms among the ITS sequences of *H. diffusa*, *H. corymbosa*, *H. pinifolia* and *H. tenelliflora* were useful to differentiate *H. diffusa*, the biological origin of the genuine medicinal materials of Baihuasheshecao, from the adulterant species and other reference species.

10.3.3 FINS Identification of Commodities

Program

- Molecular Evolutionary Genetics Analysis (MEGA, European Bioinformatics Institute, Cambridgeshire, UK)

Procedures

1. Load multiple sequence alignment of the complete ITS region in the computer program MEGA version 2.1 (Kumar, Tamura, Jakobsen & Nei, 2001).
2. Procedures of phylogenetic tree construction have been described in Chapter 4.
3. Construct a neighbour-joining tree (Figure 10.3) to reveal the identities of the seven commodity samples.

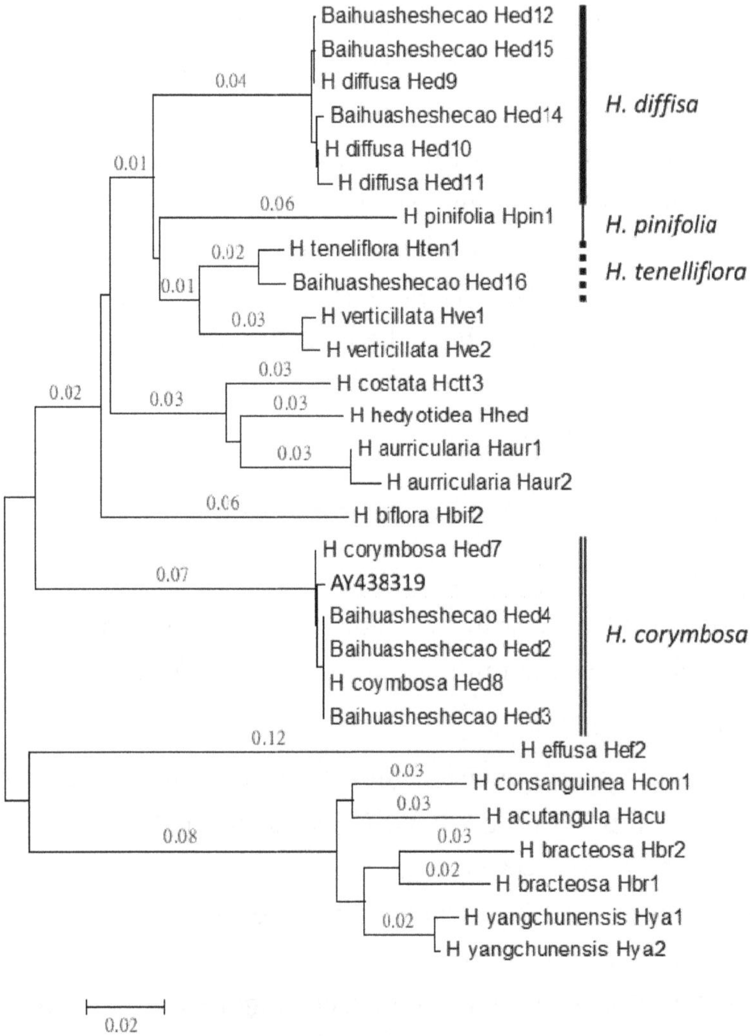

Fig. 10.3 Neighbour-joining phylogram based on the complete ITS region of the authentic *Hedyotis* samples and Baihuasheshecao commodities in this study. The numbers above branches and the scale represent the branch length, which is hidden when <0.01. The abbreviations are sample labels. Details of the samples are given in Table 10.3.

Findings

All *Hedyotis* species form distinct clades, suggesting that a neighbor-joining tree constructed based on the ITS region could successfully differentiate the *Hedyotis* species used in this study, including the genuine source species *H. diffusa* and the three commonly used adulterant species *H. corymbosa*, *H. pinifolia* and *H. tenelliflora* (Figure 10.3). Among the seven commodity samples, three samples (Hed12, Hed14 and Hed15) were clustered with *H. diffusa*, three samples (Hed2, Hed3 and Hed4) were clustered with *H. corymbose*, and one commodity (Hed16) was clustered with *H. tenelliflora*.

10.4 Conclusion

Multiple Sequence Alignment and the neighbour-joining tree demonstrated that ITS region is a good DNA locus for the differentiation of the genuine species *H. diffusa* from the adulterating species *H. corymbose*, *H. tenelliflora*, and *H. pinifolia*. The neighbour-joining tree constructed based on the ITS region can readily identify the biological origins of the seven commodity samples. Three of them are genuine Baihuasheshecao derives from *H. diffusa,* and the four other commodities belong to the closely related species *H. corymbose* and *H. tenelliflora*. None of them comes from *H. pinifolia*. In conclusion, FINS is a useful technique for the identification of Baihuasheshecao.

References

Alvarez, I., & Wendel, J. F. (2003). Ribosomal ITS sequences and plant phylogenetic inference. *Mol Phylogenet Evol, 29*, 417–434.

Baldwin, B. G., Sanderson, M. J., Porter, J. M., Wojciechowski, M. F., Campbell, C. S., & Donoghue, M. J. (1995). The ITS region of nuclear ribosomal DNA: A valuable source of evidence on angiosperm phylogeny. *Ann Mo Bot Gard, 82*, 247–277.

Bartlett, S. E., & Davidson, W. S. (1992). FINS (forensically informative nucleotide sequencing): A procedure for identifying the animal origin of biological specimens. *BioTechniques, 12*, 408–411.

Bhargava, M., & Sharma, A. (2013). DNA barcoding in plants: Evolution and applications of in silico approaches and resources. *Mol Phylogenet Evol, 67*(3), 631–641. doi:10.1016/j.ympev.2013.03.002

Cao, S., Guo, L., Luo, H., Yuan, H., Chen, S., Zheng, J., & Lin, R. (2016). Application of COI barcode sequence for the identification of snake medicine (Zaocys). *Mitochondrial DNA A DNA Mapp Seq Anal, 27*(1), 483–489. doi: 10.3109/19401736.2014.905828

CBOL Plant Working Group. (2009). A DNA barcode for land plants. *Proc Nat Acad Sci USA, 106*, 12794–12797.

Chan, W. H., Ling, K. H., Chiu, S. W., Shaw, P.C., & But, P. P. H. (2011). Molecular analyses of Cordyceps gunnii in China. *J Food Drug Anal, 19*, 18–25.

Chen, N., Zhao, S. J., & Han, L. P. (2008). DNA molecular identification of one snake crude venom used for production. *Shi Zhen Guo Yi Guo Yao, 19*, 1578–1580.

Chen, Q., Wu, X., & Zhang, D. (2020). Comparison of the abilities of universal, super, and specific DNA barcodes to discriminate among the original species of Fritillariae cirrhosae bulbus and its adulterants. *PLoS One, 15*(2), e0229181. doi:10.1371/journal.pone.0229181

Chen, S., Yao, H., Han, J., Liu, C., Song, J., Shi, L., Zhu, Y., Ma, X., Gao, T., Pang, X., Luo, K., Li, Y., Li, X., Jia, X., Lin, Y., & Leon, C. (2010). Validation of the ITS2 region as a novel DNA barcode for identifying medicinal plant species. *PLoS One, 5*, e8613.

Cheng, X. L., Liao, C. L., Liu, C. S., Bai, Z. F., Yang, Y. J., Zheng, J., & Zhang, J. (2012). DNA identification of Zijingpi's adulterant species Schisandra sphenanthera based on NCBI nucleotide database analysis. *Zhongguo Zhong Yao Za Zhi, 37*(17), 2534–2537.

Cho, Y., Mower, J. P., Qiu, Y. L., & Palmer, J. D. (2004). Mitochondrial substitution rates are extraordinarily elevated and variable in a genus of flowering plants. *Proc Nat Acad Sci USA, 101*, 17741–17746.

Chowdhury, B., & Garai, G. (2017). A review on multiple sequence alignment from the perspective of genetic algorithm. *Genomics, 109*(5–6), 419–431. doi:10.1016/j.ygeno.2017.06.007

Ding, X. Y., Wang, Z. T., Xu, H., Xu, L. S., & Zhou, K. Y. (2002). Database establishment of the whole rDNA ITS region of Dendrobium species of "fengdou" and authentication by analysis of their sequences. *Yao Xue Xue Bao, 37*, 567–573.

Essoussi, N., Boujenfa, K., & Limam, M. (2008), A comparison of MSA tools. *Bioinformation, 2*(10), 452–455. doi:10.6026/97320630002452

Forrest, A. R., & Carnegie, P. R. (1994). Identification of gourmet meat using FINS (forensically informative nucleotide sequencing). *BioTechniques, 17*, 24–26.

Girish, P. S., Anjaneyulu, A. S. R., Viswas, K. N., Anand, M., Rajkumar, N. B., Shivakumar, B. M., & Bhaskar, S. (2004). Sequence analysis of mitochondrial 12S rRNA gene can identify meat species. *Meat Sci, 66*, 551–556.

Hajibabaei, M., deWaard, J. R., Ivanova, N. V., Ratnasingham, S., Dooh, R. T., Kirk, S. L., Mackie, P. M., & Hebert, P. D. (2005). Critical factors for assembling a high volume of DNA barcodes. *Phil Trans R Soc B, 360*, 1959–1967.

Hall, T. A. (1999) BioEdit: A user-friendly biological sequence alignment editor and analysis program for Windows 95/98/NT. *Nucleic Acid Symp. 41*, 95–98.

Hebert, P. D., Cywinska, A., Ball, S. L., & deWaard, J. R. (2003). Biological identifications through DNA barcodes. *Proc Biol Sci, 270*, 313–321.

Hou, D. Y., Song, J. Y., Shi, L. C., Yang, P., Chen, S. L., & Yao, H. (2013). Molecular identification of Cynomorii herba using ITS2 DNA barcoding. *Zhongguo Zhong Yao Za Zhi, 38*(23), 4028–4032.

Hsieh, H. M., Huang, L. H., Tsai, L. C., Kuo, Y. C., Meng, H. H., Linacre, A., & Lee, J. C. (2003). Species identification of rhinoceros horns using the cytochrome b gene. *Forensic Sci Int, 136*, 1–11.

Kang, H. W., Cho, Y. G., Yoon, U. H., & Eun, M. Y. (1998). A rapid DNA extraction method for RFLP and PCR analysis from a single dry seed. *Plant Mol Bio Rep, 1998, 16*, 1–9.

Kapli, P., Yang, Z., & Telford, M. J. (2020). Phylogenetic tree building in the genomic age. *Nat Rev Genet, 21*(7), 428–444. doi:10.1038/s41576-020-0233-0

Ko, W. C. (1999). Hedyotis. In Luo, X. R. (Ed.), *Rubiaceae, Flora Republicae Popularis Sinicae. 71*(1), (pp. 32–77). Beijing: Science Press.

Kress, W. J., Wurdack, K. J., Zimmer, E. A., Weigt, L. A., & Janzen, D. H. (2005). Use of DNA barcodes to identify flowering plants. *Proc Nat Acad Sci USA, 102*, 8369–8374.

Kumar, S., Tamura, K., Jakobsen, I. B., & Nei, M. (2001) MEGA2: Molecular evolutionary genetics analysis software. *Bioinformatics, 17*(12), 1244–1245. doi:10.1093/bioinformatics/17.12.1244

Lago, F. C., Herrero, B., Vieites, J. M., & Espiñeira, M. (2011). Genetic identification of horse mackerel and related species in seafood products by means of forensically informative nucleotide sequencing methodology. *J Agric Food Chem, 59*(6), 2223–2228.

Li, M., Au, K. Y., Lam, H., Cheng, L., But, P. P. H., & Shaw, P. C. (2014). Molecular identification and in vitro cytotoxicity study of traditional Chinese medicines that are commonly confused with Aristolochia species. *Food Chem, 147*, 332–339.

Li, M., Au, K. Y., Lam, H., Cheng, L., Jiang, R. W., But, P. P. H., & Shaw, P. C. (2012a). Identification of Baiying (Herba Solani Lyrati) commodity and its toxic substitute Xungufeng (Herba Aristolochiae Mollissimae) using DNA barcoding and chemical profiling techniques. *Food Chem, 135*(3), 1653–1658.

Li, M., Cao, H., But, P. P. H., & Shaw, P. C. (2011a). Identification of herbal medicinal materials using DNA barcodes. *J Syst Evol, 49*(3), 271–283.

Li, M., Jiang, R. W., Hon, P. M., Cheng, L., Zhou, J. R., Li, L. L., P. C. Shaw, & But, P. P. H. (2010a). Authentication of the anti-tumor herb Baihuasheshecao with bioactive marker compounds and molecular sequences. *Food Chem, 119*(3), 1239–1245.

Li, M., Ling, K. H., Lam, H., Shaw, P. C., Cheng, L., Techen, N., Khan, I. A., Chang, Y. S., & But, P. P. H. (2010b). Cardiocrinum seeds as a replacement for Aristolochia fruits in treating cough. *J Ethnopharmacol, 130*, 4nn29–432.

Li, M., Wong, K. L., Chan, W. H., Li, J. X., But, P. P. H., Cao, H., & Shaw, P. C. (2012b). Establishment of DNA barcodes for the identification of the botanical sources of the Chinese 'cooling' beverage. *Food Control, 25*(2), 758–766.

Li, M., Zhang, K. Y., But, P. P., & Shaw, P. C. (2011b). Forensically informative nucleotide sequencing (FINS) for the authentication of Chinese medicinal materials. *Chin Med, 6*, 42. doi:10.1186/1749-8546-6-42

Liu, X. Z., Zhou, L. S., Liu, J. X., Jia, J., Song, J. Y., & Shi, L. C. (2017). Identification of water buffalo horn and its adulterants using COI barcode. *Yao Xue Xue Bao*, 52(3), 494–499.

Liu, Z. W., Gao, Y. Z., & Zhou, J. (2019). Molecular authentication of the medicinal species of Ligusticum (Ligustici Rhizoma et Radix, 'Gao-ben') by integrating non-coding Internal Transcribed Spacer 2 (ITS2) and its secondary structure. *Front Plant Sci, 10*, 429.

Lo, Y. T., Li, M., & Shaw, P. C. (2015). Identification of constituent herbs in ginseng decoctions by DNA markers. *Chin Med, 10*(1), 1.

Lou, S. K., Wong, K. L., Li, M., But, P. P. H., Tsui, K. W., & Shaw, P. C. (2010). An integrated web medicinal materials DNA database: MMDBD (Medicinal Materials DNA Barcode Database). *BMC Genomics, 11*(1), 402.

Lv, P., Zhou, X., You, J., Ye, B. C., & Zhang, Y. (2009). Extraction of trace amount of severely degraded DNA. *Z Naturforsch C, 64*, 581–589.

Lv, T., Teng, R., Shao, Q., Wang, H., Zhang, W., Li, M., & Zhang, L. (2015). DNA barcodes for the identification of Anoectochilus roxburghii and its adulterants. *Planta, 242*(5), 1167–1174. doi:10.1007/s00425-015-2353-x

Mitchell, S. E., Cockburn, A. F., & Seawright, J. A. (1993). The mitochondrial genome of Anopheles quadrimaculatus species A: Complete nucleotide sequence and gene organization. *Genome, 36*, 1058–1073.

Nilsson, R. H., Ryberg, M., Kristiansson, E., Abarenkov, K., Larsson, K. H., & Koljalg, U. (2006). Taxonomic reliability of DNA sequences in public sequence databases: A fungal perspective. *PLoS One,* 1, e59.

Pais, F. S., Ruy, P. C., Oliveira, G., & Coimbra, R. S. (2014). Assessing the efficiency of multiple sequence alignment programs. *Algorithms Mol Biol,* 9(1), 4. doi:10.1186/1748-7188-9-4

Pang, X., Song, J., Xu, H., & Yao, H. (2012). Using ITS2 barcode to identify ephedrae herba. *Zhongguo Zhong Yao Za Zhi, 37*(8), 1118–1121.

Pervez, M. T., Babar, M. E., Nadeem, A., Aslam, M., Awan, A. R., Aslam, N., Hussain, T., Naveed, N., Qadri, S., Waheed, U., & Shoaib, M. (2014). Evaluating the accuracy and efficiency of multiple sequence alignment methods. *Evol Bioinform, 10*, 205–217. doi:10.4137/EBO.S19199

Pharmacopoeia Commission of the Ministry of Public Health, People's Republic of China. (2005). *Pharmacopoeia of the People's Republic of China.* Beijing, China: Chemical Industry Press. pp. 29, 141–142, Appendix III p. 22.

Prendini, L., Hanner, R., & DeSalle, R. (2002). Obtaining, storing and archiving specimens and tissue samples for use in molecular studies. In DeSalle, R., Giribet, G., & Wheeler, W. C. (Eds.). *Techniques in Molecular Evolution and Systematics* (pp. 176–248). Switzerland, Basel: Birkhaeuser Verlag AG.

Rajpoot, A., Kumar, V. P., Bahuguna, A., & Kumar, D. (2017). Forensically informative nucleotide sequencing (FINS) for the first time authentication of Indian Varanus species: Implication in wildlife forensics and conservation. *Mitochondrial DNA A DNA Mapp Seq Anal, 28*(6), 892–900. doi:10.1080/24701394.2016.1202943

Sahajpal, V., & Goyal, S. P. (2009). Identification of a forensic case using microscopy and forensically informative nucleotide sequencing (FINS): A case study of small Indian civet (Viverricula indica). *Sci Justice, 50*, 94–97.

Santamaria, M., Vicario, S., Pappadà, G., Scioscia, G., Scazzocchio, C., Saccone, C. (2009). Towards barcode markers in Fungi: An intron map of *Ascomycota* mitochondria. *BMC Bioinform, 10*(Suppl 6), S15.

Schmitt, I., & Barker, F. K. (2009). Phylogenetic methods in natural product research. *Nat Prod Rep, 26*, 1585–1602.

Shao, S. G., Han, L., Ma, Y. H., Shen, J., Zhang, W. C., & Ding, X. Y. (2009). Analysis and authentication of cpDNA psbA-trnH regions of Dendrobium species of fengdous. *Yao Xue Xue Bao, 44*, 1173–1178.

Shendure, J., Balasubramanian, S., Church, G. M., Gilbert, W., Rogers, J., Schloss, J. A., & Waterston, R. H. (2019). DNA sequencing at 40: Past, present and future. *Nature, 550*(7676), 345–353. doi:10.1038/nature24286

Shi, Y., Zhao, M., Yao, H., Yang, P., Xin, T., Li, B., Sun, W., & Chen, S. (2017). Rapidly discriminate commercial medicinal Pulsatilla chinensis (Bge.) Regel from its adulterants using ITS2 barcoding and specific PCR-RFLP assay. *Sci Rep, 7*, 40000. doi:10.1038/srep40000

Singh, G., Srinivas, Y., Kumar, G. C., Singh, A., Sharma, C. P., & Gupta, S. K. (2020). Identification of selected wild felids using hair morphology and forensically informative nucleotide sequencing (FINS): Wildlife forensics prospective. *Legal Medicine* (Tokyo, Japan), *44*, 101692.doi:10.1016/j.legalmed.2020.101692

Sogin, M. L. (1990). Amplification of ribosomal RNA genes for molecular evolution studies. In Innis, M., Gelfand, D. H., Sninksky, J. (Eds.). *PCR Protocols: A Guide to Methods and Application* (p. 307). Academic Press, San Diego.

State Pharmacopoeia Commission of People's Republic of China. (2010). *Pharmacopoeia of the People's Republic of China*. China, Beijing: Chemical Industry Press.

Su, Y. Y., Li, W. J., Yang, L., Ding, D. D., & Xiang, L. (2019). Rapid identification of Cordyceps and its products using DNA barcoding method. *Zhongguo Zhong Yao Za Zhi, 44*(10), 1965–1973. doi:10.19540/j.cnki.cjcmm.20190131.002

Taberlet, P., Gielly, L., Pautou, G., & Bouvet, J. (1991). Universal primers for amplification of three non-coding regions of chloroplast DNA. *Plant Mol Biol, 17*, 1105–1109.

Techen, N., Parveen, I., Pan, Z., & Khan, I. A. (2014). DNA barcoding of medicinal plant material for identification. *Curr Opin Biotechnol, 25*, 103–110. doi:10.1016/j.copbio.2013.09.010

Teletchea, F., Maudet, C., & Hanni, C. (2005). Food and forensic molecular identification: Update and challenges. *Trends Biotechnol, 23*, 359–366.

Thakur, M., Singh, S. K., Shukla, M., Sharma, L. K., Mohan, N., Goyal, S. P., & Sathyakumar, S. (2013). Identification of Galliformes through forensically informative nucleotide sequencing (FINS) and its implication in wildlife forensics. *J Forensics Res*, *4*(4), 1–5.

Verma, S. K., & Singh, L. (2003). Novel universal primers establish identity of an enormous number of animal species for forensic application. *Mol Eco Notes, 3*, 28–31.

Vilgalys, R. (2003). Taxonomic misidentification in public DNA databases. *New Phytol, 160*, 4–5.

Wang, F. G., & Ye, H. J. (2003) Medicinal herbs of Guangdong Hedyotis species (廣東省耳草屬葯用植物資源). *Zhong Yao Cai, 26*(8), 547–548.

White, T. J., Burns, T., Lee, S., & Taylor, J. W. (1990). Amplification and direct sequencing of fungal ribosomal RNA genes for phylogenetics. In Innis, M. A., Gelfand, D. H., Sninsky, J. J., & White, T. J. (Eds.). *PCR Protocols: A Guide to Methods and Applications* (pp. 315–322). New York, NY: Academic Press.

Wolfe, K. H., Li, W. H., & Sharp, P. M. (1987). Rates of nucleotide substitution vary greatly among plant mitochondrial, chloroplast, and nuclear DNAs. *Proc Nat Acad Sci USA, 84*, 9054–9058.

Wong, K. L., Wang, J., But, P. P. H., & Shaw, P. C. (2004). Application of cytochrome b DNA sequences for the authentication of endangered snake species. *Forensic Sci Int, 139*, 49–55.

Wong, T. H., But, G. W. C., Wu, H. Y., Tsang, S. S. K., Lau, D. T. W., & Shaw, P. C. (2018). Medicinal Materials DNA Barcode Database (MMDBD) version 1.5 — one-stop solution for storage, BLAST, alignment and primer design. *Database, 2018*, 112. doi:10.1093/database/bay112

Wu, H., Wan, Q. H., Fang, S. G., & Zhang, S. Y. (2005). Application of mitochondrial DNA sequence analysis in the forensic identification of Chinese sika deer subspecies. *Forensic Sci Int, 148*, 101–105.

Xing, Y. P., Chen, S. Y., Xu, L., Liang, Y. M., Wang, J. H., Wang, B., Liu, T., & Kang, T. G. (2018). Study on high throughput sequencing identification of Fructus Arctii and five counterfeit species mix power. *Zhongguo Zhong Yao Za Zhi, 43*(19), 3862–3866. doi: 10.19540/j.cnki.cjcmm.20180703.012

Xiong, B., Zhao, Z. L., Ni, L. H., Gaawe, D., & Mi, M. (2005). DNA-based identification of Gentiana robusta and related species. *Zhongguo Zhong Yao Za Zhi, 40*(23), 4680–4685.

Yu, J., Li, M., Guo, X., Wang, R. J., Chiu, S. W., Shaw, P. C., & But, P. P. H. (2012). Value of FINS depends on choice of DNA locus as shown in Baihuasheshecao. *J Food Drug Anal, 20*(4), 879–886.

Yu, N., Wei, Y. L., Zhu, Y., Zhu, N., Wang, Y. L., Zhang, H. P., & Sun, A. D. (2018). Integrated approach for identifying and evaluating the quality of Marsdenia tenacissima in the medicine market. *PLoS One, 13*(4), e0195240. doi:10.1371/journal.pone.0195240

Zhang, G., Liu, J., Gao, M., Kong, W., Zhao, Q., Shi, L., & Wang, Q. (2020). Tracing the edible and medicinal plant pueraria montana and its products in the marketplace yields subspecies level distinction using DNA barcoding and DNA metabarcoding. *Front Pharmacol, 11*, 336. doi:10.3389/fphar.2020.00336

Zhang, G. X., Jin, Y., Jia, J., Song, J. Y., Shi, L. C., & Chen, S. L. (2016). Identification of Notopterygium seeds using DNA barcoding method. *Zhongguo Zhong Yao Za Zhi, 41*(3), 390–395. doi:10.4268/cjcmm20160305

Zhang, X. Q., Liu, C. S., Yan, X. L., Cheng, X. L., Liu, J., Wang, Q. L., Liu, K., & Wei, S. L. (2013) Sequence analysis and identification of a chloroplast matK gene in Rhei Rhizoma from different botanical origins. *Yao Xue Xue Bao, 48*(11), 1722–1728.

Zhang, Y. B., Jiang, R. W., Li, S. L., Qiao, C. F., Han, Q. B., Xu, H. X., Wong, K. L., But, P. P. H., & Shaw, P. C. (2007). Chemical and molecular characterization of Hong Dangshen, a unique medicinal material for diarrhea in Hong Kong. *J Chin Pharm Sci, 16*, 202–207.

Zhang, Y. Q., Shi, Y., Song, M., Lin, Y. H., Ma, X. X., Sun, W., Xiang, L., & Liu, X. (2014). Identification of pyrrosiae folium and its adulterants based on psbA-trnH sequence. *Zhongguo Zhong Yao Za Zhi, 39*(12), 2222–2226.

Zheng, S., Liu, D., Ren, W., Fu, J., Huang, L., & Chen, S. (2014). Integrated analysis for identifying radix astragali and its adulterants based on DNA barcoding. *Evid Based Complement Alternat Med, 2014*, 843923. doi:10.1155/2014/843923

Zhu, Y. J., Chen, S. L., Yao, H., Tan, R., Song, J. Y., Luo, K., & Lu, J. (2010). DNA barcoding the medicinal plants of the genus Paris. *Yao Xue Xue Bao, 45*, 376–382.

Chapter 11

DNA Barcoding as a Standard Molecular Authentication Technique

Hui Yao, Jian-Ping Han, Xiaohui Pang, Lin-Chun Shi, Li Xiang, Xi-Wen Li, Chao Xiong, Jing-Yuan Song & Shi-Lin Chen

11.1 Introduction

Many kinds of medicinal materials such as roots, barks, leaves, flowers, fruits and seeds can be used as Materia medica. Owing to similar morphology, medicinal materials are often confused with some closely related species or adulterants. It is urgently needed to establish an accurate and rapid identification method to distinguish medicinal materials from their adulterants.

DNA barcoding is a species identification technology based on species-specific differences in the standard short regions of nucleus and organelle DNA (Hebert, Cywinska, Ball & de Waard, 2003). Compared with the use of morphological characteristics and physiological conditions, DNA barcoding allows species identification without specialised taxonomic knowledge and is standardised by using specific DNA barcodes and universal primers. This method is beneficial for building databases and establishing a universal standard for identification. DNA barcoding can rapidly, accurately and automatedly identify species from a diverse range of raw materials. Key studies in the DNA barcoding of medicinal materials include the establishment of a DNA barcoding system for medicinal materials, key technologies of the DNA barcoding system and directions for future research on the DNA barcoding of medicinal materials (Chen *et al.*, 2014). Guidelines for DNA barcoding of Chinese Materia Medica have been initially listed in the *Pharmacopoeia of the People's Republic of China* in 2014. The DNA barcoding of medicinal materials has been listed in the British Pharmacopoeia and United States Pharmacopoeia in 2017 and 2019, respectively. Moreover, identification of crude drugs in the Japanese Pharmacopoeia using a DNA barcoding system was reported (Chen *et al.*, 2017), and a DNA barcode reference library has been established to monitor medicinal materials in the Korean Pharmacopeia (Liu *et al.*, 2017a).

The DNA sequence of each species is unique, and each position in the DNA sequence has four base choices of A, T, G and C. The 15 bp DNA sequence has 4^{15} kinds of codes that can theoretically encode all species on earth. The ideal DNA barcode should meet the following criteria: (1) It must have sufficient variability to distinguish different species that are relatively conservative within species. The sequence used as a DNA barcode must have relatively large differences between species and low sequence variation within species to ensure a clear definition of barcoding gap. (2) Standard short fragments, that is, the sequence exists in most taxa and is sufficient to complete one reaction of the sequencing work and facilitate DNA extraction and PCR amplification, especially for materials with DNA degradation (such as long-preserved wax leaf specimens). (3) The two ends of the sequence are relatively conserved to design the universal primers. In this chapter, the general principles and detailed protocols of DNA barcoding for the identification of medicinal materials are described.

11.2 Materials and Methods

11.2.1 Materials

Medicinal materials from radix et rhizome (Plant-1~Plant-3), cortex (Plant-4), whole herb (Plant-5~Plant-6), flower (Plant-7~Plant-21), fruits and seeds (Plant-22~Plant-31), materials from fungi origin (Fungi-1~Fungi-2), materials from animal origin (Animal-1~Animal-14) were collected from different places in China, United States, Canada and Mexico. Some sequences were downloaded from GenBank. Detailed information is listed in Table 11.1.

11.2.2 Total Genomic DNA Preparation

After the plant and fungi samples were ground into fine powder by using a Retsch MM 400 laboratory mixer mill (Retsch Co., Haan, Germany) at a frequency of 30 Hz, the powder was collected to extract DNA by using the Plant Genome DNA Kit (Tiangen Biotech Co., Beijing, China) in accordance with the manufacturer's instructions. Polyvinylpyrrolidone (PVP) (10%) was used to remove polyphenols.

The DNA of 93 animal horns (10 mg each of Animal-1~Animal-5) was directly extracted using the Column bone DNA out kit (Tianenze, Beijing, China). The DNA of four raw animal samples of *Bungarus multicinctus* and 37 medicinal materials of Bungarus Parvus (10 mg each of Animal-6~Animal-9) were directly extracted using the DNeasy Blood & Tissue Kit (Qiagen, Germantown). The DNA of fresh leg muscle samples of Ranae oviductus (Hamayou) and its adulterants (10 mg each of Animal-10~Animal-14) were directly extracted using the DNeasy Blood & Tissue Kit (Qiagen). For Ranae oviductus (Hamayou) and its adulterants, 5 mg of dry medicinal materials (Animal-10~Animal-14) was first

Table 11.1 Samples Information of Medicinal Materials

Sample category	Family	Species	Medicinal part	Number of sample	Place of collection
Plant-1	Araliaceae	*Panax ginseng*	Radix et rhizoma	81	Ning'an, Heilongjiang; Fusong, Ji'an, Jingyu, Dunhua, Changbai, Hunchun, Tonghua, Wangqing, Antu of Jilin province; Xinbin, Kuandian, Qingyuan of Liaoning province; Shanghai pharmacy; Hong Kong pharmacy
Plant-2	Araliaceae	*Panax quiquefolius*	Radix et rhizoma	65	Muleng, Ning'an of Heilongjiang province; Ji'an, Jingyu, Fusong, Tonghua of Jilin province; Qingyuan, Xinbin of Liaoning province; Beijing; Wendeng, Shandong, China; Canada
Plant-3	Araliaceae	*Panax notoginseng*	Radix et rhizoma	29	Wenshan, Yunnan; Tongrentang pharmacy, Beijing; Jinglongtang pharmacy, Beijing; Yong'antang pharmacy, Beijing; Zhongweishenzhou pharmacy, Beijing; Yong'antang pharmacy, Beijing; Ji'antang pharmacy, Beijing; Hongshengtang pharmacy, Beijing; Haodekuai pharmacy, Beijing

Plant-4	Araliaceae	*Eleutherococcus nodiflorus*	Dried cortex	7	Beijing; Shijiazhuang, Hebei; Tianjin; Wuhan, Hubei; Guangzhou, Guangdong
Plant-5	Campanulaceae	*Lobelia chinensis*	Dried herb	7	Anguo herbal market, Hebei; Beijing; Yulin, Guangxi
Plant-6	Labiatae	*Scutellaria barbata*	Dried herb	10	Beijing; Anguo herbal market, Hebei
Plant-7	Caprifoliaceae	*Lonicera japonica*	Flower	6	Urumqi Botanical Garden, Xinjiang; Jiaozuo, Henan; Lin'an, Zhejiang; Jilin City, Jilin
Plant-8	Caprifoliaceae	*Lonicera macranthoides*	Flower	8	Xuanen County, Hubei; Wugang, Hunan; Shaoguan, Guangdong
Plant-9	Caprifoliaceae	*Lonicera fulvotomentosa*	Flower	6	Anlong County, Guizhou; Ruili County, Yunnan
Plant-10	Caprifoliaceae	*Lonicera hypoglauca*	Flower	3	Lishui, Zhejiang
Plant-11	Caprifoliaceae	*Lonicera confusa*	Flower	2	Guangdong, Guangdong
Plant-12	Caprifoliaceae	*Lonicera caerulea*	Flower	3	Urumqi, Xinjiang
Plant-13	Caprifoliaceae	*Lonicera canadensis*	Flower	3	Maine, United States
Plant-14	Caprifoliaceae	*Lonicera fragrantissima*	Flower	3	Jinan, Shandong

(*Continued*)

Table 11.1 (*Continued*)

Sample category	Family	Species	Medicinal part	Number of sample	Place of collection
Plant-15	Caprifoliaceae	*Lonicera hirsuta*	Flower	3	Vermont, United States
Plant-16	Caprifoliaceae	*Lonicera hispida*	Flower	3	Baoji, Shaanxi, China; United States
Plant-17	Caprifoliaceae	*Lonicera involucrata*	Flower	3	Chihuahua, Mexico
Plant-18	Caprifoliaceae	*Lonicera maackii*	Flower	3	Lijiang, Yunnan; Shenyang, Liaoning
Plant-19	Caprifoliaceae	*Lonicera rupicola*	Flower	3	Shangri-La County, Yunnan; Ganzi, Sichuan; Guyuan, Ningxia
Plant-20	Caprifoliaceae	*Lonicera similis*	Flower	3	Leshan, Sichuan
Plant-21	Caprifoliaceae	*Lonicera villosa*	Flower	3	Connecticut, United States
Plant-22	Leguminosae	*Astragalus complanatus*	Seed	3	Bozhou, Anhui; Guangzhou, Guangdong; Yulin, Guangxi
Plant-23	Cruciferae	*Descurainia sophia*	Seed	3	Shiyan, Hubei; Chengdu, Sichuan; Yulin, Guangxi
Plant-24	Cruciferae	*Lepidium apetalum*	Seed	3	Urumqi, Xinjiang; Changbaishan, Jilin; Anguo, Hebei
Plant-25	Solanaceae	*Hyoscyamus niger*	Seed	26	Beijing; Xishuangbanna, Yunan; Shennongjia, Hubei

Plant-26	Balsaminaceae	*Impatiens balsamina.*	Seed	5	Shennongjia, Hubei; Guangzhou, Guangdong; Beijing
Plant-27	Plantaginaceae	*Plantago asiatica*	Seed	3	Lushan, Jiangxi; Xinglong, Hainan; Nanning, Guangxi
Plant-28	Plantaginaceae	*Plantago depressa*	Seed	3	Changbaishan, Jilin; Zhuozhou, Hebei; Beijing
Plant-29	Convolvulaceae	*Cuscuta australis*	Seed	7	Beijing; Yulin, Guangxi; Chifeng, Inner Mongolia
Plant-30	Convolvulaceae	*Cuscuta chinensis*	Seed	4	Haikou, Hainan; Wuhan, Hubei; Xingyi, Guizhou
Plant-31	Amaranthaceae	*Celosia argentea*	Seed	3	Changzhou, Jiangsu; Beijing; Lushan, Jiangxi
Fungi-1	Ophiocordycipitaceae	*Ophiocordyceps sinensis*	Whole	10	Yichang, Hubei; Hongyuan, Sichuan; Xining, Qinghai; Naqu, Tibet; Dangdui, Tibet; Kangding, Sichuan; Baqing, Tibet
Fungi-2	Polyporaceae	*Ganoderma lucidum*	Fruiting body	10	Heihe, Heilongjiang; Tianjin; Guangzhou pharmacy; Anguo herbal market, Hebei; Liaocheng, Shandong; Taiwan
Animal-1	Bovidae	*Bos grunniens*	Horn	13	Kangding, Sichuan; Xining, Qinghai; Tianzhu, Gansu
Animal-2	Bovidae	*Bos Taurus*	Horn	14	Xinxiang, Henan; Bengbu, Anhui; Jining, Shandong

(*Continued*)

Table 11.1 (*Continued*)

Sample category	Family	Species	Medicinal part	Number of sample	Place of collection
Animal-3	Bovidae	*Bubalus bubalis*	Horn	20	Liuzhou, Guangxi; Yangjiang, Guangdong; Hengyang, Hunan
Animal-4	Bovidae	*Capra hircus*	Horn	28	Xinxiang, Henan; Bengbu, Anhui; Jining, Shandong
Animal-5	Bovidae	*Ovis aries*	Horn	18	Xinxiang, Henan; Bengbu, Anhui; Jining, Shandong
Animal-6	Elapidae	*Bungarus multicinctus*	Body	46	Bozhou, Anhui; Yulin, Guangxi; Chengdu, Sichuan; GenBank
Animal-7	Elapidae	*Bungarus fasciatus*	Body	3	GenBank
Animal-8	Colubridae	*Lycodon rufozonatus*	Body	9	Yulin, Guangxi; Anguo, Hebei; Lhasa, Xizang
Animal-9	Colubridae	*Sinonatrix annularis*	Body	2	Yulin, Guangxi
Animal-10	Bufonidae	*Bufo gargarizans Cantor*	Fallopian tube	6	Shunyi, Beijing; Yancheng, Jiangsu

Animal-11	Ranidae	*Pelophylax nigromaculatus Hallowell*	Fallopian tube	3	Chengdu, Sichuan; Jixi, Heilongjiang
Animal-12	Ranidae	*Rana amurensis Boulenger*	Fallopian tube	5	Jixi, Yichun, Heilongjiang
Animal-13	Ranidae	*Rana chensinensis David*	Fallopian tube	12	Chengde, Hebei; Hulun Buir, Inner Mongolia
Animal-14	Ranidae	*Rana dybowskii Günther*	Fallopian tube	83	Haerbin, Jixi, Yichun, Heilongjiang; Baishan, Jilin city, Yanbian, Jilin; Benxi, Fushun, Yingkou, Liaoning

infiltrated with FB solution (refer to the Chinese patent: no. ZL 201610903601.2) and then homogenised using a grinding pestle.

Equipment

- Centrifuge
- Water bath
- Bead mill

Reagents

- Ethanol, 100%
- Isopropanol
- Tiangen Plant Genome DNA Kit:
    - Buffer GP1
    - Buffer GD
    - Buffer PW

Procedures

1. Pre-warm the buffer GP1 at 65°C prior to extraction. Add absolute ethanol to buffer GD and buffer PW before use.
2. After the plant and fungi samples are ground into fine powder by using a Retsch MM 400 laboratory mixer mill (Retsch Co.) at a frequency of 30 Hz, put the fine powder of materials (20 mg of Plant-1~Plant-3, 30 mg of Plant-4~Plant-6, fungi-2, 25 mg dry flower bud of Plant-7~Plant-21, 50 mg of Plant-22~Plant-31, 20–30 mg single dry stroma of fungi-1) in a 2-mL centrifuge tube. Ten percent PVP was used to remove polyphenols. Add 700 μL of 65°C preheating buffer GP1 into the centrifuge tube and mix quickly. Place the centrifuge tube in a 65°C water bath for 2 h.
3. Add 700 μL of chloroform-isoamyl alcohol (24:1), mix well and centrifuge at 12,000 rpm for 5 min.

4. Carefully transfer the upper aqueous phase from the previous step into a new centrifuge tube. Add 0.7× volume of isopropanol, mix well and let it stand at –20°C for 20 min.
5. Transfer the mixed liquid to the spin column CB3, centrifuge at 12,000 rpm for 30 s and discard the waste liquid.
6. Add 500 μL of buffer GD to the spin column CB3, centrifuge at 12,000 rpm for 30 s, discard the waste liquid and put the spin column CB3 into the collection tube.
7. Add 700 μL of buffer PW to the spin column CB3, centrifuge at 12,000 rpm for 30 s, discard the waste liquid and put the spin column CB3 into the collection tube.
8. Repeat Step 7.
9. Put the spin column CB3 into the collection tube, centrifuge at 12,000 rpm for 2 min and discard the waste liquid. Place the spin column CB3 at room temperature for a few minutes to thoroughly dry the remaining rinse solution in the adsorption material.
10. Transfer the spin column CB3 to a clean centrifuge tube, add 100 μL of distilled water to the middle of the adsorption membrane, leave at room temperature for 2 min and centrifuge at 12,000 rpm for 2 min to elute DNA.
11. Store eluted DNA at –20°C.

11.2.3 Genomic DNA Amplification

Equipment

T100™ Thermal Cycler (Bio-Rad, Hercules, CA, United States)

Reagents

- 2× PCR Master Mix (Aidlab Biotechnologies Co., Beijing, China)
- Forward primer (2.5 μmol/L)
- Backward primer (2.5 μmol/L)

Procedures

1. Prepare and mix the 25 μL PCR reaction mixture as follows: 12.5 μL of 2× PCR Master Mix, 1.0 μL of each primer (2.5 μM), 2 μL (approximately 30 ng) of DNA templates and double-distilled water.
2. Perform PCR reaction at the corresponding temperature and reaction time (Table 11.2).

The steps different from the earlier standard process are as follows: For Plant-7~Plant-21, the annealing temperature for ITS2 amplification was 58°C (Hou *et al.*, 2013). For *Ophiocordyceps*

Table 11.2 Primer Sequences and PCR Amplification Procedure

Sequence	Primer	Primer sequence (5′ to 3′)	PCR amplification procedure
ITS2	2F	ATG CGA TAC TTG GTG TGA AT	94°C 5 min; 94°C 30 sec, 56°C 30 sec, 72°C 45 sec, 40 cycles; 72°C 10 min
	3R	GAC GCT TCT CCA GAC TAC AAT	
ITS	5F	GGA AGT AAA AGT CGT AAC AAG G	97°C 1 min; 97°C 1 min, 48°C 1 min, 72°C 3 min, 30 cycles; 72°C 7 min
	4R	TCC TCC GCT TAT TGA TAT GC	
trnH-psbA	psbA	GTT ATG CAT GAA CGT AAT GCT C	94°C 5 min; 94°C 1 min, 55°C 1 min, 72°C 1.5 min, 30 cycles; 72°C 7 min
	trnH	CGC GCA TGG TGG ATT CAC AAT CC	
COI	LCO1490	GGT CAA CAA ATC ATA AAG ATA TTG G	94°C 1 min; 94°C 1 min, 45°C 1.5 min, 72°C 1.5 min, 5 cycles; 94°C 1 min, 50°C 1.5 min, 72°C 1 min, 35 cycles; 72°C 5 min
	HCO2198	TAA ACT TCA GGG TGA CCA AAA AAT CA	

sinensis (Fungi-1), the ITS region of nrDNA was amplified using an LA Taq polymerase chain reaction (PCR) kit (Takara Biotech Inc., Kusatsu, Japan) with primer pair ITS 5F/4R (Table 11.2) (Liu *et al.*, 2002). The PCR mixture contained 0.1 μL of LA Taq (5 U/μL), 2.5 μL of 10× LA Taq PCR buffer II (Mg^{2+} Plus), 1 μL of dNTP mixture (2.5 mM each), 0.6 μL of each primer (10 μM) and 1 μL of genomic DNA in a total volume of 25 μL. The samples were amplified under the following conditions: initial denaturation at 97°C for 1 min, followed by 30 cycles of denaturation at 97°C for 1 min, annealing at 48°C for 1 min, extension at 72°C for 3 min and a final elongation step at 72°C for 7 min (Liu *et al.*, 2002). One pair of primers, 156 (5′-AAC CAT CGA GTC TTT GAA CGC-3′) and 157 (5′-CCT TGT AAG TTT CTT TTC CTC C-3′), was designed for the PCR amplification of the ITS2 region of *Ganoderma* (Fungi-2) under the following conditions: 94°C for 5 min, 40 cycles of 94°C for 30 s, 50°C for 30 s and 72°C for 1 min, and a final extension at 72°C for 10 min. PCR was performed to amplify the *COI* gene of Ranae oviductus (Animal-10~Animal-14) using LWF01: 5′-TCT CTA CTA ATC ATA AAG AYA TYG G-3′ and LWR01: 5′-TAA ACT TCA GGG TGA CCA AAR AAT CA-3′ for all the samples with an expected product size of ~700 bp.

11.2.4 Data Analysis

CodonCode Aligner V5.0.2.0 (CodonCode Co., Centerville, MA, United States) software was used to assemble the original sequences. After assembling, these sequences were annotated and trimmed to obtain the complete ITS2 region by employing a hidden Markov model (Keller *et al.*, 2009). The complete ITS2 sequences were aligned using MEGA X (Kumar, Stecher, Li, Knyaz & Tamura, 2018). Kimura 2-parameter (K2P) model was used to calculate the genetic distances. HMMer software was applied to annotate the ITS2 region (Keller *et al.*, 2009). ITS1 and 5.8S sequences were retrieved according to their annotations in GenBank. The partial 18S and 28S regions were excluded from both sides of the sequences.

11.3 Results and Discussion

11.3.1 Authentication of Plant Medicines

Owing to their similar morphology, *Panax ginseng* and *P. quinquefolius* are easily confused with one another. However, single-nucleotide polymorphism (SNP) is an accurate identification method to distinguish them. For both species, the interspecific nucleotide diversity in the ITS2 at position 32 and 43 would represent two typical SNP sites (Table 11.3). Analytical results for the experimental sequences of *P. ginseng* and *P. quinquefolius* revealed that these two SNP sites were stable between all sequences as verified by their published GenBank sequences. For *P. ginseng*, C and T exist stably at positions 32 and 43, respectively, and T and C exist in *P. quinquefolius*. In particular, nucleotide T at position 32 is exclusive to *P. quinquefolius* (other *Panax* species have C at this site). This uniqueness could be helpful to discriminate *P. quinquefolius* from other *Panax* species. For *P. notoginseng*, the three SNPs

Table 11.3 Five Stable SNPs in ITS2 as a Unique Marker of Three *Panax* Species

Species name	28 bp	32 bp	43 bp	140 bp	207 bp	GenBank accession number
P. ginseng	C	C	T	A	C	JX996141
P. quinquefolius	C	T	C	A	C	JX996142
P. notoginseng	T	C	C	T	T	JX996143

at positions 28, 140 and 207 (T/T/T) could be used to distinguish it from all the other *Panax* species (Table 11.3). However, according to the ITS2 sequences of *P. ginseng*, *P. quinquefolius* and *P. notoginseng*, their intraspecific divergence was surprisingly low. No variation in ITS2 was observed in the 81 samples of *P. ginseng* or the 65 samples of *P. quinquefolius*, though they were collected from different locations, such as Canada, Korea and three provinces in Northern China. A high level of sequence diversity was observed in *P. notoginseng* with four variation sites, namely, 83, 160, 175 and 216 C-T mutations (Chen *et al.*, 2013).

The ITS2 region of all samples was successfully amplified. All the PCR products were successfully sequenced, and the high-quality bidirectional sequences were obtained. The length of the ITS2 sequences belonging to seven *Eleutherococcus nodiflorus* samples was 230 bp, and the GC content was 62.4% on average. Three sites of nucleotide variation and three ITS2 haplotypes were detected (Zhao, Chen, Song, Pang & Chen, 2015). Detailed information about the three ITS2 haplotypes from *E. nodiflorus* is provided in Figure 11.1. According to the K2P model, the maximum interspecific distance of *E. nodiflorus* was 0.0132, and the minimum was 0.

All seven samples of *L. chinensis* were successfully amplified. The average sequence length of the ITS2 region was 246 bp. The GC content of all samples ranged from 66.3% to 67.2%. Three interspecies variable sites were found in the ITS2 region at positions of 26 (T-C), 94 (C-G) and 242 (G-T) (Figure 11.2). The intraspecific genetic distances of *L. chinensis* were ranged from 0 to 0.0124 (Zhao, Pang, Song & Chen, 2014).

The PCR amplification, sequencing success rate and sequence acquisition rate of all experimental samples of *Scutellaria barbata* were 100%. The ITS2 sequences of *S. barbata* were 241 bp in length. The GC content ranged from 68.9% to 69.3%.

```
                                           1 1111111112 2222222223 3333333334 4444444445 5555555556
                                  1234567890 1234567890 1234567890 1234567890 1234567890 1234567890
Eleutherococcus nodiflorus YC0123MT02   CGCATCGCGT CGCCCCCCAA CCATGCACTC TCTCACGGGA GTCATGACTG AGGGGCGGAT
Eleutherococcus nodiflorus YC0123MT14   .......... .......... .......... C......... .......... ..........
Eleutherococcus nodiflorus YC0123MT18   .......... .......... .......... C......... .......... ..........

                                                                                  1 1111111111 1111111111
                                  6666666667 7777777778 8888888889 9999999990 0000000001 1111111112
                                  1234567890 1234567890 1234567890 1234567890 1234567890 1234567890
Eleutherococcus nodiflorus YC0123MT02   ACTGGCCTCC CGTGTCTCAC CGCGCGGTTG GCCCAAATGT GAGTCCTTGG CGACGGGCGT
Eleutherococcus nodiflorus YC0123MT14   .......... .......... .......... .......... .......... ..........
Eleutherococcus nodiflorus YC0123MT18   .......... .......... .......... .......... .......... ..........

                                  1111111111 1111111111 1111111111 1111111111 1111111111 1111111111
                                  2222222223 3333333334 4444444445 5555555556 6666666667 7777777778
                                  1234567890 1234567890 1234567890 1234567890 1234567890 1234567890
Eleutherococcus nodiflorus YC0123MT02   CACGACAAGT GGTGGTTGTA AAAAGCCCTC TTCTCCTGTC GTGCGGTGGA CCGTCGCCAA
Eleutherococcus nodiflorus YC0123MT14   .......... .......... .......... .......... .......... .........G
Eleutherococcus nodiflorus YC0123MT18   .......... .......... .......... .......... .......... .........T

                                  1111111111 1111111112 2222222222 2222222222 2222222222
                                  8888888889 9999999990 0000000001 1111111112 2222222223
                                  1234567890 1234567890 1234567890 1234567890 1234567890
Eleutherococcus nodiflorus YC0123MT02   CAAAAGCTCA TGTGACCCTG TTGTGCCGTC CTCGACGAGC ACTCCGACCG
Eleutherococcus nodiflorus YC0123MT14   .......... .........T .......... .......... ..........
Eleutherococcus nodiflorus YC0123MT18   .......... .......... .......... .......... ..........
```

Fig. 11.1 Variable sites in the ITS2 sequences of *Eleutherococcus nodiflorus*.

```
                                   1 1111111112 2222222223 3333333334 4444444445 5555555556 6666666667 7777777778 8888888889 99999
                          1234567890 1234567890 1234567890 1234567890 1234567890 1234567890 1234567890 1234567890 1234567890 12345
Lobelia chinensis BABL0001   CGCATCGCGT CGCTCCCCCC GAGCATAC-- ATATATATAT GTGCACGGGG GAAGCGGATA CTGGCCTCCC GTGCCCCTCG CGGACGCGGC TGGGT
Lobelia chinensis BABL0004   .......... .......... ........-- .......... .......... .......... .......... .......... .......... ...C.
Lobelia chinensis BABL0006   .......... .......... .....C..-- .......... .......... .......... .......... .......... .......... ...C.
Lobelia chinensis BABL0007   .......... .......... ........AT .......... .......... .......... .......... .......... .......... ...C.

                              111111 1111111111 1111111111 1111111111 1111111111 1111111111 1111111111 1111111111 1111111111 11111
                          9999000000 0000111111 1111222222 2222333333 3333444444 4444555555 5555666666 6666777777 7777888888 88889
                          6789012345 6789012345 6789012345 6789012345 6789012345 6789012345 6789012345 6789012345 6789012345 67890
Lobelia chinensis BABL0001   CAAAACGGAG TCCCCGACGG AGGACGCACG ACAAGTGGTG GTGGTTTTAC AAAAGCACTC GCGTCGTGTC GTGCGCGCGT CCTGCGCCGG TGCCG
Lobelia chinensis BABL0004   .......... .......... .......... .......... .......... .......... .......... .......... .......... .....
Lobelia chinensis BABL0006   .......... .......... .......... .......... .......... .......... .......... .......... .......... .....
Lobelia chinensis BABL0007   .......... .......... .......... .......... .......... .......... .......... .......... .......... .....

                          1111111112 2222222222 2222222222 2222222222 2222222222 222222
                          9999999990 0000000001 1111111112 2222222223 3333333334 444444
                          1234567890 1234567890 1234567890 1234567890 1234567890 123456
Lobelia chinensis BABL0001   GCTCGCGTGA CCCTCTTGCG CCTCCCTCGC TCCCGCGACG GACGGTGCTT CTACCG
Lobelia chinensis BABL0004   .......... .......... .......... .......... .......... .G....
Lobelia chinensis BABL0006   .......... .......... .......... .......... .......... .G....
Lobelia chinensis BABL0007   .......... .......... .......... .......... .......... .G....
```

Fig.11.2 Variable sites in the ITS2 sequence of *Lobelia chinensis*.

Two variation sites within *S. barbata* were found at positions 59 (G-A) and 229 (G-A). Detailed information about the three ITS2 haplotypes from *S. barbata* is provided in Figure 11.3. The minimum genetic distance within the *S. barbata* ITS2 sequence was 0, and the maximum was 0.0084 (Guo, Ren, Chen & Pang, 2016).

The ITS2 sequence lengths of *L. japonica* samples were 228 bp. A nucleotide variation site was found at the 27th base and was

```
                                    1 1111111112 2222222223 3333333334 4444444445 5555555556 6666666667 7777777778 8
                           1234567890 1234567890 1234567890 1234567890 1234567890 1234567890 1234567890 1234567890 1
Scutellaria barbata BAZL0001 CGCATCGCGT CGCCCCCCGC ACGCATCGCC TCGAGCGACG CCGATGTCGG GGGCGGAGA TTGGCCTCCC GTGCGCCCCG G
Scutellaria barbata BAZL0003 .......... .......... .......... .......... .......... .......... .......... .......... .
Scutellaria barbata BAZL0010 .......... .......... .......... .......... .......... ........A. .......... .......... .

                                   11 1111111111 1111111111 1111111111 1111111111 1111111111 1111111111 1
                           8888888899 9999999900 0000000011 1111111122 2222222233 3333333344 4444444455 5555555566 6
                           2345678901 2345678901 2345678901 2345678901 2345678901 2345678901 2345678901 2345678901 2
Scutellaria barbata BAZL0001 CGCGCGGCCG GCCCAAATGC GATCCCCCGG CGACGCACGC CCCGACAAGT GGTGGTTGAG CCTTCAACTC GCGTGCTGTC G
Scutellaria barbata BAZL0003 .......... .......... .......... .......... .......... .......... .......... .......... .
Scutellaria barbata BAZL0010 .......... .......... .......... .......... .......... .......... .......... .......... .

                           1111111111 1111111111 1111111111 1111111222 2222222222 2222222222 2222222222 222222222
                           6666666777 7777777888 8888888999 9999999000 0000000111 1111111222 2222222333 333333344
                           3456789012 3456789012 3456789012 3456789012 3456789012 3456789012 3456789012 345678901
Scutellaria barbata BAZL0001 GGCGCCAAGG CGTCGTCCGT TCGGGAGAAA CACATCGATC GATGTTGGAC CCAACGGCCC TTAATAGAGC CATCGACCG
Scutellaria barbata BAZL0003 .......... .......... .......... .......... .......... .......... ......A... .........
Scutellaria barbata BAZL0010 .......... .......... .......... .......... .......... .......... .......... .........
```

Fig. 11.3 Variable sites in the ITS2 sequence of *Scutellaria barbata.*

identified as the substitution of C/T. The ITS2 sequence length of Flos Lonicerae was 228 bp. A total of 81 variation sites and 29 insertion/deletion (or missing sites) mutations were detected in 55 ITS2 sequences. Except that of *L. japonica,* the ITS2 regions of the other *Lonicera* species can be divided into six haplotypes. A phylogenetic tree was constructed using the NJ method with 1,000 bootstrap replicates for the ITS2 sequence (Figure 11.4). The results showed that *L. japonica* samples were into one clade that could be distinguished successfully from its closely related species.

A total of 192 samples representing 64 species were obtained following the operating procedure for the DNA barcoding of medicinal plants (Xiong *et al.*, 2018). The ITS2 fragment was efficiently amplified from most of the samples using the universal ITS2 primers, with the exception of 15 samples from three seed medicines: Arecae Semen (seeds of *Areca catechu* L.), Myristicae Semen (seeds of *Myristica fragrans* Houtt.) and Pruni Semen (seeds of *Prunus pedunculata* Maxim., *P. japonica* Thunb. and *P. humilis* Bge.). Owing to the difficulty of amplifying the ITS2 region in these species, the successfully amplified *psbA-trnH* region was employed as a supplementary identification marker. The ITS2 sequence lengths ranged from 190 to 280 bp, and their GC content was between 43% and 77%. The average length and GC content

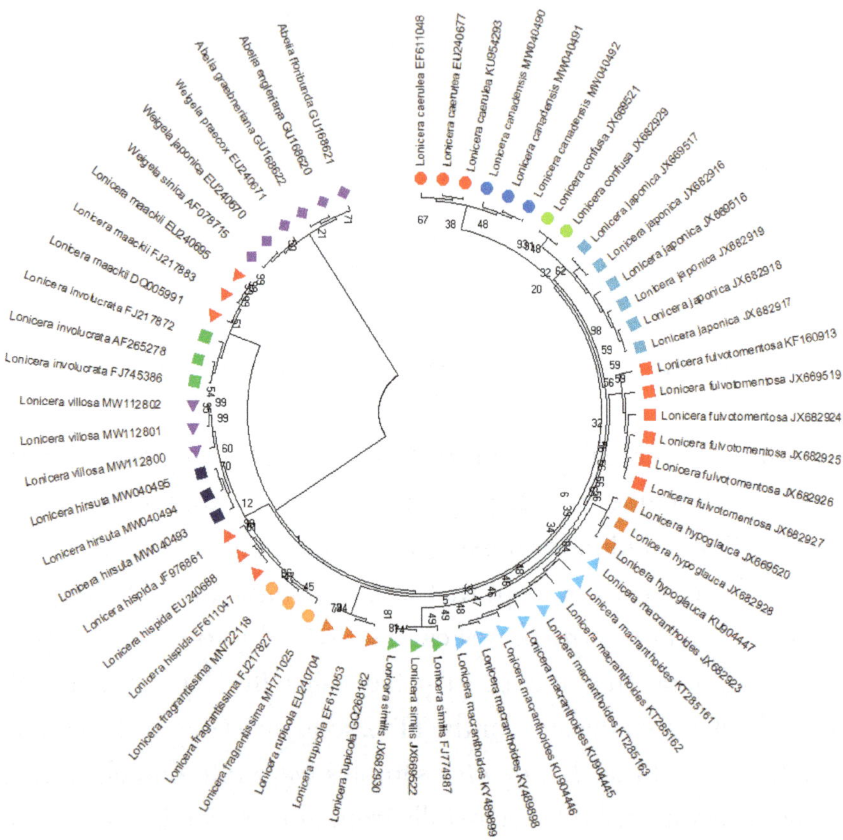

Fig. 11.4 Phylogenetic tree of Flos Lonicerae Japonicae and its closely related species constructed with the ITS2 sequences by the NJ method using three *Weigela* and three *Abelia* species as an outgroup.

were 220 bp and 61%, respectively. Tree-building analysis using the genetic distances method was recommended and employed in species discrimination. The tree includes 177 ITS2 sequences representing 59 species found in 48 kinds of medicinal materials. The tree analysis comprised a hierarchical clustering tree (ML) with Kimura 2-parameter and 1,000 bootstrap replicates to test the support for each branch. The results showed that the ITS2 sequences of the 48 kinds of seed traditional Chinese medicines (TCMs; not species) can be differentiated from each other and formed distinct, non-overlapping groups in the ML tree (Figure 11.5). Similar results were obtained for the other 15 *psbA-trnH* sequences by using the same tree construction method (Figure 11.6). DNA barcoding can also be used for the rapid, highly accurate authentication of some seed TCMs from its common adulterants. For instance, *Hyoscyamus niger* can be distinguished from its adulterants *Hygrophila salicifolia, Astragalus complanatus, Cuscuta australis, Cuscuta chinensis* and *Impatiens balsamina*.

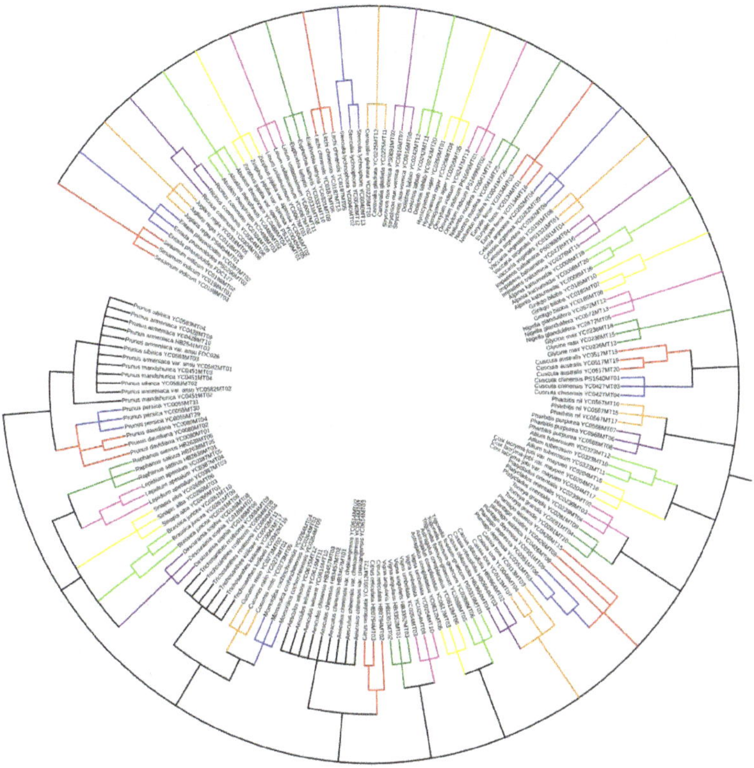

Fig. 11.5 Unrooted tree of the species in 48 seed TCMs constructed from the ITS2 sequences using the ML method (Xiong *et al.*, 2018). Note: Bootstrap 1,000 repetitions, only branches with support ≥50% are shown.

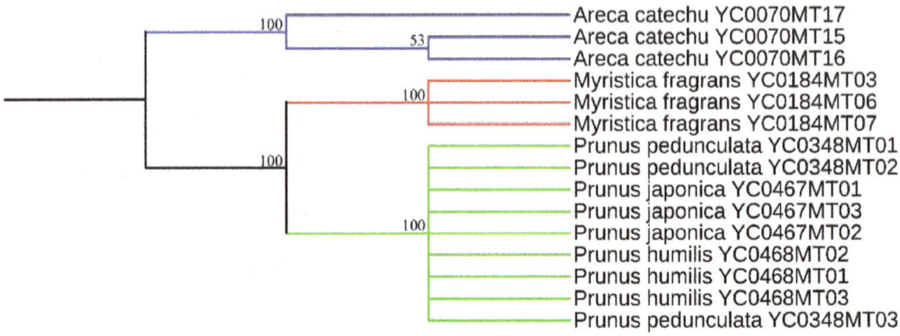

Fig. 11.6 Unrooted tree of species in three seed TCMs constructed from the *psbA-trnH* sequences using the ML method (Xiong *et al.*, 2018). Note: Bootstrap 1000 repetitions, only branches with support ≥50% are shown.

11.3.2 Authentication of Fungal Medicines

The sequence length of *O. sinensis* was 493 bp, and the average GC content was 65%. Twenty-nine nucleotide variation sites were detected in the ITS region: 20 T/C (9); A/G (11) transitions; and 9 G/C (2), A/C (4), T/G (1) and T/A (2) transversions (Xiang *et al.*, 2013). The following deletions were detected: 1 bp deletion within the ITS regions of three samples at sites 62, 341 (3), 462 and 469 (Figure 11.7) (Xiang *et al.*, 2013).

The PCR product size of *Ganoderma* (Lingzhi) was approximately 500 bp. The length of ITS2 was 195 bp after the deletion of the 5.8S and 28S rDNA. The average G-C and A-T contents of this region were 49% and 51%, respectively (Liao *et al.*, 2015). The following seven intraspecific variable sites were found among the 10 samples: 8 (T/C), 33 (G/C), 67 (C/G), 105 (C/T), 122 (T/G), 139 (C/T) and 158 (G/A) (Figure 11.8).

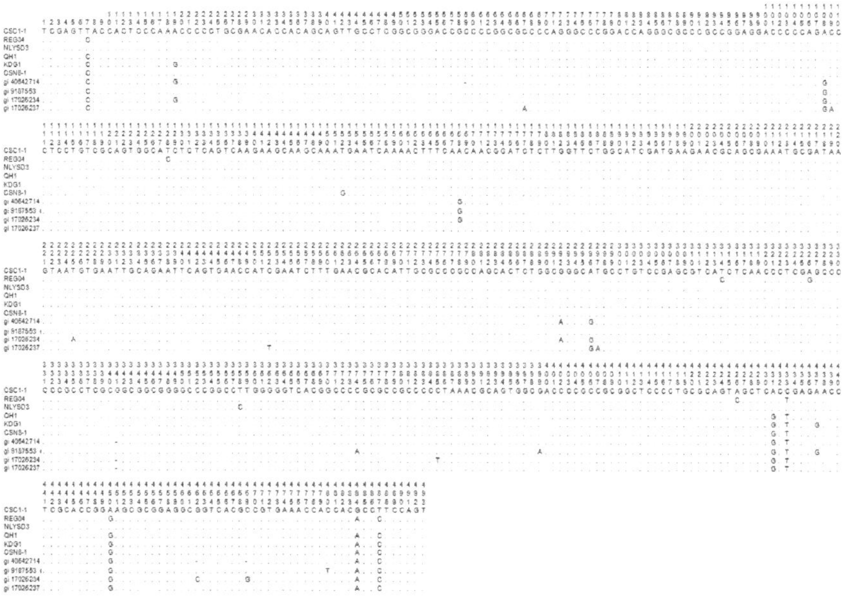

Fig. 11.7 Variable sites in the ITS sequence of *Ophiocordyceps sinensis*.

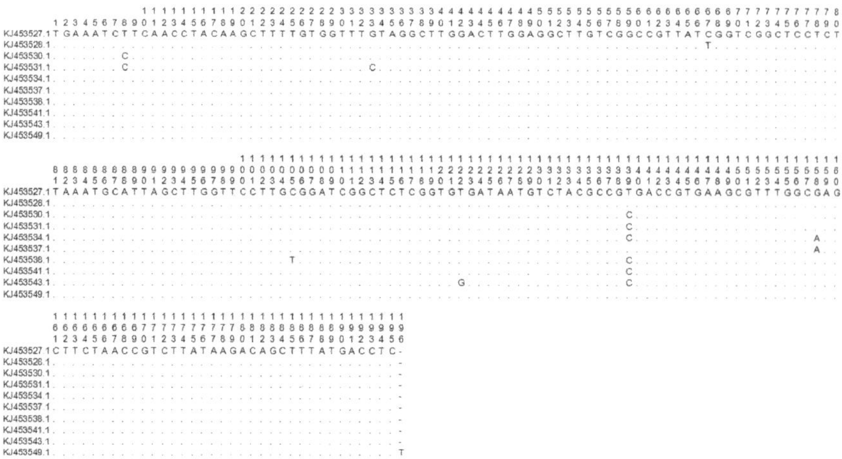

Fig. 11.8 Variable sites in the ITS2 sequence of *Ganoderma lucidum*.

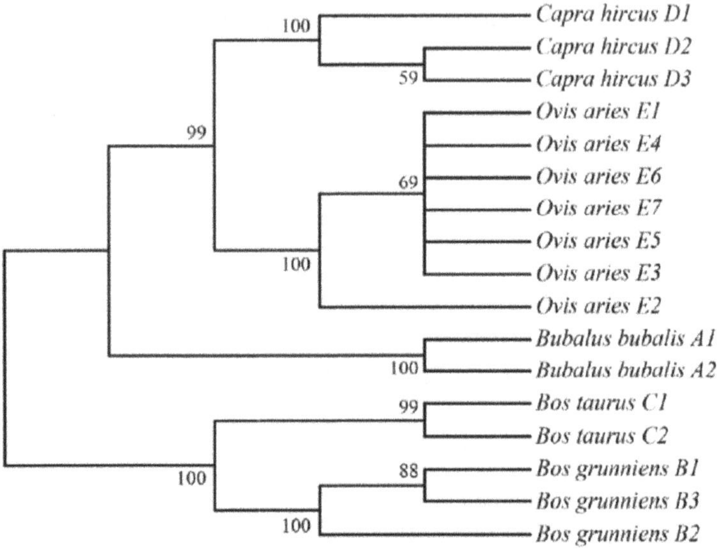

Fig. 11.9 NJ tree of *COI* haplotype sequences from *Bubalus bubalis*, *Bos grunniens*, *Bos taurus*, *Capra hircus* and *Ovis aries*. Bootstrap values of >50% are indicated at the nodes (Liu *et al.*, 2017b).

11.3.3 Authentication of Animal Medicines

The concentration of extracted DNA of *Bubali cornu* ranged from 50 to 100 ng/μL, and the A260/A280 values of DNA were between 1.65 and 1.80. The maximum K-2P distances for the five animal species were all less than 0.015, and the average K-2P distances within the species were all less than 0.008. The NJ phylogenetic tree constructed based on the haplotype of the original animal shows that the five original animals are clustered into one group with a bootstrap value of 100 and can be distinguished from each other (Figure 11.9) (Liu *et al.*, 2017b).

The maximum genetic distance within the species of the *B. multicinctus* was 0.0201, and the average genetic distance within the species was 0.0014±0.0038. Compared with that of *B. fasciatus*, the minimum genetic distance between species

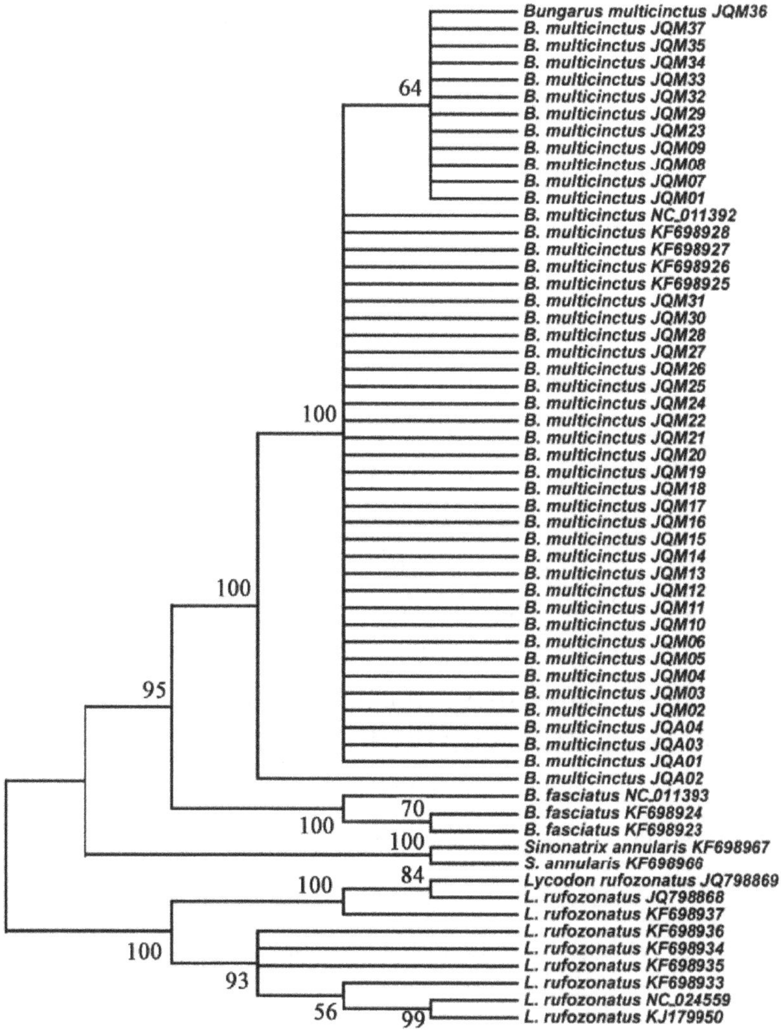

Fig. 11.10 Neighbour-joining phylogenetic tree constructed using the *COI* sequences of Bungarus Parvus and its adulterants (Shi *et al.*, 2018).

was 0.1561, and the average genetic distance between species was 0.1569±0.0008. Compared with that of *L. rufozonatus*, the minimum genetic distance between species was 0.2088, and the average genetic distance between species was 0.2143±0.0032. Compared with that of *S. annularis*, the minimum genetic distance between species was 0.2093, and the average genetic distance between species was 0.2119±0.0009. *B. multicinctus*, *B. fasciatus*, *L. rufozonatus* and *S. annularis* are clustered into different branches on the NJ tree and can be clearly distinguished from each other (Figure 11.10) (Shi *et al.*, 2018).

Ranae oviductus (Hamayou) is a rare and precious Chinese medicine; however, its identification faces many challenges, such as the presence of many adulterants and the controversy over its origin. The main adulterants of Ranae oviductus (Hamayou) are *R. dybowskii* Günther, *Pelophylax nigromaculatus* and *Bufo gargarizans* Cantor. The official original species for Ranae oviductus (Hamayou) is *R. chensinensis* David, according to the *Pharmacopoeia of the People's Republic of China* (2020). However, many studies pointed out that the correct original species for Ranae oviductus (Hamayou) should be *R. dybowskii* Günther (Li *et al.*, 2003). Furthermore, DNA extraction and PCR amplification for Ranae oviductus (Hamayou) still have difficulties. The NJ phylogenetic tree was constructed using the complete mitochondrial genome sequence (Figure 11.11). *R. chensinensis*, *R. kukunoris*,

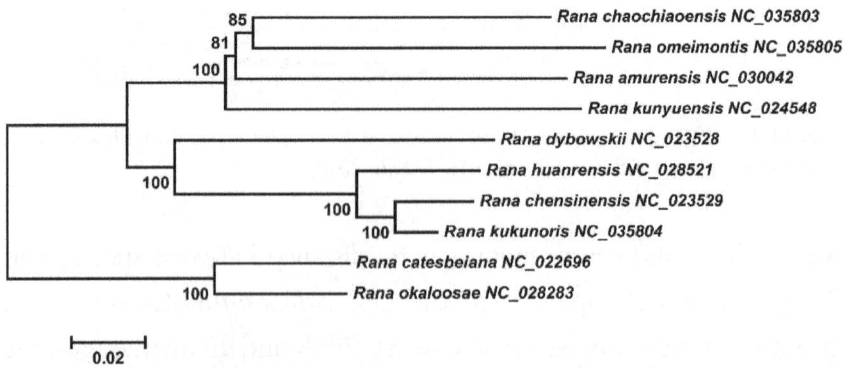

Fig. 11.11 Neighbour-joining phylogenetic tree constructed using whole mitochondrial genomes of *Rana* species distributed in North China (Shi *et al.*, 2019).

R. huanrenensis and *Rana dybowskii* are clustered into a large branch with a bootstrap value of 100. *R. chensinensis* and *R. kukunoris* exhibit a close relationship and are clustered into a small branch inside the above large branch with a bootstrap value of 100. *R. chaochiaoensis, R. omeimontis, R. kunyuensis* and *R. amurensis* are clustered into another large branch with a bootstrap value of 100. On the basis of the molecular phylogenetic relationship based on the whole mitochondrial genome, *R. amurensis*, *R. chensinensis* and *R. dybowskii* are all accepted species. After pre-treatment with demucosification solution, a supernatant of more than 400 μL was obtained. The concentration of extracted DNA was more than 50 ng/μL, and the ratio of A260/A280 was between 1.6 and 2.0. LWF01/LWR01 was used to amplify the samples of muscle and medicinal materials to obtain clear, bright and single bands. The maximum intraspecific genetic distances of *R. amurensis*, *R. chensinensis* and *R. dybowskii* were substantially smaller than the minimum interspecific distance between each other, and clear boundaries were present between species (Shi *et al.*, 2019).

11.4 Conclusion

Rapid and accurate identification of medicinal materials is very important for drug safety. There are many research studies of medicinal materials using DNA barcoding. Here, the intra- and interspecific genetic distance and identification efficiency of the DNA barcoding sequence for authentication of the medicinal materials mentioned earlier were discussed. ITS2 barcode has shown good identification efficiency in numerous medicinal plants (Chen *et al.*, 2010, 2013; Gu *et al.*, 2013; Hou *et al.*, 2013; Pang *et al.*, 2011; Xiang *et al.*, 2013; Xin *et al.*, 2013; Yao *et al.*, 2010). Our results showed in this chapter also illustrate that ITS2 is effective in differentiating selected important medicinal materials, including *P. ginseng*, *Eleutherococcus nodiflorus*, *Lobelia chinensis*, *Scutellaria barbata*, *Lonicera japonica*, *Ganoderma lucidum* and seed medicines in Chinese Pharmacopoeia from its closely related species. For animal species, *COI* is a common DNA barcode. We illustrated that *COI* is the preferred DNA barcode sequence for identifying *Bubalus bubalis*, *Bungarus multicinctus* and *Rana chensinensis* from its adulterants.

Acknowledgements

This work was supported by the National Natural Science Foundation of China (81874339) and Chinese Academy of Medical Sciences (CAMS) Innovation Fund for Medical Sciences (CIFMS) (NO. 2016-I2M-3-016).

References

Chen, S., Yao, H., Han, J., Liu, C., Song, J., Shi, L., Zhu, Y., Ma, X., Gao, T., Pang, X., Luo, K., Li, Y., Li, X., Jia, X., Lin, Y., & Leon, C. (2010). Validation of the ITS2 region as a novel DNA barcode for identifying medicinal plant species. *PLoS One*, *5*, e8613.

Chen, S. L., Pang, X. H., Song, J. Y., Shi, L. C., Yao, H., Han, J. P., & Leon, C. (2014). A renaissance in herbal medicine identification from morphology to DNA. *Biotechnol Adv*, *32*, 1237–1244.

Chen, X. C., Liao, B. S., Song, J. Y., Pang, X. H., Han, J. P., & Chen, S. L. (2013). A fast SNP identification and analysis of intraspecific variation in the medicinal *Panax* species based on DNA barcoding. *Gene*, *530*, 39–43.

Chen, X. C., Xiang, L., Shi, L. C., Li, G., Yao, H., Han, J. P., Lin, Y., Song, J., & Chen, S. L. (2017). Identification of crude drugs in the Japanese pharmacopoeia using a DNA barcoding system. *Sci Rep*, *7*, 42325.

Gu, W., Song, J. Y., Cao, Y., Sun, Q. W., Yao, H., Wu, Q. N., Chao, J., Zhou, J., Xue, W., & Duan, J. A. (2013). Application of the ITS2 region for barcoding medicinal plants of Selaginellaceae in Pteridophyta. *PLoS One, 8*, e67818.

Guo, M., Ren, L., Chen X., & Pang, X. (2016). Identification of *Scutellaria barbata* and its adulterants using ITS2 barcode. *World Chin Med, 11*, 796–800.

Hebert, P. D. N., Cywinska, A., Ball, S. L., & de Waard, J. R. (2003). Biological identifications through DNA barcodes. *Proc Royal Soc B Biol Sci, 270*, 313–321.

Hou, D. Y., Song, J. Y., Shi, L. C., Ma, X. C., Xin, T. Y., Han, J. P., Xiao, W., Sun, Z. Y., Cheng, R. Y. & Yao, H. (2013). Stability and accuracy assessment of identification of traditional Chinese materia medica using DNA barcoding, a case study on Flos Lonicerae Japonicae. *Biomed Res Int, 2013*, 549037.

Keller, A., Schleicher, T., Schultz, J., Müller, T., Dandekar, T., & Wolf, M. (2009). 5.8S-28S rRNA interaction and HMM-based ITS2 annotation. *Gene, 430*(1–2), 50–57.

Kumar, S., Stecher, G., Li, M., Knyaz, C., & Tamura, K. (2018). MEGA X: Molecular evolutionary genetics analysis across computing platforms. *Mol Biol Evol, 35*, 1547–1549.

Li, Y., Zhang, J., Li, M., Liu, C., Jiang, D., & Deng, M. (2003). Study on the origin for oviduetus Ranae. *China J Chin Mat Medica, 28*, 11–17.

Liao, B. S., Chen, X. C., Han, J. P., Dan, Y., Wang, L. L., Jiao, W. J., Song, J. Y., & Chen, S. L. (2015). Identification of commercial *Ganoderma* (*Lingzhi*) species by ITS2 sequences. *Chin Med, 10*, 22.

Liu, J. X., Shi, L. C., Song, J. Y., Sun, W., Han, J. P., Liu, X., Hou, D. Y., Yao, H., Li, M. Y., & Chen, S. L. (2017a). BOKP: A DNA barcode reference library for monitoring herbal drugs in the Korean pharmacopeia. *Front Pharmacol, 8*, 931.

Liu, X., Zhou, L., Liu, J., Jia, J., Song, J., & Shi, L. (2017b). Identification of water buffalo horn and its adulterants using COI barcode. *Acta Pharm Sin, 52*, 494–499.

Liu, Z., Liang, Z., Liu, A., Yao, Y., Hyde, K. D., & Yu, Z. (2002). Molecular evidence for teleomorph–anamorph connections in Cordyceps based on ITS-5.8S rDNA sequences. *Mycol Res, 106*, 1100–1108.

Pang, X. H., Song, J. Y., Zhu, Y. J., Xu, H. X., Huang, L. F., & Chen, S. L. (2011). Applying plant DNA barcodes for Rosaceae species identification. *Cladistics, 27*, 165–170.

Shi, L., Liu, J., Tang, X., Liu, J., Yao, H., Zhang, L., Li Xiang, Zhang, Q., Xie, C., Song, J. (2019). Herbalogical studies of Ranae oviductus (Hamayou) and its species identification using DNA barcoding method. *Sci Sin Vitae, 49*, 1032–1040.

Shi, L., Tang, X., Hu, Z., Zhao, C., Feng, L., & Liu, J. (2018). Investigation of medicinal sources for Bungarus Parvus by DNA barcoding technology. *Chin J Exp Trad Med Form, 24*, 16–22.

Xiang, L., Song, J. Y., Xin, T. Y., Zhu, Y. J., Shi, L. C., Xu, X. L., Pang, X. H., Yao, H., Li, W. J., & Chen, S. L. (2013). DNA barcoding the commercial Chinese caterpillar fungus. *FEMS Microbiol Let, 347*, 156–162.

Xin, T. Y., Yao, H., Gao, H. H., Zhou, X. Z., Ma, X. C., Xu, C. Q., Chen, J., Han, J. P., Pang, X. H., Xu, R., Song, J. Y., & Chen, S. L. (2013). Super food *Lycium barbarum* (Solanaceae) traceability via an internal transcribed spacer 2 barcode. *Food Res Int, 54*, 1699–1704.

Xiong, C., Sun, W., Li, J. J., Yao, H., Shi, Y. H., Wang, P., Huang, B. S., Shi, L. C., Liu, D., Hu, Z. G., & Chen, S. L. (2018). Identifying the species of seeds in Traditional Chinese Medicine using DNA barcoding. *Front Pharmacol,* 9, 701.

Yao, H., Song, J. Y., Liu, C., Luo, K., Han, J. P., Li, Y., Pang, X. H., Xu, H. X., Zhu, Y. J., Xiao, P. G., & Chen, S. L. (2010). Use of ITS2 region as the universal DNA barcode for plants and animals. *PLoS One, 5*, e13102.

Zhao, S., Chen, X., Song, J., Pang, X., & Chen, S. (2015). Internal transcribed spacer 2 barcode: A good tool for identifying Acanthopanacis cortex. *Front Plant Sci, 6*, 840.

Zhao, S., Pang, X., Song, J., & Chen, S. (2014). Identification of albiziae cortex, albiziae flos and their adulterants using ITS2 barcoding. *China J Chin Mat Med, 39*(12), 2164–2168.

Chapter 12

Authentication of Medicinal Products by Adaptor Ligation-Mediated Polymerase Chain Reaction and Metabarcoding

Yat-Tung Lo, Mavis Hong-Yu Yik & Xiao Lin

12.1 Introduction

The use of DNA barcoding for species identification (please refer to Chapter 11 for a detailed discussion) is a common laboratory practice in molecular authentication nowadays. Standard DNA barcode regions or genes with length between 500 and 800 bp are amplified by polymerase chain reaction (PCR) and sequenced for species identification. Instead of designing species-specific primers, the use of universal primers simplifies the identification work on unknown species as sequence information of the target species is not a prerequisite (Moon *et al.*, 2016). However, the use of universal primers is successful only for raw materials as PCR amplification of full-length DNA barcode often fails in medicinal products due to DNA degradation. For instance, our previous studies have revealed that DNA in decoctions (Lo, Li & Shaw, 2015) and concentrated Chinese medicine granules (CCMG) (Jiang, Lo,

Chen & Shaw, 2016) are fragmented. Other studies have also found that DNA fragments with a size larger than 200 bp were rare in archival specimens (Song, Dong, Zhang, Liu & Sun, 2017) and herbal supplements (Little, 2014). Although the use of 'DNA mini-barcode' may be a possible solution with a shortened amplicon size (Little, 2014; Meusnier *et al.*, 2008; Song, Dong, Zhang, Liu & Sun, 2017), it is difficult to design conserved primers within the standard barcode region due to sequence variation. Also, matching between primers and target sequences is critical to the success of PCR amplification and subsequent sequence data analysis.

Adaptor ligation-mediated PCR utilises a specially designed synthetic adaptor (double-stranded oligonucleotides) ligated with the sticky end of sample DNA, followed by PCR amplification using only one end of the universal primer and adaptor-specific primer (Figure 12.1). The DNA fragments with variable length

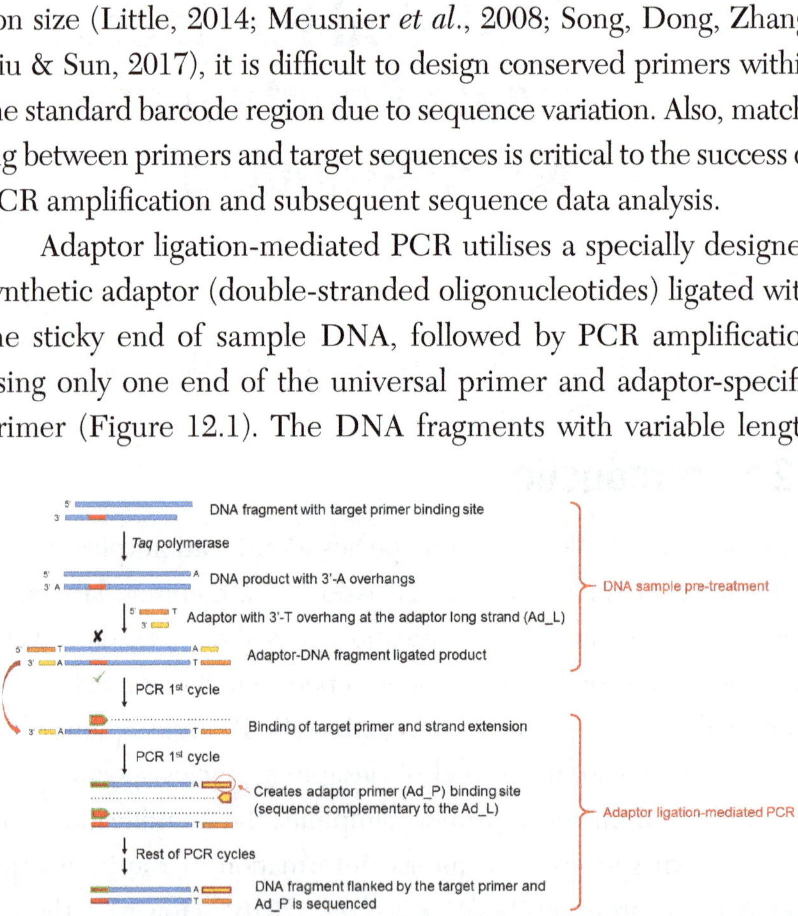

Fig. 12.1 The principle of the modified adaptor ligation-mediated PCR. A pool of sample DNA fragments was ligated to the adaptor and only those fragments with a target primer binding site are amplified by PCR. Adaptors are first ligated to the pool of DNA fragments, then a universal primer and an adaptor-specific primer are used to amplify the pool of ligated DNA fragments. Since these 'adaptor-tags' have already provided the specific starting position for amplification, DNA fragments of various length with the presence of the target DNA barcode region can be amplified (Figure adapted from [Lo & Shaw, 2018]).

are ligated to the adaptors and only those fragments with the target sequence are selectively amplified. It allows selective amplification of various DNA fragments simultaneously without prior knowledge of sequence information. This technique has been used for DNA sequencing, genome mapping and DNA footprinting (Guilfoyle, Leeck, Kroening, Smith & Guo, 1997; O'Malley, Alonso, Kim, Leisse & Ecker, 2007; Smith, 1992).

In order to reveal all the amplified PCR products on the barcoding region after adaptor ligation-mediated PCR, next generation sequencing (NGS) (i.e., metabarcoding) is used, which gives massive parallelisation of sequencing reaction to generate multiple reads and determine genomic sequences, regardless of the relative amount of DNA sequence in the sample (Nyren, 2007; Ronaghi, Uhlen & Nyren, 1998); thus great species coverage is given with sensitive determination of 1% plant or animal taxa in a complex mixture (Arulandhu *et al.*, 2017). The use of NGS for the authentication and quality control of medicinal products have been published by different groups. Cheng *et al.* (2014) performed metagenomic analysis on a medicinal product known as Liuwei Dihuang Wan to find the biological ingredients involved. From the NGS data, it was also found that the quality and stability are significantly different among manufacturers and some are affected by biological contaminations. Study on Ruyi Jinhuang powder showed that high-quality read ranged from 50 to 500 bp was produced with the identity score of up to 97%. The use of NGS allowed comprehensive ingredient profiling and effective determination of whether adulterant *Pinellia pedatisecta* was present in the powder (Li *et al.*, 2018). When 78 *Hypericum perforatum* medicinal products were analysed by amplicon metabarcoding, it was found that the highest amplification success rate was obtained for herbal teas (97% for nrITS1 and 88% for nrITS2), followed by capsules (62% for nrITS1 and 62% for nrITS2), tablets (43% for nrITS1 and 45% for nrITS2) and extracts (27% for nrITS1 and 40% for nrITS2) (Raclariu *et al.*, 2017). Coghlan *et al.* (2012) used NGS to determine the ingredients of 15 medicinal products in the form of powder, capsule, tablet and herbal teas. Targeting both the p-loop region of the plastid *trnL* gene and the mitochondrial 16S ribosomal RNA gene, over 49,000 amplicon sequence reads were generated, and 78% of the samples showed unlabelled species on the packaging.

Detection of endangered species involved in medicinal products can also be performed by NGS. For instance, trade-restricted species listed within the appendices in the Convention on International Trade in Endangered Species of Wild Fauna and Flora (CITES) were identified using NGS platforms (Arulandhu *et al.*, 2017; Coghlan *et al.*, 2015). NGS is especially useful to authenticate animal-derived products with the lack of effective markers for chemical and protein analysis (Yeung *et al.*, 2006; Zhou & Wang, 2004). By using the NGS techniques to reveal the species composition in complex and highly processed products and supplements, the quality and stability of products among different manufacturers can be revealed. In addition, accurate and reliable sequences can be obtained for better species determination since NGS produces independent repeat results with low cost and high throughput (Jia, Xu, Xin, Shi & Song, 2017), thus it can be adopted by the Good Manufacturing Practice (GMP) factory for quality control regulation and determination of contaminant and species composition in processed products (Coissac, Hollingsworth, Lavergne & Taberlet, 2016). The recent advance in NGS technologies further decreases the sequencing cost.

Hedyotis, investigated in this study, is a genus with about 500 species in the family Rubiaceae. They are annual or perennial herbs that are mainly distributed in tropical and subtropical regions (Chen & Taylor, 2011). *Hedyotis diffusa* Willdenow (colloquially Baihuasheshecao) is one of the well-known *Hedyotis* species possessing anti-oxidation, anti-tumour and anti-inflammatory properties (Yan *et al.*, 2017), which is considered as folk medicine for maintaining good health. Chinese herbal tea (Liang Cha) is one of the most common *H. diffusa*–containing products in the market (Yik *et al.*, 2021a). Owing to the plaguing taxonomic and lectotypification problems, the morphological characteristics description of *H. diffusa* and its closely related species are confusing (Siu, Yik, Boufford, Shaw & Lau, 2021) and subsequently lead to intentional or inadvertent adulteration. To further enhance the quality assurance and quality control of medicinal products in the industry, we aim to reveal the *Hedyotis* identity in different *Hedyotis*-containing products by using adaptor ligation-mediated PCR with metabarcoding (Yik *et al.*, 2021b).

12.2 Materials and Methods

The key procedures involved in the study are illustrated in Figure 12.2.

12.2.1 *Hedyotis* Samples

Three medicinal products claimed as 'Baihuasheshecao' on their labels were collected from China and Thailand (Table 12.1).

12.2.2 DNA Extraction

Modified column kit extraction method was used for DNA extraction, which is the combined use of Cetyltrimethylammonium Bromide (CTAB) extraction and the DNeasy Plant Pro kit (Qiagen, Hilden, Germany).

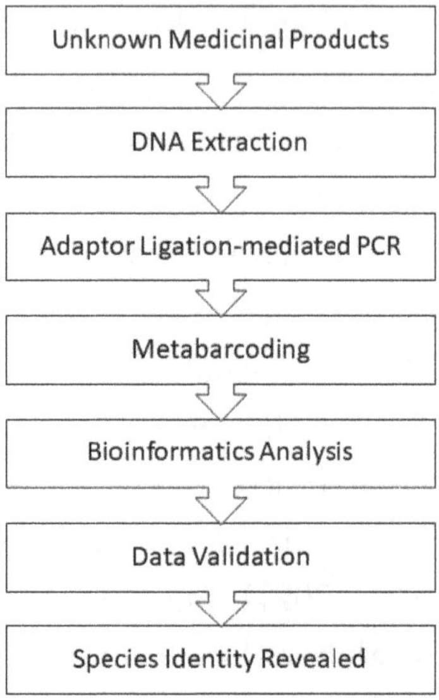

Fig. 12.2 Experimental flow chart of this study.

Table 12.1 List of Samples Studied

Sample voucher	Sample name	Location of sample collected
T4794	Baihuasheshecao powder	Anhui, China
T4795	Baihuasheshecao powder	Guangdong, China
T4286	Baihuasheshecao tablet	Bangkok, Thailand

Equipment

- Benchtop centrifuge

Reagents

- 2× CTAB buffer
    - 100 mM Tris-HCl (pH 8.0)
    - 1.4 M NaCl
    - 20 mM ethylenediaminetetraacetic acid (EDTA)
    - 2% CTAB
    - 1% PVP-360
    - 0.2% 2-mercaptoethanol

- Extraction buffer
    - 200 mM Tris-HCl (pH 8.0)
    - 200 mM NaCl
    - 25 mM EDTA
    - 0.5% sodium dodecyl sulfate (SDS)
- DNeasy Plant Pro kit (Qiagen)

Procedures

CTAB extraction part:

1. Weigh 50 mg samples of each product for DNA extraction and place each sample in a microcentrifuge tube.
2. Add 400 μL of extraction buffer to the samples.
3. Incubate the mixture at 65°C for 30 min.
4. Centrifuge the dissolved samples for 5 min at 11,336 ×g to obtain a clear supernatant.
5. Add 400 μL of 2× CTAB buffer to the supernatant and incubate on ice for 30 min.
6. Centrifuge the mixture for 5 min at 11,336 ×g to obtain a clear supernatant.

DNeasy Plant Pro Kit extraction part:

7. Add 500 μL APP buffer to the clear supernatant and vortex for 5 s.
8. Place an MB spin column in a 2-mL collection tube.
9. Add the mixture to the MB spin column and centrifuge for 1 min at 12,100 ×g.
10. Discard the flow-through and place the MB spin column back to the same collection tube.
11. Repeat Step 9 and 10 until all the mixture from Step 7 has passed through the MB spin column.
12. Place the MB spin column into a clean 2-mL collection tube.

13. Add 650 µL AW1 buffer to the MB spin column and centrifuge for 1 min at 12,100 ×g.
14. Discard the flow-through and place the MB spin column back to the same collection tube.
15. Add 650 µL AW2 buffer to the MB spin column and centrifuge for 1 min at 12,100 ×g.
16. Discard the flow-through and place the MB spin column back to the same collection tube.
17. Centrifuge the empty MB spin column for 2 min at 16,000 ×g.
18. Place the MB spin column back in a new 1.5-mL microcentrifuge tube.
19. Add 50 µL EB buffer to the centre of the spin column membrane. Let the column stand for 1 min and then centrifuge for 1 min at 12,100 ×g to obtain the purified DNA extract.

12.2.3 Modified Adaptor Ligation-Mediated PCR

12.2.3.1 *Adaptor Assembly and Pre-Treatment of DNA Sample*

Equipment

- Thermocycler

Reagents

- PCR buffer, 10×
- $MgCl_2$, 25 mM
- Deoxynucleoside triphosphates (dNTPs), 2.5 mM
- *Taq* DNA polymerase, 5 U/µL

Procedures

1. Prepare and mix well 5 µM adaptor long strand (AL1) and short strand (AS1) (Table 12.2) and incubate at 96°C for 2 min, followed by a 5% ramp rate of decreasing temperature to 20°C.

Table 12.2 Oligonucleotides for Adaptor Assembly and Primers for Adaptor Ligation–Mediated PCR

Oligonucleotide/Primer name	Sequence (5′ to 3′)
Long strand adaptor (AL1)	ACT ATT CAG GCG GTA ATA ACG TAT CGG GCT GTG CTA T
Short strand adaptor (AS1)	Phosphate — TAG CAC AGC CCG — Amino C7
Adaptor primer (AP1)	ACT ATT CAG GCG GTA ATA ACG
Barcoding primer on *psbA-trnH* region (fwd)	GTT ATG CAT GAA CGT AAT GCT C

2. Incubate the DNA samples at 96°C for 2 min, followed by a 5% ramp rate of decreasing temperature to 20°C for better base pairing.
3. Create a single 3′-adenine (A) overhang on DNA samples for adaptor ligation (Section 12.2.3.2) according to the following temperature and reaction time profile:

Reagent	Reaction volume	Reaction temperature and period
Double-distilled water	12.5 μL	72°C for 15 min
PCR buffer	2.5 μL	
$MgCl_2$	2.5 μL	
dNTPs	2.3 μL	
Taq DNA polymerase	0.2 μL	
Treated DNA sample	5 μL	

12.2.3.2 *Adaptor Ligation–Mediated PCR*

Equipment

- Thermocycler

Reagents

- Rapid Ligation Buffer, 2× (Promega, Madison, WI)
- T4 DNA Ligase, 3 Weiss unit/µL (Promega)
- PCR buffer, 10×
- $MgCl_2$, 25 mM
- dNTPs, 2.5 mM
- *Taq* DNA polymerase, 5 U/µL

Procedures

1. Ligate the assembled adaptor pairs and pre-treated DNA samples in Section 12.2.3.1 according to the following temperature and reaction time profile:

Reagent	Reaction volume	Reaction temperature and period
Rapid ligation buffer	5 µL	25°C for 2 h (ligation); 96°C for 5 min (post-ligation ligase denaturation)
Adaptor pairs	2 µL	
T4 DNA Ligase	1 µL	
Pre-treated DNA sample	2 µL	

2. Perform PCR reaction according to the following temperature and reaction time profile:

Reagent	Reaction volume	Reaction temperature and period
Double-distilled water	12.1 µL	94°C for 3 min; 35 cycles of 94°C for 30 s, 55°C for 20 s and 72°C for 30 s; 72°C for 5 min
PCR buffer	2.5 µL	
$MgCl_2$	2.5 µL	
dNTPs	2.5 µL	
Adaptor primer (AP1)	1.5 µL	
Barcoding primer (fwd)	1.5 µL	
Taq DNA polymerase	0.4 µL	
Ligated product	2 µL	

12.2.4 Next Generation Sequencing

The PCR products (around 1.5 μg amount) obtained after adaptor ligation-mediated PCR were sent for library construction and NGS. This involves four major steps: (1) Original sample quality control (QC): The quantity of DNA was determined by fluorescence-based quantification, which employed double-stranded DNA (dsDNA)-specific dye to quantitate dsDNA specifically and accurately, even in the presence of many common contaminants. On the other hand, the UV-spectrometer-based method, which relies on the absorbance at 260 nm, was prone to overestimating the DNA concentration due to the presence of RNA and other contaminants commonly found in DNA preparations. Electrophoresis was then conducted to reveal the DNA condition, such as smearing of DNA bands, nicking or any other DNA damage. The size range of DNA fragments were then checked by a 2100 Bioanalyzer (Agilent, Santa Clara, CA). (2) Library construction: The sequencing library was prepared using a TruSeq DNA Sample prep Kit following the manufacturer's instruction: TruSeq DNA Sample Preparation Guide, Part # 15026486 Rev. C for 5′ and 3′ library adaptor ligation. The library adaptor-ligated fragments were then PCR amplified with gel purified, followed by library QC. (3) Sequencing: Illumina HiSeqXTen Sequencing Platform was used, by which the library was loaded into a flow cell where fragments were captured on a lawn of surface-bound oligos, which were complementary to the library adaptors. Each fragment was then amplified into distinct, clonal clusters through bridge amplification. When cluster generation was completed, the templates were then sequenced by the reversible terminator-based method that detected single bases as they incorporated into DNA template strands. (4) Generation of raw data: The raw images generated by

Illumina sequencing were analysed by an integrated primary analysis software, Real-Time Analysis (RTA), which is a sequencing control software for system control and base calling through. The BCL (base calls) binary was converted into raw data in FASTQ format utilising the Illumina package bcl2fastq.

12.2.5 Bioinformatics Analysis

The raw sequencing data in FASTQ format were compressed by GZIP. Quality control steps were performed before proceeding to data analysis using FastQC (https://www.bioinformatics.babraham.ac.uk/projects/fastqc/). The sequencing quality of each base, lengths, GC contents and sequencing adaptor contamination of the reads were checked. Usually, the raw sequencing data were not perfect, e.g., contaminated by the sequencing adaptor. In this protocol, we recommend Trimmomatic (Bolger, Lohse & Usadel, 2014) to perform the adaptor trimming step. The data quality was improved after the adaptor trimming, confirmed by FastQC. The trimmed read data were then mapped to the reference database. The BWA aligner (https://arxiv.org/abs/1303.3997) was chosen in this protocol to perform the mapping step, and Samtools (https://samtools.github.io/) was used to handle the alignment file generated by BWA. Finally, to count the number of reads being mapped to each reference sequence, HTSeq (Anders, Pyl & Huber, 2015) was used for generating the read counts.

12.2.5.1 *Preparation of Computational Environment*

This protocol was designed for using a computer with Linux systems, such as Ubuntu with a command line terminal. Depending on the size of the raw sequencing data, the minimal requirement of RAM should be between 16 and 32 G. There was no requirement for the number of CPU threads. But, usually, more CPUs would speed up the process of analysis. Conda environment (https://docs.conda.io/en/latest/) was also used in this protocol, which is a virtual environment for the convenient management of bioinformatics software.

12.2.5.2 *Setting Up the Conda Environment and Installing Required Bioinformatics Software*

1. *Installation of Miniconda*

Minicoanda was downloaded from https://docs.conda.io/en/latest/miniconda.html. Miniconda is a minimised version of the regular Conda, Anaconda, containing only a small number of useful packages required for daily operation. The Linux installer was downloaded in this protocol. The instructions at https://conda.io/projects/conda/en/latest/user-guide/install/linux.html were followed to install Miniconda.

2. *Create the Conda environment and install the required bioinformatics software*

A Conda environment, with a user-defined name, was created by following the Managing environments session at https://conda.io/projects/conda/en/latest/user-guide/getting-started.html. In the newly created Conda environment, fastqc, trimmomatic, bwa, samtools, cd-hit and htseq were installed following the instructions at https://conda.io/projects/conda/en/latest/user-guide/getting-started.html and the Managing packages session. The following analyses were performed in the activated Conda environment.

12.2.5.3 *Reference Database Construction*

Database with the feature of species 'Plant', sequencing type 'Nucleotide' and barcoding region '*psbA-trnH*' was downloaded from GenBank in FASTA format for read alignment. The respective database in GFF3 format was also downloaded as the HTSeq reference. In this protocol, the FASTA and GFF3 file were named as raw_database.fasta and raw_database.gff3, respectively. The respective Cluster Database at High Identity with Tolerance (CD-HIT) program (Fu, Niu, Zhu, Wu & Li, 2012) should be used for collapsing reference sequences that were similar, by which the data of the downloaded database were clustered by the following command:

cd-hit-est -i <raw_database.fasta> -o <ref_database.fasta> -c 0.95 -n 10

12.2.5.4 *Quality Control of Sequencing Read Data*

Assuming the sequencing read data were paired-end, named as read1.fastq.gz and read2.fastq.gz, FastQC could be run using the following command:

fastqc <read1.fastq.gz> <read2.fastq.gz>

There were usually two output files generated for each read file, i.e., read1_fastqc.zip and read1_fastqc.html; and read2_fastqc.zip and read2_fastqc.html. The '.html' file is usually sufficient for visualising the result, whereas the '.zip' file contains all the source data and images present in the html file.

After checking the quality of the read data, adaptor trimming was usually performed. Adaptor sequence of the sample was required before trimming. The information of the adaptor sequence should be specified by the sequencing library kit.

The adaptor sequence and its reverse complement were saved in a FASTA file, e.g., adaptors.fasta, with contents as follows:

>adaptor
Adaptor sequence *
>adaptor_RC
Adaptor sequence (in reverse complement) #

* The sequence of the adaptor used in the ligation step.
# The reverse complementary sequence of the adaptor used in the ligation step.

Trimmomatic was then used to perform adaptor trimming using the following command:

trimmomatic PE -trimlog <read.log> <read1.fastq.gz> <read2.fastq.gz> <read1_paired.fastq.gz> <read1_unpaired.fastq.gz> <read2_paired.fastq.gz> <read2_unpaired.fastq.gz> ILLUMINACLIP:adaptors.fa:2:30:10 MINLEN:36

The above command instructs Trimmomatic to trim off the adaptor sequence, as well its reverse complement, as specified in adaptors.fa. At least 36 nucleotides were retained for any trimmed read, otherwise the read pairs were discarded. The successfully trimmed read pairs were in read1_paired.fastq.gz and read2_paired.fastq.gz, whereas the discarded pairs were in read1_unpaired.fastq.gz and read2_unpaired.fastq.gz. The read.log file contains the information of how the reads were trimmed. It is highly recommended to read the Trimmomatic manual (http://www.usadellab.org/cms/?page=trimmomatic) to know more about the parameters and outputs. An additional quality control step using FastQC was performed to check the data quality after the trimming step.

12.2.5.5 *Read Mapping to the Reference Database*

After data trimming, the clean read data were ready for mapping to the reference database. To perform the mapping step, index files of the database were generated using BWA with the following command:

bwa index <ref_database.fasta>

There were five index files being generated, including the following:

ref_database.fasta.amb
ref_database.fasta.ann
ref_database.fasta.bwt
ref_database.fasta.fai
ref_database.fasta.pac
ref_database.fasta.sa

Read mapping was then performed using the following command:

bwa mem <ref_database.fasta> <read1_paired.fastq.gz> <read2_paired.fastq.gz> | samtools view -bS - | samtools sort - > <read.bam>

In this step, the read pairs were mapped to the reference sequences using the BWA-MEM algorithm. It first generated the result in SAM format (https://samtools.github.io/hts-specs/SAMv1.pdf), which was then passed to Samtools for converting to BAM format and sorting. BAM is a compressed binary format of the SAM format, which contains the information of how each read mapped to the reference sequences. The BAM files were viewed using the following command:

samtools view <read.bam>

12.2.5.6 *Read Counting to Reference Sequences*

Since the reads were mapped to the reference sequences, the number of reads mapped to each reference sequence was counted for quantifying the abundance of reference sequences in the amplicon library. The following command was used for read counting:

htseq-count -t region -i Dbxref <read.sam> <raw_database.gff3> **>** <read_count.txt>

Multiple BAM files could be supplied to HTSeq, which should precede the GFF3 file, to perform read counting for multiple samples simultaneously. The output file is a table, with the row indicating each reference sequence and the column summarising the read count in each sample. For comparing the abundance of reference sequences in different samples, the read count of each reference sequence was normalised, e.g., divided by the total number of mapped reads in the corresponding sample.

12.2.6 Result Validation

Primers were designed for the validation of the *Hedyotis* species revealed from the HTSeq analysis (Table 12.3). Target DNA was amplified by PCR. The PCR product was purified and sequenced (BGI Hong Kong). The identities of the obtained sequences were compared by the Basic Local Alignment Search Tool (BLAST),

Table 12.3 Sequences and Parameters of the Designed Primers for Data Validation

Target species	Primer name	DNA locus	Primer sequence (5′ to 3′)	Annealing temp. (°C)	Amplicon size (bp)
Hedyotis diffusa, *H. corymbosa* and *H. tenelliflora*	ITS_F1	*ITS*	CGG AAA GCG CCA AGG ACT AC	58	138
	ITS_R1		TCA CGG GAT TCT GCA ATT CAC		

National Center for Biotechnology Information (NCBI) with the consideration of different parameters, including query cover, E-value, score and identity (%). Query sequences were identified with the top hit of similarity.

12.3 Results

12.3.1 Data Quality after Adaptor Ligation-Mediated PCR

The modified DNA extraction method removed colour pigments and relative metabolites effectively and resulted in high-quality DNA extracts. DNA concentration and A260/A280 measurements of DNA extracts are shown in Table 12.4.

12.3.2 Database Construction

GenBank from NCBI was used as the reference database. The database downloaded with 28,688 sequences at barcoding region '*psbA-trnH*' was clustered by CD-HIT, with nearly 85% repeated sequences discarded, and only 4,398 sequences remained.

Table 12.4 DNA Concentration and A260/A280 Measurements of the Three Samples Studied

Sample voucher	DNA concentration (ng/μL)	A260/A280
T4794	110.2	1.95
T4795	115.8	1.86
T4286	114.3	1.90

Table 12.5 FastQC Results of the Three Samples Before and After Adaptor Trimming

Sample voucher		T4794	T4795	T4286
Before adaptors trimming	Total reads	18,028,408	11,418,002	11,695,814
	Sequence length	101	101	101
	GC (%)	41	42	42
After adaptors trimming	Total reads	313,418	508,726	507,574
	Sequence length	36–101	36–101	36–101
	GC (%)	41	41	42
Sequence retained (%)		1.74%	4.46%	4.34%

12.3.3 Adaptor Trimming

The general sequence information of the three samples before and after adaptor trimming by Trimmomatic are summarised in Table 12.5.

12.3.4 Read Mapping

The algorithm, BWA-MEM, from the BWA tool was chosen, which was best suited for 70–100 bp Illumina reads. The mapping statistics showed the number of mapped reads of T4794, T4795 and T4286 were 41.6%, 12.38% and 4.17%, respectively. The mapping results were in universal SAM format, which can be manipulated by SAMtools.

12.3.5 Read Counting

HTSeq was used to count the number of reads against a provided list of plant species features. The top 10 plant species with corresponding reads number obtained are shown in Table 12.6.

Table 12.6 Identification Results with Matched Species in HTSeq. The Top 10 Matched Species Are Shown in the Descending Order of Relative Abundance

	T4794		T4795		T4286	
	Species	**# Matched**	**Species**	**# Matched**	**Species**	**# Matched**
1	*Hedyotis diffusa**	2415	*Hedyotis corymbosa**	2308	*Crotalaria podocarpa*	1682
2	*Spermacoce alata*	1473	*Crotalaria podocarpa*	1197	*Hedyotis corymbosa**	531
3	*Cichorium intybus*	1217	*Hedyotis tenelliflora**	1186	*Sinomenium acutum*	359
4	*Hedyotis corymbosa**	955	*Trigonella foenum-graecum*	502	*Steganotaenia araliacea*	81
5	*Magnolia champaca*	925	*Melilotus officinalis*	292	*Andrographis paniculata*	71
6	*Justicia gendarussa*	482	*Cuscuta reflexa*	259	*Elephantopus scaber*	42
7	*Hedyotis tenelliflora**	366	*Leptodermis ovata*	227	*Thymus pulegioides*	32
8	*Senna alexandrina*	284	*Hedyotis diffusa**	91	*Centratherum australianum*	30
9	*Bryum argenteum*	1174	*Trigastrotheca stricta*	73	*Cyperus lancastriensis*	28
10	*Sambucus nigra*	122	*Glycyrrhiza glabra*	54	*Cuscuta reflexa*	21

*Species belongs to genus *Hedyotis*.

12.3.6 Validation of Identified Species from NGS Data

The BLAST results revealed the top identical species with 100% query coverage and identity. It showed that T4794 was most likely to be *H. diffusa*, and T4795 and T4286 were most likely to be *H. corymbosa*.

12.4 Discussion

12.4.1 Adaptor Ligation-Mediated PCR

Adaptor ligation-mediated PCR utilises an adaptor-specific primer with one of the universal primers to amplify target DNA fragments. In contrast with diagnostic PCR, no prior knowledge about the target DNA sequence is required. This technique is widely used for genomic footprinting (Mueller & Wold, 1989; Steigerwald, Pfeifer & Riggs, 1990), amplifying genomic DNA fragments (Fors, Saavedra & Hood, 1990; Riley *et al.*, 1990; Roux & Dhanarajan, 1990) and low-abundance cDNA (Chaudhary *et al.*, 1990; Huang & Stollar, 1991; Ko, 1990; Timblin, Battey & Kuehl, 1990). In this study, we adopt the adaptor ligation-mediated PCR modified from O'Malley, Alonso, Kim, Leisse & Ecker (2007), which is used to determine the T-DNA insertion site, to amplify DNA barcode in degraded DNA.

After the adaptor ligation step, three major types of DNA products were formed: (A) Adaptor — Sample DNA with target primer binding site — Adaptor, (B) Adaptor — Sample DNA without target primer binding site — Adaptor and (C) Non-ligated sample DNA or adaptor only. The formation of (B) and (C) without the target site may interfere with the subsequent sequence analysis.

The design of asymmetric strands and terminal modification (Figure 12.3) for the adaptor maximises the amplification of (A) while prohibits the non-target amplification of (B) and (C). The non-paired region on adaptor long strand (AL1) has exactly the same oligonucleotide sequence as the adaptor-specific primer (AP1), i.e., no complementary binding between AL1 and AP1. Successful PCR amplification will only occur after the complementary strand of AL1 (i.e., the AP1 binding site) is synthesised by strand extension during the first PCR cycle, which is initiated by the

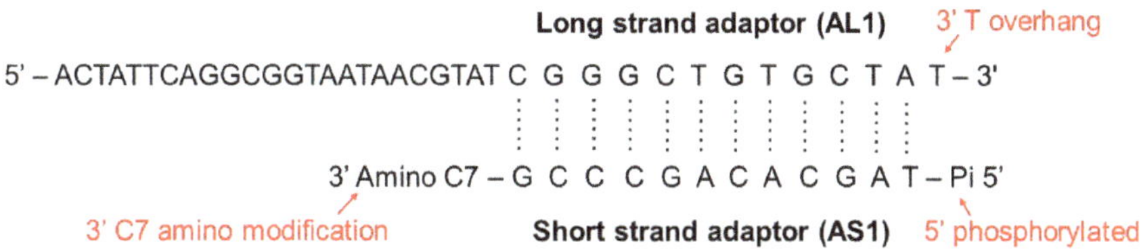

Fig. 12.3 Design of the adaptor. It consists of a long strand (AL1) and a short strand (AS1) with modifications. Both strands share a short complementary region for the assembly of the adaptor. The long strand contains a 3′-T overhang, which corresponds to the 3′-A overhang in the *Taq* polymerase-treated DNA sample.

binding of the barcoding primer with the presence of the target site (fwd). Moreover, the 3′-C7 amino modification at the adaptor short strand (AS1) prevents self-strand extension beyond the 3′ end of AS1 to create a latent AP1 binding site. The formation of the latent binding site will cause non-specific amplification for adaptor-flanked templates, even without the target site. Since this 'adaptor-tag' DNA sample only needs one end of the barcoding primer for amplification, various lengths of DNA fragments with a target site (fwd) will be amplified. On the other hand, the 3′-thymine (T) overhang at AL1 facilitates the sticky-end ligation to the 3′-adenine (A) overhang in the *Taq* polymerase-treated DNA sample and prevents self-ligation of adaptors, which may decrease the efficiency of adaptor ligation.

DNA from medicinal products is usually degraded and universal primers are not applicable for PCR. Another common practice of using mini-barcode primers for PCR followed by cloning is time-consuming and expensive. Moreover, the adulterant DNA may be missed if insufficient clones are picked for sequencing. Our developed adaptor ligation-mediated PCR with metabarcoding method overcomes these problems. The amplicons generated with different sizes facilitate the subsequent high-throughput sequencing and results in abundant raw data information for analysis.

12.4.2 Bioinformatics Analysis

The protocol developed in this study mapped the sequencing reads to a reference database and counted the number of reads mapped to the reference sequences by various bioinformatics software (Table 12.7). BWA is an accurate and fast read mapper. HTSeq takes the mapping results and performs read counting. For reads that cannot be uniquely mapped to the reference, they will not be counted for any feature. Instead, these reads will be counted in rows, including __no_feature, __ambiguous, __too_low_aQual, __not_aligned and __alignment_not_unique. These non-uniquely mapped reads should be better handled in the future. For example, they can be given different weights to the mapped reference sequences by some probabilistic models.

To reveal that all the suspected plant species existed in an unknown product, it is necessary to construct an informative reference database before the read mapping steps. In this project, we used GenBank from NCBI as the reference database. The database downloaded with 28,688 sequences was first clustered by CD-HIT with nearly 85% repeated sequences discarded, and only 4,398 sequences remained. The CD-HIT program enhanced the subsequent mapping and reads counting performance by reducing sequence redundancy.

Success of species identification relies on the DNA sequence information obtained. If the size of the amplicon is too short or the DNA region selected for amplification is too conserved, it may fail to differentiate closely related species with low sequence resolution. To increase the accuracy in authentication, a validated DNA sequence database as reference is needed.

Table 12.7 Bioinformatics Software Used in the Study

Software	Description	Function	Reference
FastQC	A quality control software	To validate the data quality with detailed summary graphs and tables as reference	(Wingett & Andrews, 2018)
Trimmomatic	A trimming tool	To process paired-end data and to trim Illumina adaptor sequences, self-designed adaptor sequences and poor-quality sequences	(Bolger, Lohse & Usadel, 2014)
CD-HIT	A database clustering program	To construct an informative reference database by reducing sequence data redundancy	(Fu, Niu, Zhu, Wu & Li, 2012)
BWA	A local aligner	To map read sequences to the clustered nucleotide database	(Li & Durbin, 2010)
SAMtools	A high-throughput sequencing data manipulation utility	To manipulate alignments in the SAM, BAM and CRAM formats, including sorting, merging, indexing, etc.	(Li *et al.*, 2009)
HTSeq	A high-throughput sequencing data analyser	To count the number of reads overlapping with genomic features given. It possesses a non-redundant counting feature. Reads aligned with more than one gene features are discarded	(Anders, Pyl & Huber, 2015)

12.5 Conclusion

In conventional DNA barcoding, species identification work is carried out by PCR amplification followed by DNA sequencing using universal primers. However, it is difficult to amplify the full-length DNA barcodes in processed products due to DNA degradation. The adaptor ligation-mediated PCR is a promising universal method for species identification in highly processed food and medicinal products. With the support of prevailing bioinformatics technologies, NGS becomes the newly emerged cost-effective and high-throughput sequencing platform for the identification and authentication of medicinal products. The combination of adaptor ligation-mediated PCR with NGS allows the amplification of degraded DNA by massively sequencing the PCR products. Besides extending this approach to other medicinal products, we may apply it on (1) adulterant/contaminant discovery and (2) semi-quantification of products with multi-ingredients.

References

Anders, S., Pyl, P. T., & Huber, W. (2015). HTSeq — a Python framework to work with high-throughput sequencing data. *Bioinformatics, 31*(2), 166–169. doi:10.1093/bioinformatics/btu638

Arulandhu, A. J., Staats, M., Hagelaar, R., Voorhuijzen, M. M., Prins, T. W., Scholtens, I., Costessi, A., Duijsings, D., Rechenmann, F., Gaspar, F. B., Crespo, M. T. B., Holst-Jensen, A., Birck, M., Burns, M., Haynes, E., Hochegger, R., Klingl, A., Lundberg, L., Natale, C., Niekamp, H., Perri, E., Barbante, A., Rosec, J. P., Seyfarth, R., Sovová, T., Moorleghem, C. V., Ruth, S. V., Peelen, T., & Kok, E. (2017). Development and validation of a multi-locus DNA metabarcoding method to identify endangered species in complex samples. *Gigascience, 6*(10), 1–18. doi:10.1093/gigascience/gix080

Bolger, A. M., Lohse, M., & Usadel, B. (2014). Trimmomatic: A flexible trimmer for Illumina sequence data. *Bioinformatics, 30*(15), 2114–2120. doi:10.1093/bioinformatics/btu170

Chaudhary, V. K., Batra, J. K., Gallo, M. G., Willingham, M. C., FitzGerald, D. J., & Pastan, I. (1990). A rapid method of cloning functional variable-region antibody genes in Escherichia coli as single-chain immunotoxins. *Proc Nat Acad Sci USA, 87*(3), 1066–1070. doi:10.1073/pnas.87.3.1066

Chen, T., & Taylor, C. M. (2011). Hedyotis. In Z. Y. Wu, P. H. Raven, & D. Y. Hong (Eds.), *Flora of China* (Vol. 19, pp. 147–174). Beijing, Louis: Science Press, Missouri Botanical Garden Press.

Cheng, X., Su, X., Chen, X., Zhao, H., Bo, C., Xu, J., Bai, H., & Ning, K. (2014). Biological ingredient analysis of traditional Chinese medicine preparation based on high-throughput sequencing: The story for Liuwei Dihuang Wan. *Sci Rep, 4*, 5147. doi:10.1038/srep05147

Coghlan, M. L., Haile, J., Houston, J., Murray, D. C., White, N. E., Moolhuijzen, P., Bellgard, B. I., & Bunce, M. (2012). Deep sequencing of plant and animal DNA contained within traditional Chinese medicines reveals legality issues and health safety concerns. *PLoS Genet, 8*(4), e1002657. doi:10.1371/journal.pgen.1002657

Coghlan, M. L., Maker, G., Crighton, E., Haile, J., Murray, D. C., White, N. E., Byard, R. W., Bellgard, M. I., Mullaney, I., Trengove, R., Allcock, R. J. N., Nash, C., Hoban, C., Jarrett, K., Edwards, R., Musgrave, I. F., & Bunce, M. (2015). Combined DNA, toxicological and heavy metal analyses provides an auditing toolkit to improve pharmacovigilance of traditional Chinese medicine (TCM). *Sci Rep, 5*, 17475. doi:10.1038/srep17475

Coissac, E., Hollingsworth, P. M., Lavergne, S., & Taberlet, P. (2016). From barcodes to genomes: Extending the concept of DNA barcoding. *Mol Ecol, 25*(7), 1423–1428. doi:10.1111/mec.13549

Fors, L., Saavedra, R. A., & Hood, L. (1990). Cloning of the shark Po promoter using a genomic walking technique based on the polymerase chain reaction. *Nucleic Acids Res, 18*(9), 2793–2799. doi:10.1093/nar/18.9.2793

Fu, L., Niu, B., Zhu, Z., Wu, S., & Li, W. (2012). CD-HIT: Accelerated for clustering the next-generation sequencing data. *Bioinformatics, 28*(23), 3150–3152. doi:10.1093/bioinformatics/bts565

Guilfoyle, R. A., Leeck, C. L., Kroening, K. D., Smith, L. M., & Guo, Z. (1997). Ligation-mediated PCR amplification of specific fragments from a class-II restriction endonuclease total digest. *Nucleic Acids Res, 25*(9), 1854–1858. doi:10.1093/nar/25.9.1854

Huang, C., & Stollar, B. D. (1991). Construction of representative immunoglobulin variable region cDNA libraries from human peripheral blood lymphocytes without in vitro stimulation. *J Immunol Methods, 141*(2), 227–236. doi:10.1016/0022–1759(91)90149-a

Jia, J., Xu, Z., Xin, T., Shi, L., & Song, J. (2017). Quality control of the traditional patent medicine Yimu Wan based on SMRT sequencing and DNA barcoding. *Front Plant Sci, 8*, 926. doi:10.3389/fpls.2017.00926

Jiang, L. L., Lo, Y. T., Chen, W. T., & Shaw, P. C. (2016). DNA authentication of animal-derived concentrated Chinese medicine granules. *J Pharm Biomed Anal, 129*, 398–404. doi:10.1016/j.jpba.2016.07.030

Ko, M. S. (1990). An 'equalized cDNA library' by the reassociation of short double-stranded cDNAs. *Nucleic Acids Res, 18*(19), 5705–5711. doi:10.1093/nar/18.19.5705

Li, H., & Durbin, R. (2010). Fast and accurate long-read alignment with Burrows-Wheeler transform. *Bioinformatics, 26*(5), 589–595. doi:10.1093/bioinformatics/btp698

Li, H., Handsaker, B., Wysoker, A., Fennell, T., Ruan, J., Homer, N., Marth, G., Abecasis, G., Durbin, R., & Genome Project Data Processing Subgroup (2009). The sequence alignment/map format and SAMtools. *Bioinformatics, 25*(16), 2078–2079. doi:10.1093/bioinformatics/btp352

Li, Q., Sun, Y., Guo, H., Sang, F., Ma, H., Peng, H., Zheng, N., and Xu, L. (2018). Quality control of the traditional Chinese medicine Ruyi jinhuang powder based on high-throughput sequencing and real-time PCR. *Sci Rep, 8*(1), 8261. doi:10.1038/s41598–018-26520-3

Little, D. P. (2014). A DNA mini-barcode for land plants. *Mol Ecol Resour, 14*(3), 437–446. doi:10.1111/1755-0998.12194

Lo, Y. T., Li, M., & Shaw, P. C. (2015). Identification of constituent herbs in ginseng decoctions by DNA markers. *Chin Med, 10*(1), 1. doi:10.1186/s13020-015-0029-x

Lo, Y. T., & Shaw, P. C. (2018). DNA barcoding in concentrated Chinese medicine granules using adaptor ligation-mediated polymerase chain reaction. *J Pharm Biomed Anal, 149*, 512–516. doi:10.1016/j.jpba.2017.11.048

Meusnier, I., Singer, G. A., Landry, J. F., Hickey, D. A., Hebert, P. D., & Hajibabaei, M. (2008). A universal DNA mini-barcode for biodiversity analysis. *BMC Genomics*, 9, 214. doi:10.1186/1471-2164-9-214

Moon, B. C., Kim, W. J., Ji, Y., Lee, Y. M., Kang, Y. M., & Choi, G. (2016). Molecular identification of the traditional herbal medicines, Arisaematis Rhizoma and Pinelliae Tuber, and common adulterants via universal DNA barcode sequences. *Genet Mol Res, 15*(1), gmr7064. doi:10.4238/gmr.15017064

Mueller, P. R., & Wold, B. (1989). In vivo footprinting of a muscle specific enhancer by ligation mediated PCR. *Science, 246*(4931), 780–786. doi:10.1126/science.2814500

Nyren, P. (2007). The history of pyrosequencing. *Methods Mol Biol, 373*, 1–14. doi:10.1385/1-59745-377-3:1

O'Malley, R. C., Alonso, J. M., Kim, C. J., Leisse, T. J., & Ecker, J. R. (2007). An adapter ligation-mediated PCR method for high-throughput mapping of T-DNA inserts in the Arabidopsis genome. *Nat Protoc, 2*(11), 2910–2917. doi:10.1038/nprot.2007.425

Raclariu, A. C., Paltinean, R., Vlase, L., Labarre, A., Manzanilla, V., Ichim, M. C., Crisan, G., Brysting, A. K., & de Boer, H. (2017). Comparative authentication of Hypericum perforatum herbal products using DNA metabarcoding, TLC and HPLC-MS. *Sci Rep, 7*(1), 1291. doi:10.1038/s41598-017-01389-w

Riley, J., Butler, R., Ogilvie, D., Finniear, R., Jenner, D., Powell, S., Anand, R., Smith, J. C., & Markham, A. F. (1990). A novel, rapid method for the isolation of terminal sequences from yeast artificial chromosome (YAC) clones. *Nucleic Acids Res, 18*(10), 2887–2890. doi:10.1093/nar/18.10.2887

Ronaghi, M., Uhlen, M., & Nyren, P. (1998). A sequencing method based on real-time pyrophosphate. *Science, 281*(5375), 363, 365. doi:10.1126/science.281.5375.363

Roux, K. H., & Dhanarajan, P. (1990). A strategy for single site PCR amplification of dsDNA: Priming digested cloned or genomic DNA from an anchor-modified restriction site and a short internal sequence. *BioTechniques, 8*(1), 48–57. Retrieved from https://www.ncbi.nlm.nih.gov/pubmed/2322453

Siu, T. Y., Yik, M. H. Y., Boufford, D. E., Shaw, P. C., & Lau, D. T. W. (2021). (2813) Proposal to conserve the name Hedyotis diffusa (Oldenlandia diffusa, Scleromitrion diffusum) (Rubiaceae) with a conserved type. *TAXON, 70*(2), 443–444. doi:https://doi.org/10.1002/tax.12488

Smith, D. R. (1992). Ligation-mediated PCR of restriction fragments from large DNA molecules. *PCR Methods Appl, 2*(1), 21–27. doi:10.1101/gr.2.1.21

Song, M., Dong, G. Q., Zhang, Y. Q., Liu, X., & Sun, W. (2017). Identification of processed Chinese medicinal materials using DNA mini-barcoding. *Chin J Nat Med, 15*(7), 481–486. doi:10.1016/S1875-5364(17)30073-0

Steigerwald, S. D., Pfeifer, G. P., & Riggs, A. D. (1990). Ligation-mediated PCR improves the sensitivity of methylation analysis by restriction enzymes and detection of specific DNA strand breaks. *Nucleic Acids Res, 18*(6), 1435–1439. doi:10.1093/nar/18.6.1435

Timblin, C., Battey, J., & Kuehl, W. M. (1990). Application for PCR technology to subtractive cDNA cloning: Identification of genes expressed specifically in murine plasmacytoma cells. *Nucleic Acids Res, 18*(6), 1587–1593. doi:10.1093/nar/18.6.1587

Wingett, S. W., & Andrews, S. (2018). FastQ Screen: A tool for multi-genome mapping and quality control. *F1000Res, 7*, 1338. doi:10.12688/f1000research.15931.2

Yan, Z., Feng, J., Peng, J., Lai, Z., Zhang, L., Jin, Y., Yang, H., Chen, W., & Lin, J. (2017). Chloroform extract of Hedyotis diffusa Willd inhibits viability of human colorectal cancer cells via suppression of AKT and ERK signaling pathways. *Oncol Lett, 14*(6), 7923–7930. doi:10.3892/ol.2017.7245

Yeung, C. Y., Lee, H. C., Lin, S. P., Yang, Y. C., Huang, F. Y., & Chuang, C. K. (2006). Negative effect of heat sterilization on the free amino acid concentrations in infant formula. *Eur J Clin Nutr, 60*(1), 136–141. doi:10.1038/sj.ejcn.1602279

Yik, M. H., Kong, B. L., Siu, T. Y., Lau, D. T., Cao, H., & Shaw, P. C. (2021a). Differentiation of Hedyotis diffusa and common adulterants based on chloroplast genome sequencing and DNA barcoding markers. *Plants (Basel), 10*(1). doi:10.3390/plants10010161

Yik, M. H., Lo, Y. T., Lin, X., Sun, W., Chan, T. F., & Shaw, P. C. (2021b). Authentication of Hedyotis products by adaptor ligation-mediated PCR and metabarcoding. *J Pharm Biomed Anal, 196*, 113920. doi:10.1016/j.jpba.2021.113920

Zhou, J. L., & Wang, Y. S. (2004). *Analysis of Concentrated Medicinal Granules: A Thin Layer Chromatography Atlas*. Nanjing, China: Jiangsu Science and Technology Publishing House.

Chapter 13

Super-Barcoding of Medicinal Materials Based on Complete Plastid Genomes and Nuclear Ribosomal DNA

Hyun-Seung Park, Padmanaban Mohanan & Tae-Jin Yang

13.1 Introduction

The chloroplast is the most popular form of the plastid in plant cells and is an essential organelle for photosynthesis and metabolism (Jensen & Bassham, 1966; Wang & Benning, 2012). Plastid contains their own genome with a well-conserved circular structure across the plant lineages (Li *et al.*, 2019). Owing to the advancement in sequencing technology, a massive number of plastid genomes (plastome) have been reported. Up to now, around 8,269 complete plastid genomes from 3,289 species, which belong to angiosperm, gymnosperm, and green algae, are publicly available in GenBank, National Center for Biotechnology Information (NCBI).

Since the first idea of DNA barcoding, several universal barcoding regions based on the plastome and 'nuclear 45S ribosomal DNA' (45S nrDNA) regions were applied. The intergenic region of *trnH-GUG*, *psbA-trnH*, *rbcL*, *matK* in plastome, and internal transcribed spacer 2 (ITS2) in 45S nrDNA, have been the most commonly used regions for DNA barcoding (Chen *et al.*, 2010; Group *et al.*, 2009). The concept and protocol for universal DNA barcoding are standardised by the International Consortium for the Barcode of Life (CBOL) and applied to many studies for genetic diversity, genetic authentication and environmental meta-barcoding (García-Robledo, Erickson, Staines, Erwin & Kress, 2013; Li *et al.*, 2015). However, in concern with a recent burst of plastome sequences, there has been an attempt to use whole plastid genome itself as a barcode, called a super-barcode (Coissac, Hollingsworth, Lavergne & Taberlet, 2016; Li *et al.*, 2015), and many studies have been published applying this concept to medicinal or resource plants (Chen *et al.*, 2018; Kim *et al.*, 2015a; Lee *et al.*, 2017; Lee *et al.*, 2020; Li *et al.*, 2019; Nguyen *et al.*, 2017, 2020; Park *et al.*, 2020; Zhang, Zhang, Song, Guan & Ma, 2019). In this chapter, we reviewed the current status of super-barcoding by whole plastome and nrDNAs, the practical application method, and the characteristics of plastome to be considered to make an error-free precise DNA barcoding.

13.2 Genome Information for Barcoding Targets

DNA barcoding uses the genome information in plant cells. The nucleus contains the most abundant genomic materials that vary in size and the number of protein-coding genes because of frequent genome recombination and duplication. Finding a common set of nuclear protein-coding genes conserved through plant lineage has been a challenging task for DNA barcoding, since protein-coding genes should be conserved through diverse plant species (Hollingsworth, Graham & Little, 2011; Jayakodi *et al.*, 2020; Paterson, Freeling, Tang & Wang, 2010). Meanwhile, three other kinds of genomes are available for barcoding, namely nrDNA, plastome and mitochondrial genome (mitogenome) (Figure 13.1). The 45S

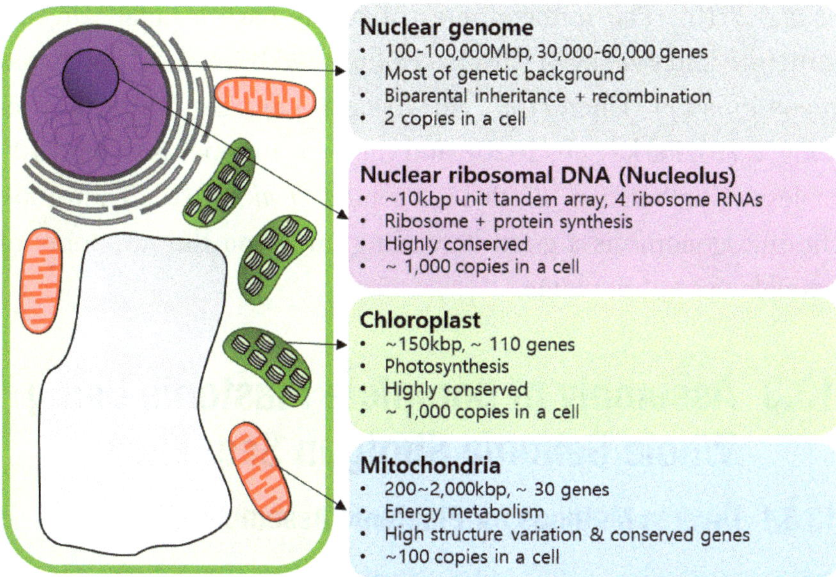

Fig. 13.1 Characteristics of the three genomes in a plant cell.

or 5S nrDNA are well conserved across the species and remain as a highly repetitive tandem array of more than several thousands of copies in the nucleolus (Baldwin *et al.*, 1995; Cloix *et al.*, 2000; Rosato, Kovař, Garilleti & Rossell, 2016). The ITS1, ITS2 and 5.8S rDNA or ITS2 itself are mainly used for barcoding target for the plants, animals and fungi (Chen *et al.*, 2010; Hillis & Dixon, 1991; Hollingsworth, 2011; Kress, Wurdack, Zimmer, Weigt & Janzen, 2005; Schoch *et al.*, 2012; Yao *et al.*, 2010).

Two cellular organelles, plastids and mitochondria, harbour their own independent genetic information separated from nuclear genomes in plants (McFadden, 1999). Plastomes are well conserved with a circular structure of around 150 kb in size and show high sequence similarity across the lineage in land plants (Li *et al.*, 2019) with around 1,000 or more, depending on the tissue type and developmental stage (Sakamoto & Takami, 2018; Takami *et al.*, 2018). The mitogenomes of plants have a highly diverse structure and size, even within a cell formed by a repeat-mediated recombination (Chen *et al.*, 2017; Park, Lee, Lee, Choi, Kim & Yang, 2013; Park *et al.*, 2020), and the copy number is around 100 or less (Gualberto *et al.*, 2014; Preuten *et al.*, 2010). Therefore, the mitogenome is a good barcoding target on the taxonomy of animals but not in plants.

13.3 Assembly of Complete Plastome Using Whole Genome Shotgun Sequence

13.3.1 Diverse Methods for Plastome Assembly

Diverse plastome assembly pipelines have been developed using second and third-generation sequencing platforms. Whole genome shotgun sequence (WGS) data are obtained based on the well-known genome assemblers such as SOAPdenovo2, SPAdes or CLC Genomics Workbench. Other approaches developed for the assembly of organelle genome are Novoplasty (Dierckxsens, Mardulyn & Smits, 2017), Interactive Organellar Genome Assembly pipeline (Bakker *et al.*, 2016) and GetOrganelle (Jin *et al.*, 2020). Those methods are open-source software publicly available and have been cited more than several hundred times for their fast and accurate assembly of organelle genome with efficient memory requirement.

13.3.2 *De novo* Assembly Using Low-Coverage Whole Genome Shotgun Sequence (dnaLCW)

The *de novo* assembly using low-coverage whole genome shotgun sequence (dnaLCW) is a high-throughput method to obtain the organelle genomes and nrDNA units simultaneously (Figure

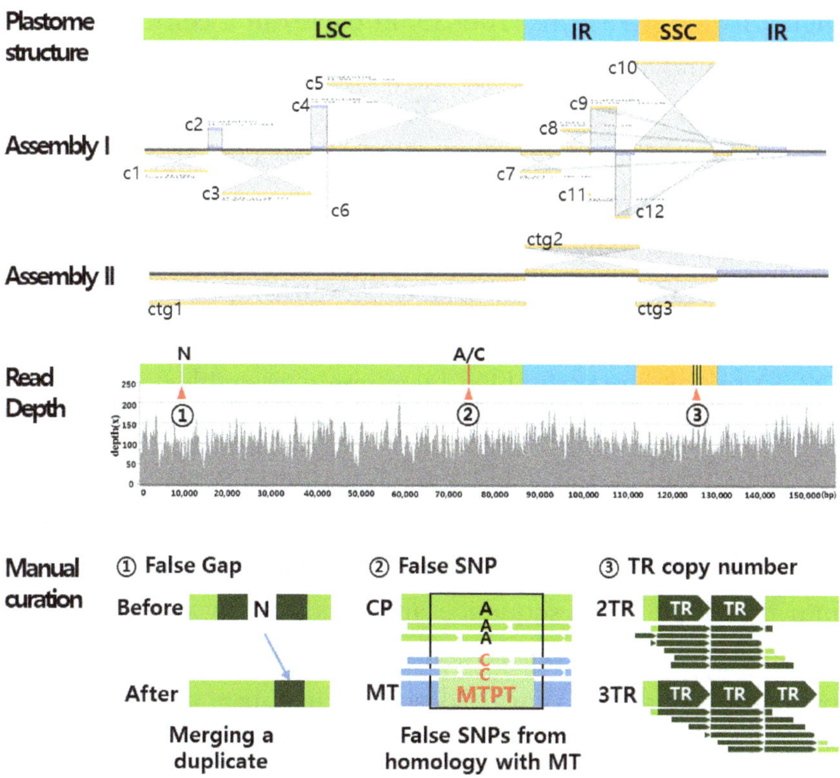

Fig. 13.2 Overview of complete plastome assembly and error corrections by dnaLCW. Plastome: The general plastome structure is represented. Assembly I: 12 basic contigs were obtained using 20 Gbp of Illumina paired-end (PE) reads. Assembly II: Three basic contigs representing LSC, IR and SSC were obtained by dnaLCW (1 Gbp of Illumina PE reads). Mapping depth: Mapping of raw PE reads on the assembled contigs showed approximately 100× coverage. Manual curation: Three assembly errors are marked with red triangles, and methods for manual curation are schematically presented. (1) The false gap can be curated by removing one of the duplicated regions marked with dark green boxes. (2) The false single nucleotide polymorphisms (SNPs) derived from MTPT or NUPT. (3) The misassembly derived from the copy number variation of tandem repeat (TR).

13.2). This method requires only one to three Giga base pairs (Gbp) of Illumina platform WGS reads. Even though the low-coverage WGS reads (LCW) represent around 1× or less coverage for nuclear genomes in diverse plants, it represents high depth coverage for plastome, mitogenomes and nrDNA because of their highly repetitive nature (100~1,000 copies in a cell). Therefore, the LCW provides enough sequencing depth for good assembly (Assembly-II in Figure 13.2). Too many of WGS reads do not provide a good assembly because of unexpected interruption of homologous sequences in other genomic sections, such as mitochondrial plastid DNA (MTPT) and nuclear plastid DNA (NUPT) (Assembly-I in Figure 13.2) Kim *et al.*, (2015b).

First, high-quality trimmed PE next generation sequencing (NGS) reads were assembled by genome assembler, and gaps in initial contigs were filled using the Gapcloser program. The plastid, mitochondria and nrDNA-related contigs were captured by Mummer using a reference genome sequence of relative species as bait. The captured contigs were aligned, ordered and merged into the single draft sequence and validated by remapping the whole genome reads on to themselves. Detailed procedures and parameters of dnaLCW were described in Kim *et al.*, (2015b).

Procedures

1. Preparing NGS raw data file in FASTQ format: You can generate the data by direct sequencing or download the Sequence Read Archive (SRA) data from National Center for Biotechnology Information (NCBI). Here, we used Illumina sequencing data as an example.
2. Raw data filtering: Removing poor quality reads from the raw data (Phred scores of 20 or less) using filtering software such as Trimmomatic or Quality trim tool in CLC assembly cell package.

    clc_quality_trim -r -i <file1> <file2> -f 33 -p <paired file> -o <unpaired file>

3. *De novo* assembly: Assemble the low-coverage NGS data based on plastid genome coverage under 200× using genome assemblers like SOAPdenovo2, SPAdes or CLC assembly cell.

    clc_novo_assemble -p fb ss <distance> -q <paired file> -p no <unpaired file> -o <output file>

    The '<distance>' includes both the reads and the sequence between them, which could be adjusted based on your NGS library size (default is '180 250').

4. Gap filling: Fill the sequence gaps using Gapcloser included in the SOAP package.

    GapCloser -b <library info file> -a <assembled contigs file> -o <output FASTA file>

    You can find an example of the library info file at SOAPdenovo manual (Appendix A). Changing the maximal read length in the library info file based on your NGS raw data will improve the gap filling result.

5. Retrieving plastid- or nrDNA-related contigs: BLAST or Nucmer can be used for finding plastid-related sequence from gap-filled FASTA file. Plastomes or nrDNA of closely related species are recommended to use as a reference.
    The order and direction of contigs consisting plastome or nrDNA are decided at this step and connected into a single draft sequence.

    nucmer *–p <PREFIX> <Reference sequence> < gap-filled FASTA file>*
    show-coords <"PREFIX".delta>

    This command will print the nucmer data to the screen.

6. Sequence validation and curation: Align the raw read onto the single draft sequence using read mapping program. Here, we used clc_mapper in CLC assembly cell package.

   clc_mapper -o mapping.cas -q <Paired file> -p no <Unpaired file> -p fb ss <distance> -d <single draft sequence>

   The '<distance>' here has the same meaning with the one used at de novo assembly and could also be adjusted based on your NGS library size (default is '180 250')
   The cases for manual curation are described in detail in Sections 13.3.2.1–13.3.2.3.

From 2015 to 2020, our group conducted NGS analysis on more than 500 species and published 66 papers about the complete chloroplast, mitochondrial genome, or nrDNA using the dnaLCW methods. We studied major food crops like rice (Kim *et al.*, 2015b), pepper (Park, Lee, Lee, Yang & Yoon, 2016), Brassica species (Kim *et al.*, 2018) as well as diverse medicinal or resource plants such as *Panax*, *Artemisia*, *Taraxacum*, *Epimedium*, *Hydrangea*, *Euonymus*, *Eclipta* and *Ilex* (Kim *et al.*, 2017a, 2017c; Kong *et al.*, 2021; Lee *et al.*, 2016, 2019a, 2020; Nguyen *et al.*, 2020) and completed mitogenomes of *Cynanchum*, *Platycodon grandifloras*, *Codonopsis lanceolate*, *Panax ginseng*, *Senna occidentalis*, *Solanum commersonii* and mushroom *Wolfiporia cocos* (Cho *et al.*, 2018; Jang *et al.*, 2020; Kang, Lee, Ahn & Kim, 2019; Lee *et al.*, 2018, 2019b; Park *et al.*, 2020). The validation and assembly error corrections are the crucial step for our assembly pipeline. The initially ordered draft plastome sequences are validated by aligning raw PE reads and manual curation. We summarised representative cases of unexpected false gaps, misassembly caused by paralogous and/or homologous DNAs, or slippage mediated by TR copy number errors that were frequently faced during sequence validation

(Figure 13.2). These regions were typically recognised by the accumulation of discordantly mapped reads or huge read depth at visualisation software.

13.3.2.1 *False Gaps*

This type of error is frequently found at ambiguous 'N' in the initially assembled contigs. The upstream and downstream sequences of an 'N' are simply duplicated, causing an unexpected gap. The gap can be corrected by merging duplicated common sequences flanking the gap. Removing one copy of the duplicate will show clear assembly by read mapping on the contigs.

13.3.2.2 *False SNPs*

DNA fragments homologous to the plastid genome are ubiquitous in mitochondrial and nuclear genomes of the plant, called MTPT and NUPT (Matsuo, Ito, Yamauchi & Obokata, 2005; Park *et al.*, 2020). These promiscuous DNA can interfere with the plastid DNA during plastome assembly, leading to false SNPs. Each false SNP could be corrected by following the nucleotide with the highest depth because the copy number of plastid DNA is much higher than those of mitochondria or nuclear DNA (Figure 13.1). For example, in a complete assembly of the organelle genome of *Cynanchum* species, the read depth mapped to the mitogenome was around 10% for those on plastome, representing the copy number difference of organelle genome within a cell (Kim *et al.*, 2015b; Park *et al.*, 2020).

13.3.2.3 *TR Copy Number Error*

The copy number error is a major challenge for *de novo* assembly using short reads (Treangen & Salzberg, 2012). When repeats are shorter than the read length, increasing the k-mer value above the

TR unit length can reduce misassembly. Copy number errors in the assembly can be identified and manually edited by abundant mismapped reads coupled with abnormal high read depth at the TR compared to the flanking region. Since most of the TRs in plastome are simple and less than 100 bp, such an error tends to be decreased by using long-read NGS platforms.

13.4 Genomics Perspective of Super-Barcoding Based on Plastome

13.4.1 Advantage and Disadvantage of Universal Barcode Primer

Traditional universal barcodes have been widely studied to diverse plant species, and the sequence database has been accumulated by the global scale projects such as BARCODE 500K or BIOSCAN by the international Barcode of Life consortium (iBOL) (Hobern & Hebert, 2019; Ratnasingham & Hebert, 2007). The easy accessibility through a standardised protocol, a simple sequencing step, a less computational requirement and the meta genome application are the major advantages of universal barcodes. The iBOL unveils the huge diversity for life, but short-sequence information obtained by polymerase chain reaction (PCR) amplification might have a limitation for understanding the deep depth of genome diversity and complexity. The ITS regions in 45S nrDNA are heterogeneous and provide some confusion in some plants (Kim *et al.*, 2018).

13.4.2 Plastome Diversity and Database

Compared to a short barcoding region, plastome can provide a wide range of interspecific variation, even in closely related species. Nucleotide variation occurs at the entire plastome, although certain genes or regions show suppressed or elevated variation, which may vary from species to species. Therefore, comparing the whole plastomes provides more opportunity to discover the concrete species-specific or genus-specific variations, and is particularly effective for reliable authentication. Additionally, more than 8,000 plastomes have been stored in public databases, and rapidly increase, which makes it easier to apply the concept of super-barcoding for the identification or authentication of plant samples.

For example, a comparison of the whole plastomes of seven *Panax* species, *P. ginseng*, *P. trifolius*, *P. stipuleanatus*, *P. vietnamensis*, *P. japonicus*, *P. notoginseng* and *P. quinquefolius*, detected 1,783 SNPs, including 1,128 located in the CDS regions. We also identified a number of intraspecific variations among multi-plastomes and mitogenomes in *P. ginseng* (Giang, Hyun-Seung, Nguyen, Park & Yang, 2021; Kim *et al.*, 2015a; Nguyen *et al.*, 2020) (Figure 13.3). The SNPs were distributed in most of the protein-coding genes, except the seven conserved genes, *psaJ*, *psbN*, *rpl23*, *psbF*, *psbL*, *rps18* and *rps7*, with no variation. Multiple markers developed from species-specific SNPs can clearly discriminate each of the seven *Panax* species. Another comparative analysis of chloroplast genome is a study of six Korean *Taraxacum* genus coupled with metabolomics. Interspecific variations were not only distributed at conventional barcoding regions but also the entire plastome and were frequently found at intergenic regions than CDS with three divergent hotspots of *trnM(CAU)-aptE*, *rbcL-psaI* and *trnL(UAG)-ccsA* (Lee *et al.*, 2020).

13.4.3 Intraspecific Plastome Diversity

The plastomes of multiple collections have enabled the identification of intraspecific diversity. False authentication can be induced

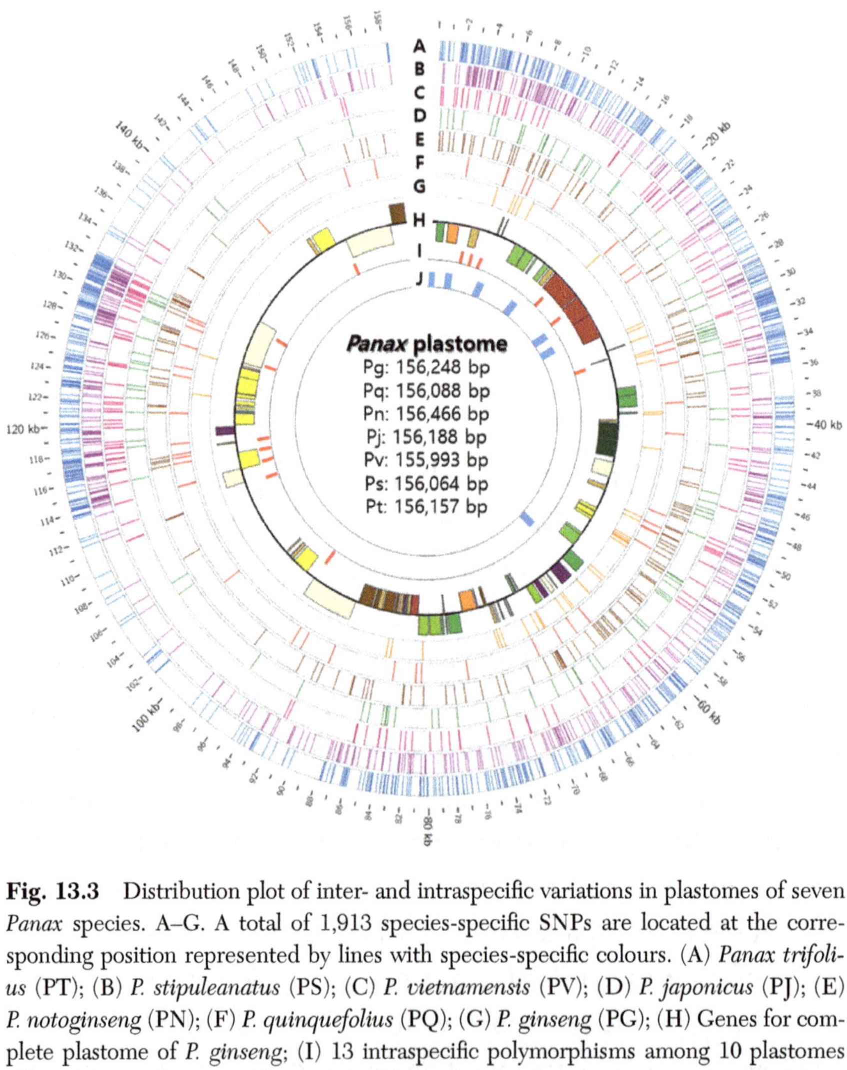

Fig. 13.3 Distribution plot of inter- and intraspecific variations in plastomes of seven *Panax* species. A–G. A total of 1,913 species-specific SNPs are located at the corresponding position represented by lines with species-specific colours. (A) *Panax trifolius* (PT); (B) *P. stipuleanatus* (PS); (C) *P. vietnamensis* (PV); (D) *P. japonicus* (PJ); (E) *P. notoginseng* (PN); (F) *P. quinquefolius* (PQ); (G) *P. ginseng* (PG); (H) Genes for complete plastome of *P. ginseng*; (I) 13 intraspecific polymorphisms among 10 plastomes of *P. ginseng* collections; (J) 7 universal barcoding targets. Figures were modified from previous papers (Kim *et al.*, 2015a; Nguyen *et al.*, 2020).

between closely related species because of the intraspecific variation within the same species. The fundamental basis of DNA barcoding using plastome is based on highly conserved characteristics across species and genus level. Nevertheless, intraspecific diversity still

(A)

Marker	*Panax ginseng* accessions										PQ
	ChP	YP	GU	GO	SU	SP	CS	SH	JK	HS	
Pgycf1	1	2	2	2	2	2	2	2	2	1	3
Pgcp137	2	2	2	2	2	2	2	1	2	2	2
Pgcpd02	2	2	1	2	2	2	1	2	2	2	2
Pgcpd01*	1	2	2	2	2	2	2	2	2	2	1

(B)

Marker	*Cynanchum wilfordii* accessions										Ca
Ca_i_6	1	2	1	1	2	1	2	1	1	2	3
Ca_i_7	2	3	2	2	3	2	3	2	2	3	2
Ca_i_8	2	2	1	1	3	1	3	2	3	1	2

(C)

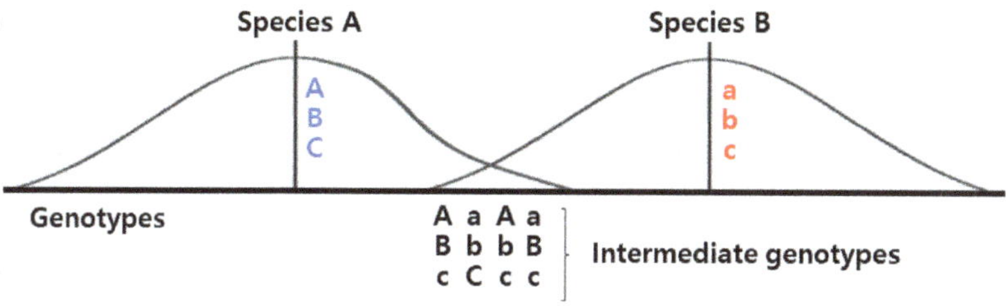

Fig. 13.4 Genotype data of several plastid markers showing intraspecific diversity among collections of *Panax ginseng* and *Cynanchum wilfordii*. Both figures were retrieved and modified from previously published papers (Kim *et al.*, 2015a; Park *et al.*, 2020). (A) Genotype data of four intraspecific markers from *P. ginseng* applied to 10 cultivars and natural accession of *P. ginseng* and 1 *P. quinquefolius* (PQ). 'ChP' is an abbreviation of the *P. ginseng* cultivar 'Chunpoong'. (B) Genotype data for the three InDel markers applied to 10 *C. wilfordii* collections and 1 *C. auriculatum* (Ca) collection. (C) Distribution of natural genetic diversity of three different marker genotypes. Putative genotypes for three loci are denoted with the alphabet.

exists in plant populations and cannot be avoided because of the abundant genetic diversity. This diversity is even much higher in the wild resource plants, which are used as a medicinal source by wildcrafting or cultivation of wild resources. The genotype found from intraspecific diversity can be the same with the closely related species (Figure 13.4). It is important to develop the genuine authentication markers by not taking the region with intraspecific diversity into account by comparing multiple plastomes of the same species, as well as screening of the candidate markers against a large population.

The plastomes of 10 *P. ginseng* cultivars presented a total of 12 intraspecific variations, including 4 genic SNPs, 2 intergenic SNPs, 1 genic InDels, and 5 intergenic InDels (Kim *et al.*, 2015a). The cultivar 'Chunpoong' (ChP) had a specific SNP distinct to other 10 cultivars in *rpoC1* gene. The ChP genotype is the same as *P. quinquefolius, the American ginseng*. Similar situation was also found from three intraspecific markers designed using diversity among five plastomes of *Cynanchum wilfordii* (Cw). Several Cw collections have the same genotypes as those of *C. auriculatum* (Ca) (Figure 13.4A and B). Three practically applied authentication markers also detected false positive among large Cw collections (Kim *et al.*, 2013, 2017b; Park *et al.*, 2020). Some plants might have confused intermediate genotypes from multiple markers because of the intraspecific diversity. An international guideline will be necessary for the authentication of these plant samples with intermediate genotypes derived from multiple markers (Figure 13.4C).

13.4.4 MTPT and DNA Barcoding Paradox

Since the first report at 1980s, the presence of MTPTs (Lonsdale, Hodge, Howe & Stem, 1983) has been confirmed by whole mitogenome sequences of diverse plants (Park *et al.*, 2020; Sloan & Wu, 2014; Wang, Chen, Yang & Liu, 2018). Investigation of MTPT from reported mitochondrial genomes showed dynamic and lineage-specific distribution (Figure 13.5). In general, the nucleotide substitution rate of mitochondrial genes is slower than those of plastid genes (Palmer & Herbon, 1988). Once the fragments from plastid genome have been inserted within the mitochondrial genome, the mutation rate is slower in the mitogenome compared

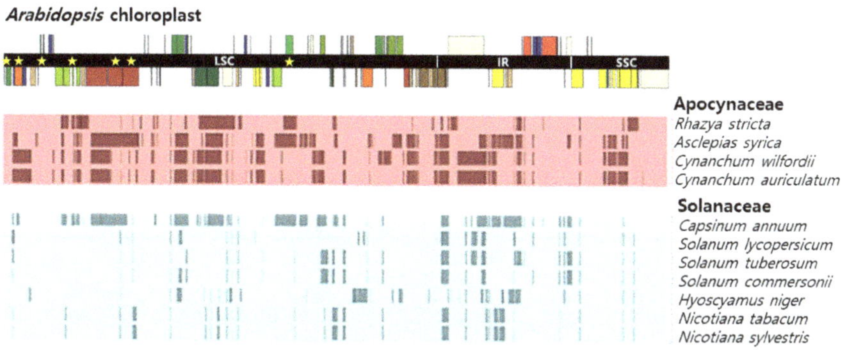

Fig. 13.5 Distribution of MTPTs from reported mitochondrial genomes of Apocynaceae and Solanaceae. MTPT regions (grey blocks) of each species were detected by comparing to the chloroplast genome of *Arabidopsis thaliana* and aligned on the linear chloroplast genome map of *A. thaliana*. Seven universal plant barcoding regions (Group *et al.*, 2009) were marked with yellow stars on the map.

to the plastome (Park *et al.*, 2020). Therefore, if plastome markers are designed from plastome that has MTPT homologs, false-positive detection could happen, coupled with co-amplification of the plastid target as well as the MTPT target in closely related species. Other promiscuous DNA such as the NUPT can also affect DNA barcoding but the possibility might be lower than MTPT because of the relatively low depth of the nuclear genome in a single cell compared to the organelle genomes (Kim *et al.*, 2015b).

The DNA barcoding research of two *Cynanchum* species is a representative example showing how the co-amplified MTPT can induce false-positive barcoding results. The complete plastome and mitogenomes of two *Cynanchum* species were assembled from low-coverage NGS data (Figure 13.6). The plastome of each species was in the length of 161,241 bp for Cw and 160,840 bp for Ca, and they showed the conserved structure of typical quadripartite with 97.5% similarity at the sequence level. However, the mitogenomes showed structural rearrangement, whereas

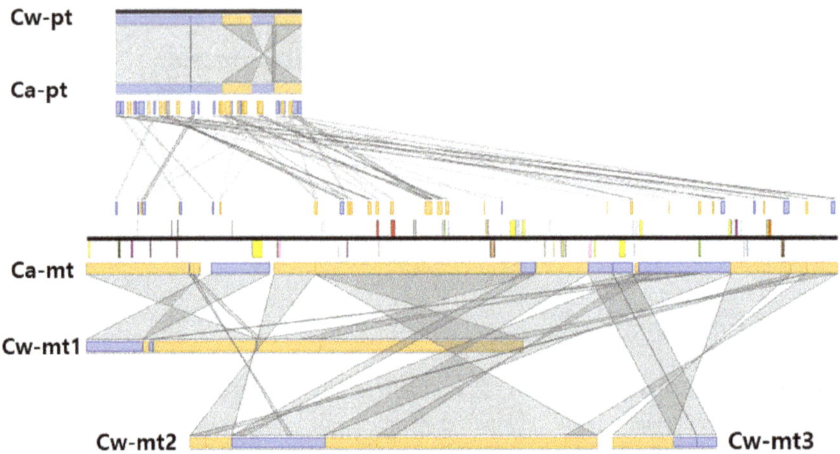

Fig. 13.6 Comparison of plastome and mitogenome showing genome flux in the *Cynanchum* species. The overall plastid (pt) and mitochondria (mt) genome structures of *Cynanchum wilfordii* (Cw) and *C. auriculatum* (Ca) were compared by BLAST. Blue and yellow rectangles under the linear map of pt and mt represent homology blocks with forward and reverse direction, respectively.

their sequence did overall collinearity with high similarity, and the sequence of all the protein-coding genes were identical except for the copy number of the *atp9* gene. Approximately 35% of plastomes showed homology with mitogenomes and 36 out of 75 plastid protein-coding genes were found in mitogenomes (Figure 13.6). For example, the whole *matK* gene, one of the well-known universal DNA barcoding genes, was identified as MTPTs in both species. The MTPT of *matK* were highly conserved between species, even more similar than the current plastid *matK*. An SNP marker was developed from this target to authenticate Cw and Ca (Figure 13.7A) (Kim *et al.*, 2017b), which had been practically used for a while until the regulatory stop of Cw products in Korea. The marker may provide precise authentication results under precise PCR cycles and the DNA template amount but resulted in false-positive authentication by increasing PCR cycles or the template DNA amount (Figure 13.7B and 13.7C). We revealed that

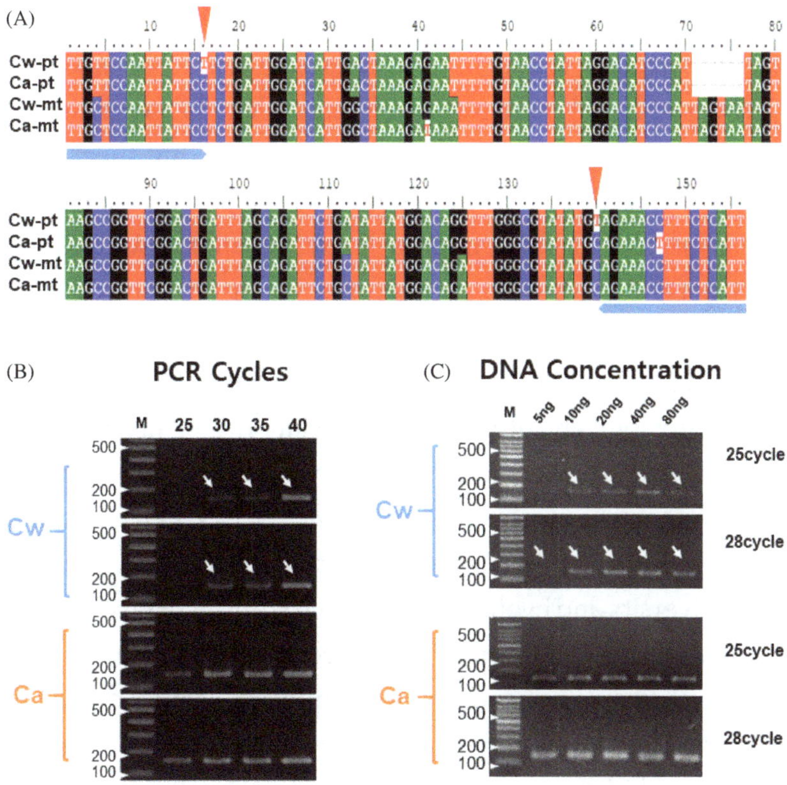

Fig. 13.7 An example to show a DNA marker paradox derived from the mitochondrial plastid DNA (MTPT) target. (A) PCR amplicons of SNP-dominant marker specific to *Cynanchum auriculatum*. Cw, *C. wilfordii*; Ca, *C. auriculatum*; pt, plastid genome; mt, MTPT segment in the mitogenome. Primer regions and target SNP for detection of Cw and Ca are marked with the blue box and red triangle, respectively. Sequential electrophoresis of PCR products under (B) different PCR cycles and (C) different template DNA amounts. The bands amplified from MTPT regions are denoted by white arrows.

these phenomena were mediated by MTPT fragments that can also be found in any plant species (Park *et al.*, 2020).

13.4.5 Nuclear Ribosomal DNAs

From the low-coverage NGS data, the complete nrDNA unit can be assembled simultaneously with plastome via dnaLCW. The RNA coding regions and ITS regions in 45S and 5S nrDNA can be obtained by dnaLCW, but the intergenic spacer regions between each transcription unit are still challenging due to diverse repeat sequences or high heterogeneous features. The ITS regions in 45S nrDNA are popular universal barcoding targets, but their heterogeneous forms often provide confusion for practical application (Song *et al*., 2012). NGS approach can assemble multiple forms of 45S nrDNA and easily retrieve the major type to reduce the possibility of mis-authentication (Kim *et al*., 2015b). Moreover, a combined phylogenetic relationship using both plastome and 45S nrDNA provides an integrated understanding of taxonomic and evolutionary context because the nrDNA reflects the biparentally inherited genome information (Kim *et al*., 2015b; Lee *et al*., 2020).

The maternal inheritance of plastome is a big advantage for genetic diversity and evolutionary lineage study in plants. However, it can provide biased information. We compared the plastomes and nrDNAs of two representative rice cultivars, 'Tongil' and 'M23', which are bred by inter-subspecies hybrids. Although the nuclear genotype and phenotype of both cultivars are followed predominantly of the *indica*-type rice, the cultivar 'Tongil' contains *indica*-type plastome but the 'M23' contains *japonica*-type plastome (Kim *et al*., 2015b). If only plastome was used for identification, these two cultivars might be concluded as different subspecies. The nuclear gene and the ribosomal gene, as well as the phenotypes, show that the two varieties are both *indica*-like cultivars (Kim *et al*., 2014, 2015b). The plastome genotype is determined by the maternal parent during interspecific or inter-subspecific hybridisation, even though many rounds of self-crossing are followed in the breeding of 'Tongil' and 'M23' cultivars. Therefore, it is very important to consider both plastome and nrDNAs together for super-barcoding for characterising genetic diversity.

13.5 Integrated Interspecific Authentication System Based on Super-Barcode

DNA barcoding has been widely applied from raw materials to highly processed commercial products (Figure 13.8A) (Jung, Kim, Yang, Bang & Yang, 2014; Parveen, Gafner, Techen, Murch & Khan, 2016).

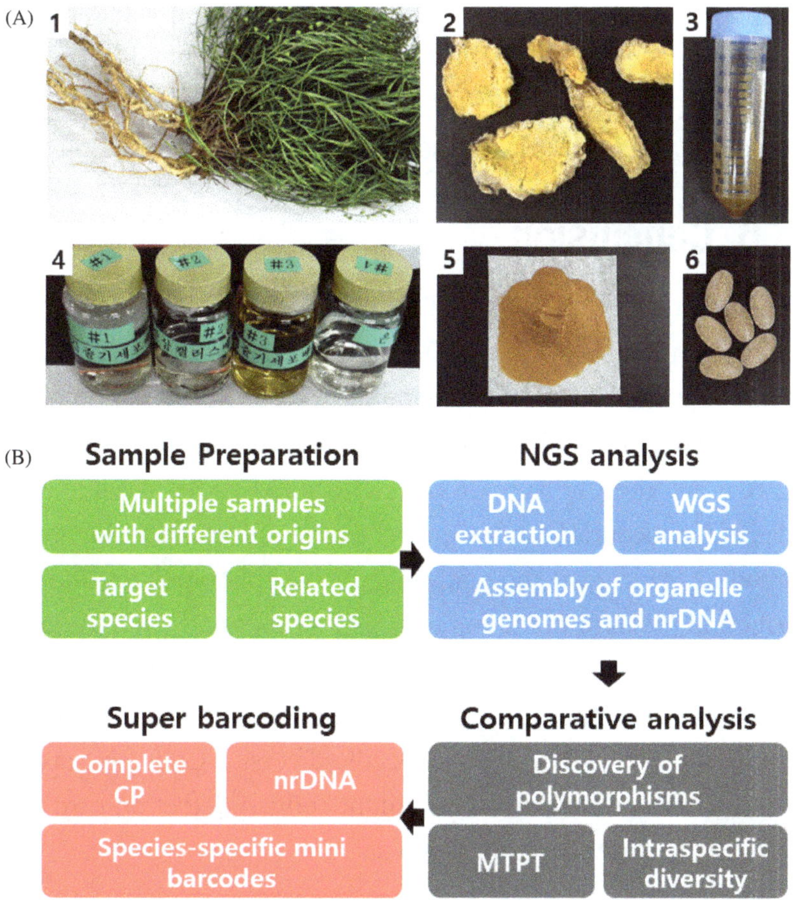

Fig. 13.8 Super-barcoding pipeline for integrated authentication for diverse plant samples. (A) Diverse medicinal materials from raw plants to processed commercial products. (B) A super-barcoding pipeline for medicinal materials using dnaLCW.

The practical application of DNA barcoding can be useful for the identification of raw ingredients for preventing adulteration and protecting the industry. However, most of the medicinal materials are heterogeneous because of the natural diversity. The information and characteristics of the plant genome are complex. DNA barcoding and molecular markers are powerful and useful tools, but it should be carefully applied to avoid errors. Therefore, it is necessary to establish a barcoding system based on the multi-plastomes, genome complexity and genome diversity in plant species (Figure 13.8B). DNA barcoding paradox should be considered, and multiple DNA markers should be used for precise authentication of plant species.

13.6 Conclusion

The plastid genome provides essential information for genetic diversity and authentication. Owing to the advances in sequencing technology, the assembly of a complete plastome has become more accessible. Compared with the traditionally used universal barcoding regions, the entire plastome data called super-barcoding provides more accurate and comprehensive information for genetic barcoding. Here, we show advanced assembly pipelines and error correction tools for obtaining entire plastomes and nrDNA concurrently, based on dnaLCW. However, plastid markers occasionally make false detection caused by genome complexity such as mitochondrial plastid DNA or intraspecific diversity. Collective application of plastomes and nrDNAs might reduce detection errors and increase the super-barcoding power.

References

Bakker, F. T., Lei, D., Yu, J., Mohammadin, S., Wei, Z., van de Kerke, S., Gravendeel, B., Nieuwenhuis, M., Staats, M., Alquezar-Planas, D. E., &

Holmer, R. (2016). Herbarium genomics: Plastome sequence assembly from a range of herbarium specimens using an Iterative Organelle Genome Assembly pipeline. *Biol J Linn Soc, 117*, 33–43.

Baldwin, B. G., Sanderson, M. J., Porter, J. M., Wojciechowski, M. F., Campbell, C. S., & Donoghue, M. J. (1995). The ITS region of nuclear ribosomal DNA: A valuable source of evidence on angiosperm phylogeny. *Ann Mo Bot Gard*, 247–277, Vol. 82, No. 2.

CBOL Plant Working Group (2009). A DNA barcode for land plants. *Proc Nat Acad Sci USA, 106*, 12794–12797.

Chen, S., Yao, H., Han, J., Liu, C., Song, J., Shi, L., Zhu, Y., Ma, X., Gao, T., Pang, X., Luo, K., Li, Y., Li, X., Jia, X., Lin, Y., & Leon, C. (2010). Validation of the ITS2 region as a novel DNA barcode for identifying medicinal plant species. *PLoS One, 5*, e8613.

Chen, X., Zhou, J., Cui, Y., Wang, Y., Duan, B., & Yao, H. (2018). Identification of Ligularia herbs using the complete chloroplast genome as a super-barcode. *Front Pharmacol, 9*, 695.

Chen, Z., Zhao, N., Li, S., Grover, C. E., Nie, H., Wendel, J. F., & Hua, J. (2017). Plant mitochondrial genome evolution and cytoplasmic male sterility. *Crit Rev Plant Sci, 36*, 55–69.

Cho, K. S., Cho, J. H., Im, J. S., Choi, J. G., Park, Y. E., Hong, S. Y., & Park, T. H. (2018). Mitochondrial genome sequence of tuber-bearing wild potato, *Solanum commersonii* Dunal. *Mitochondrial DNA B Resour, 3*, 198–199.

Cloix, C., Tutois, S., Mathieu, O., Cuvillier, C., Espagnol, M., Picard, G., & Tourmente, S. (2000). Analysis of 5S rDNA arrays in *Arabidopsis thaliana*: physical mapping and chromosome-specific polymorphisms. *Genome Res, 10*, 679–690.

Coissac, E., Hollingsworth, P. M., Lavergne, S., & Taberlet, P. (2016). From barcodes to genomes: Extending the concept of DNA barcoding. *Mol Ecol, 25*, 1423–1428.

Dierckxsens, N., Mardulyn, P., & Smits, G. (2017). NOVOPlasty: de novo assembly of organelle genomes from whole genome data. *Nucleic Acids Res, 45*, e18–e18.

García-Robledo, C., Erickson, D. L., Staines, C. L., Erwin, T. L., & Kress, W. J. (2013). Tropical plant–herbivore networks: reconstructing species interactions using DNA barcodes. *PLoS One, 8*, e52967.

Giang, V. N. L., Hyun-Seung, P., Nguyen, V. B., Park, J. H., & Yang, T. J. (2021). Genotypic characterization of Panax collections in Vietnam and Southern China based on multi plastomes and application of SNP. *In progress*.

Gualberto, J. M., Mileshina, D., Wallet, C., Niazi, A. K., Weber-Lotfi, F., & Dietrich, A. (2014). The plant mitochondrial genome: Dynamics and maintenance. *Biochimie, 100*, 107–120.

Hillis, D. M., & Dixon, M. T. (1991). Ribosomal DNA: Molecular evolution and phylogenetic inference. *Q Rev Biol, 66*, 411–453.

Hobern, D., & Hebert, P. (2019). BIOSCAN-revealing eukaryote diversity, dynamics, and interactions. *Biodivers Inf Sci Stand, 3*, e37333.

Hollingsworth, P. M. (2011). Refining the DNA barcode for land plants. *Proc Nat Acad Sci USA, 108*, 19451–19452.

Hollingsworth, P. M., Graham, S. W., & Little, D. P. (2011). Choosing and using a plant DNA barcode. *PLoS One, 6*, e19254.

Jang, W., Lee, H. O., Kim, J. U., Lee, J. W., Hong, C. E., Bang, K. H., Chung, J. W., & Jo, I. H. (2020). Complete mitochondrial genome and a set of 10 novel kompetitive allele-specific PCR markers in ginseng (Panax ginseng CA Mey.). *Agronomy, 10*, 1868.

Jayakodi, M., Padmarasu, S., Haberer, G., Bonthala, V. S., Gundlach, H., Monat, C., Lux, T., Kamal, N., Lang, D., Himmelbach, A., Ens, J., Zhang, X. Q., Angessa, T. T., Zhou, G. F., Tan, C., Hill, C., Wang, P. H., Schreiber, M., Boston, L. B., Plott, C., Jenkins, J., Guo, Y., Fiebig, A., Budak, H., Xu, D. D., Zhang, J., Wang, C. C., Grimwood, J., Schmutz, J., Guo, G. G., Zhang, G. P., Mochida, K., Hirayama, T., Sato, K., Chalmers, K. J., Langridge, P., Waugh, R., Pozniak, C. J., Scholz, U., Mayer, K. F. X., Spannagl, M., Li, C. D., Mascher, M., & Stein, N. (2020). The barley pan-genome reveals the hidden legacy of mutation breeding. *Nature, 588*, 284–289.

Jensen, R., & Bassham, J. (1966). Photosynthesis by isolated chloroplasts. *Proc Nat Acad Sci USA, 56*, 1095.

Jin, J. J., Yu, W. B., Yang, J. B., Song, Y., DePamphilis, C. W., Yi, T. S., & Li, D. Z. (2020). GetOrganelle: A fast and versatile toolkit for accurate de novo assembly of organelle genomes. *Genome Biol*, 21(1), 1–31.

Jung, J., Kim, K. H., Yang, K., Bang, K. H., & Yang, T. J. (2014). Practical application of DNA markers for high-throughput authentication of *Panax ginseng* and *Panax quinquefolius* from commercial ginseng products. *J Ginseng Res, 38*, 123–129.

Kang, S. H., Lee, H. O., Ahn, B. O., & Kim, C. K. (2019). The complete mitochondrial genome sequence of *Senna occidentalis* (Fabales: Fabaceae). *Mitochondrial DNA B Resour, 4*, 85–86.

Kim, B., Kim, D. G., Lee, G., Seo, J., Choi, I. K., Choi, B. S., Yang, T. J., Kim, K. S., Lee, J., Chin, J. H., & Koh, H. J. (2014). Defining the genome structure of Tongil'rice, an important cultivar in the Korean "Green Revolution". *Rice, 7*, 1–9.

Kim, C. K., Seol, Y. J., Perumal, S., Lee, J., Waminal, N. E., Jayakodi, M., Lee, S. C., Jin, S., Choi, B. S., Yu, Y., Ko, H. C., Choi, J. W., Ryu, K. Y., Sohn, S. H., Parkin, I., & Yang, T. J. (2018). Re-exploration of U's triangle Brassica species based on chloroplast genomes and 45S nrDNA sequences. *Sci Rep, 8*, 1–11.

Kim, I., Park, J. Y., Lee, Y., Lee, H. O., Park, H. S., Jayakodi, M., Waminal, N., Kang, J. H., Lee, T. J., Sung, S. H., Kim, K. Y., & Yang, T. J. (2017b). Discrimination and authentication of *Eclipta prostrata* and *E. alba* based on the complete chloroplast genomes. *Plant Breed Biotechnol, 5*, 334–343.

Kim, J. H., Moon, J. C., Kang, T. S., Kwon, K., & Jang, C. S. (2017a). Development of cpDNA markers for discrimination between *Cynanchum wilfordii* and *Cynanchum auriculatum* and their application in commercial *C. wilfordii* food products. *Appl Biol Chem, 60*, 79–86.

Kim, K., Lee, S. C., Lee, J., Lee, H. O., Joh, H. J., Kim, N. H., Park, H. S., & Yang, T. J. (2015a). Comprehensive survey of genetic diversity in chloroplast genomes and 45S nrDNAs within *Panax ginseng* species. *PLoS One, 10*, e0117159.

Kim, K., Lee, S. C., Lee, J., Yu, Y., Yang, K., Choi, B, Koh, H. J., Waminaly, N. E., Choi, H. I., Kim, N. H., Jang, W., Park, H. S., Lee, J., Lee, H. O., Joh, H. J., Lee, H. J., Park, J. Y., Perumal, S., Jayakodi, M., Lee, Y. S., Kim, B., Copetti, D., Kim, S., Kim, S., Lim, K. B., Kim, Y. D., Lee, J., Cho, K. S., Park, B. S., Wing, R. A., & Yang, T. J. (2015b). Complete chloroplast and ribosomal sequences for 30 accessions elucidate evolution of Oryza AA genome species. *Sci Rep, 5*, 15655.

Kim, K., Nguyen, V. B., Dong, J., Wang, Y., Park, J. Y., Lee, S. C., & Yang, T. J. (2017c). Evolution of the Araliaceae family inferred from complete chloroplast genomes and 45S nrDNAs of 10 Panax-related species. *Sci Rep, 7*, 4917.

Kim, M., Wang, H., Kim, Y., Sathiyamoorthy, S., Kwon, W., & Yang, D. (2013). Molecular authentication by multiplex-PCR of three similar medicinal plant species: *Cynanchum wilfordii, Cynanchum auriculatum* and *Polygonum multiflorum* (*Fallopia multiflorum*). *J Med Plants Res, 7*, 2584–2589.

Kong, B. L. H., Park, H. S., Lau, T. W. D., Lin, Z., Yang, T. J., & Shaw, P. C. (2021). Comparative analysis and phylogenetic investigation of Hong Kong Ilex chloroplast genomes. *Sci Rep, 11*, 5153.

Kress, W. J., Wurdack, K. J., Zimmer, E. A., Weigt, L. A., & Janzen, D. H. (2005). Use of DNA barcodes to identify flowering plants. *Proc Nat Acad Sci USA, 102*, 8369–8374.

Lee, H. O., Choi, J. W., Baek, J. H., Oh, J. H., Lee, S. C., & Kim, C. K. (2018). Assembly of the mitochondrial genome in the campanulaceae family using Illumina low-coverage sequencing. *Genes, 9*, 383.

Lee, J., Joh, H. J., Kim, N. H., Lee, S. C., Jang, W., Choi, B. S., Yu, Y., & Yang, T. J. (2017). High-throughput development of polymorphic simple sequence repeat markers using two whole genome sequence data in peucedanum japonicum. *Plant Breed Biotechnol, 5*, 134–142.

Lee, J., Kang, S. J., Shim, H., Lee, S. C, Kim, N., Jang, W., Park, J. Y., Kang, J., Lee, W., Lee, T., Nah, G., & Yang, T. J. (2019a). Characterization of chloroplast genomes, nuclear ribosomal DNAs, and polymorphic SSR markers using whole genome sequences of two *Euonymus hamiltonianus* phenotypes. *Plant Breed Biotechnol, 7*, 50–61.

Lee, J., Lee, S. C., Joh, H. J., Lee, H., Sung, S. H., Kang, J. H., & Yang, T. J. (2016). The complete chloroplast genome sequence of a Korean indigenous ornamental plant *Hydrangea serrata* for. *fertilis* Nakai (Hydrangeaceae). *Mitochondrial DNA B Resour, 1*, 27–28.

Lee, S. H., Lee, H. O., Park, H. S., Ryu, H. J., Kim, J. W., Choi, S. H., Park, J. Y., & Yang, T. J. (2019b). The complete mitochondrial genome of *Wolfiporia cocos* (Polypolales: Polyporaceae). *Mitochondrial DNA B Resour, 4*, 1010–1011.

Lee, Y. S., Kim, J., Woo, S., Park, J. Y., Park, H. S., Shim, H., Choi, H. I., Kang, J. H., Lee, T. J., Sung, S. H., Yang, T. J., & Kang, K. B. (2020). Assessing the genetic and chemical diversity of Taraxacum species in the Korean Peninsula. *Phytochemistry, 181*, 112576.

Li, H. T., Yi, T. S., Gao, L. M., Ma, P. F., Zhang, T., Yang, J. B., Gitzendanner, M. A., Fritsch, P. W., Cai, J., Luo, Y., Wang, H., van der Bank, M., Zhang, S. D., Wang, Q. F., Wang, J., Zhang, Z. R., Fu, C. N., Yang, J., Hollingsworth, P. M., Chase, M. W., Soltis, D. E., Soltis, P. S., & Li, D. Z. (2019). Origin of angiosperms and the puzzle of the Jurassic gap. *Nat Plants, 5*, 461–470.

Li, X., Yang, Y., Henry, R. J., Rossetto, M., Wang, Y., & Chen, S. (2015). Plant DNA barcoding: From gene to genome. *Biol Rev, 90*, 157–166.

Lonsdale, D. M., Hodge, T. P., Howe, C. J., & Stem, D. B. (1983). Maize mitochondrial DNA contains a sequence homologous to the ribulose-1, 5-bisphosphate carboxylase large subunit gene of chloroplast DNA. *Cell, 34*, 1007–1014.

Matsuo, M., Ito, Y., Yamauchi, R., & Obokata, J. (2005). The rice nuclear genome continuously integrates, shuffles, and eliminates the chloroplast genome to cause chloroplast–nuclear DNA flux. *Plant Cell, 17*, 665–675.

Mcfadden, G. I. (1999). Endosymbiosis and evolution of the plant cell. *Curr Opin Plant Biol, 2*, 513–519.

Nguyen, V. B., Giang, V. N. L., Waminal, N. E., Park, H. S., Kim, N. H., Jang, W., Lee, J., & Yang, T. J. (2020). Comprehensive comparative analysis of chloroplast genomes from seven Panax species and development of an authentication system based on species-unique SNP markers. *J Ginseng Res*. 44(1), 135–144.

Nguyen, V. B., Park, H. S., Lee, S. C., Lee, J., Park, J. Y., & Yang, T. J. (2017). Authentication markers for five major Panax species developed via comparative analysis of complete chloroplast genome sequences. *J Agric Food Chem, 65*, 6298–6306.

Palmer, J. D., & Herbon, L. A. (1988). Plant mitochondrial DNA evolved rapidly in structure, but slowly in sequence. *J Mol Evol, 28*, 87–97.

Park, H. S., Jayakodi, M., Lee, S. H., Jeon, J. H., Lee, H. O., Park, J. Y., Moon, B. C., Kim, C. K., Wing, R. A., Newmaster, S. G., Kim, J. Y., & Yang, T. J. (2020). Mitochondrial plastid DNA can cause DNA barcoding paradox in plants. *Sci Rep, 10*, 1–12.

Park, H. S., Lee, J., Lee, S. C., Yang, T. J., & Yoon, J. B. (2016). The complete chloroplast genome sequence of *Capsicum chinense* Jacq.(Solanaceae). *Mitochondrial DNA B Resour, 1*, 164–165.

Park, J. Y., Lee, Y. P., Lee, J., Choi, B. S., Kim, S., & Yang, T. J. (2013). Complete mitochondrial genome sequence and identification of a candidate gene responsible for cytoplasmic male sterility in radish (*Raphanus sativus L.*) containing DCGMS cytoplasm. *Theor Appl Genet, 126*, 1763–1774.

Parveen, I., Gafner, S., Techen, N., Murch, S. J., & Khan, I. A. (2016). DNA barcoding for the identification of botanicals in herbal medicine and dietary supplements: Strengths and limitations. *Planta Med, 82*, 1225–1235.

Paterson, A. H., Freeling, M., Tang, H., & Wang, X. (2010). Insights from the comparison of plant genome sequences. *Ann Rev Plant Biol, 61*, 349–372.

Preuten, T., Cincu, E., Fuchs, J., Zoschke, R., Liere, K., & Brner, T. (2010). Fewer genes than organelles: Extremely low and variable gene copy numbers in mitochondria of somatic plant cells. *Plant J, 64*, 948–959.

Ratnasingham, S., & Hebert, P. D. (2007). BOLD: The barcode of life data system. *Mol Ecol Notes, 7*, 355–364. Retrieved from http://www.barcodinglife.org

Rosato, M., Kovařik, K. A., Garilleti, R., & Rossell, J. A. (2016). Conserved organisation of 45S rDNA sites and rDNA gene copy number among major clades of early land plants. *PLoS One, 11*, e0162544.

Sakamoto, W., & Takami, T. (2018). Chloroplast DNA dynamics: Copy number, quality control and degradation. *Plant Cell Physiol, 59*, 1120–1127.

Schoch, C. L., Seifert, K. A., Huhndorf, S., Robert, V., Spouge, J. L., Levesque, C. A., Chen, W., & Fungal Barcoding Consortium (2012). Nuclear ribosomal internal transcribed spacer (ITS) region as a universal DNA barcode marker for Fungi. *Proc Nat Acad Sci USA, 109*, 6241–6246.

Sloan, D. B., & Wu, Z. (2014). History of plastid DNA insertions reveals weak deletion and AT mutation biases in angiosperm mitochondrial genomes. *Genome Biol Evol, 6*, 3210–3221.

Song, J., Shi, L., Li, D., Sun, Y., Niu, Y., Chen, Z., Luo, H., Pang, X., Sun, Z., Liu, C., Lv, A., Deng, Y., Larson-Rabin, Z., Wilkinson, M., & Chen, S. (2012). Extensive pyrosequencing reveals frequent intra-genomic variations of internal transcribed spacer regions of nuclear ribosomal DNA. *PLoS One, 7*, e43971.

Takami, T., Ohnishi, N., Kurita, Y., Iwamura, S., Ohnishi, M., Kusaba, M., Mimura, T., & Sakamoto, W. (2018). Organelle DNA degradation contributes to the efficient use of phosphate in seed plants. *Nat Plants, 4*, 1044–1055.

Treangen, T. J., & Salzberg, S. L. (2012). Repetitive DNA and next-generation sequencing: Computational challenges and solutions. *Nat Rev Genet, 13,* 36–46.

Wang, X.-C., Chen, H., Yang, D., & Liu, C. (2018). Diversity of mitochondrial plastid DNAs (MTPTs) in seed plants. *Mitochondrial DNA A, 29,* 635–642.

Wang, Z., & Benning, C. (2012). Chloroplast lipid synthesis and lipid trafficking through ER–plastid membrane contact sites. *Biochem Soc Trans, 40,* 457–463.

Yao, H., Song, J., Liu, C., Luo, K., Han, J., Li, Y., Pang, X., Xu, H., Zhu, Y., Xiao, P., & Chen, S. (2010). Use of ITS2 region as the universal DNA barcode for plants and animals. *PLoS One, 5,* e13102.

Zhang, Z., Zhang, Y., Song, M., Guan, Y., & Ma, X. (2019). Species identification of Dracaena using the complete chloroplast genome as a super-barcode. *Front Pharmacol, 10,* 1441.

Part V
Advanced Applications and Outlook of Molecular Authentication Techniques

Chapter 14

Rapid Detection of CITES-Listed Shark Species Using Loop-Mediated Isothermal Amplification

Grace Wing-Chiu But, Hoi-Yan Wu,
Kwang-Tsao Shao & Pang-Chui Shaw

14.1 Introduction

Different DNA techniques have been developed and applied for the identification of medicinal materials. Amplification of a specific region in genomic DNA by conventional polymerase chain reaction (PCR) is a widely used approach. Although it enables quick verification and the cost is relatively low, it requires a thermal cycler and gel electrophoresis system with a long amplification time. Recently, several rapid isothermal amplification techniques have been developed, which include strand displacement amplification (SDA), rolling circle amplification (RCA), helicase-dependent amplification (HDA), recombinase polymerase amplification (RPA) and loop-mediated isothermal amplification (LAMP).

HDA is based on the double-stranded DNA unwinding activity of a DNA helicase separating the strands. After unwinding, the target region of the separated DNA strand is coated by single-stranded DNA-binding protein (SSB). Then, specific primers bind to the single-stranded DNA and extend with the help of strand-displacing DNA polymerase to generate a double-stranded DNA at 65°C. HDA has been applied for differentiating Asian ginseng (*Panax ginseng*) from American ginseng (*P. quinquefolius*) (Jiang, Liu, Wong, Nip & Shaw, 2015). For RPA, it is a single-tube technique that employs three types of protein: recombinase, SSB and strand-displacing polymerase. Recombinase–primer complex is first formed by recombinase and specific primers, and the primers are inserted to the target site by strand-displacement activity of the recombinase. SSB binds to the displaced DNA strands, and strand-displacing polymerase extends to generate a double-stranded DNA at a constant temperature of 37–42°C. RPA has been applied for identifying *Ficus hirta* (Tian, Liu, Ye, Li & Chao, 2017) and differentiating *Ginkgo biloba* from *Sophora japonica* (Liu, Wang, Wei, Gao & Han, 2018). Both of HDA and RPA can be applied for on-site detection in room temperature and the result can be observed by real-time analysis, gel electrophoresis and lateral flow strips. Although the design of primers for HDA and RPA is relatively simple, their low reaction temperature (60°C or below) leads to the formation of primer-dimers and unwanted hybrid, resulting in the increase of background and a decrease of sensitivity and accuracy (Yang *et al.*, 2015). LAMP, on the other hand, is simple in procedure and allows easy end-product detection; thus, it is more widely applied to rapid identification of medicinal materials. Principles of LAMP techniques and application of LAMP techniques on the identification of shark species, which is a kind of material used in traditional Chinese medicine, listed in Appendix II of the Convention on International Trade in Endangered Species of Wild Fauna and Flora (CITES, also known as the Washington Convention), will be discussed in the following section.

14.2 General Principles of LAMP

In the early 2000's, the LAMP technique was developed as a rapid and simple detection method. It is performed using DNA polymerase with strand displacement activity at a single temperature within an hour (Nagamine, Hase & Notomi, 2002; Notomi *et al.*, 2000). In LAMP reaction, at least two pairs of specific primers are designed to target six distinct regions of target DNA to generate loop-formed DNA. Loop-formed products generated increase in sensitivity and specificity when compared to conventional PCR (Kim, Jeong, Kim, Kim & Cho, 2015). Under a constant temperature (60–70°C), one of the LAMP primers is bound to the complementary sequence of the double-stranded DNA, and the DNA sequence is amplified by extension with, most typically, *Bst* polymerase, or *Bsm* polymerase and *BcaBEST* polymerase. They have single-strand displacement activity, of which a single-stranded DNA is displaced and released (Figure 14.1) (Tomita, Mori, Kanda & Notomi, 2008; Wang *et al.*, 2017). The four LAMP primers include the forward outer primer (F3), backward outer primer (B3), forward inner primer (FIP) and backward (BIP). FIP and BIP are hybrid primers that consist of two parts, namely, F1c and F2 for FIP, and B1c and B2 for BIP. As shown in Figure 14.1A, the sequence of F1c is complementary to that of F1, so as F2c to F2, F3c to F3, B1c to B1, B2c to B2, and B3c to B3. The F2 region binds to the F2c region and starts the extension with the help of *Bst* polymerase. After that, F3 primer binds to the F3c region and *Bst* polymerase starts single-strand displacement DNA synthesis. DNA synthesised using the FIP primer is then displaced and released. Since the F1c and F1 regions are complementary to one another (Figure 14.1B),

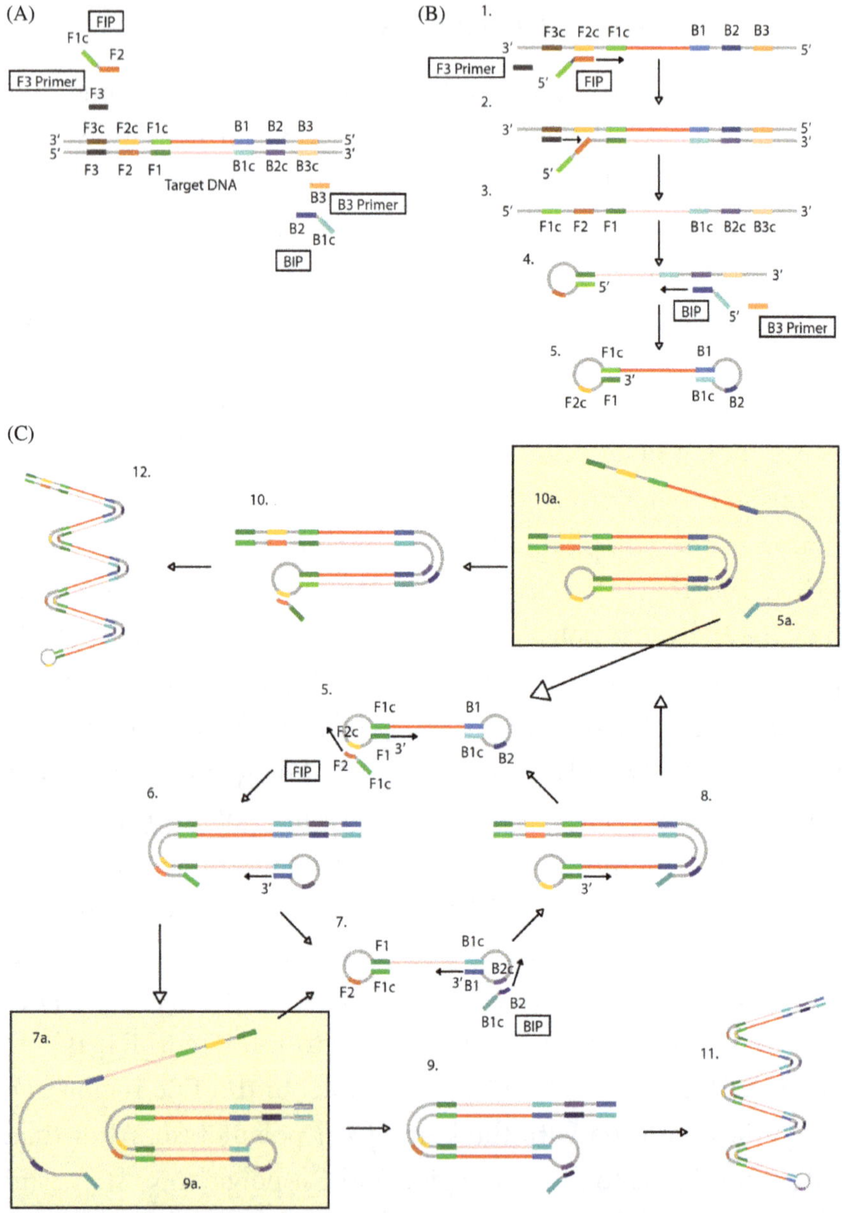

Fig. 14.1 Schematic diagram on loop-mediated isothermal amplification (LAMP) (Tomita, Mori, Kanda & Notomi, 2008). (A) Two pairs of LAMP primers targeting six distinct regions of the sequence. (B) The DNA sequence is amplified by extension with *Bst* polymerase and forms a looped product. (C) Cycling amplification continues the amplified looped intermediate, resulting in a large amount of the long and looped product.

they hybridise and form a loop structure. DNA synthesis proceeds at the other end of the DNA strand, and a loop structure is formed at both ends. The DNA with the loop structure at both ends then acts as template and is bound by another FIP primer (Figure 14.1C). As cycling amplification goes on, a lot of long and looped DNA strands are formed, hence increasing the sensitivity of detection.

Besides having high specificity by targeting six distinct regions with two pairs of primers and high sensitivity due to the large amount of looped products generated, LAMP detection is also favourable for on-site detection since it does not require a thermal cycler and it can be detected by visual observation of fluorescence by adding DNA binding dye such as SYBR Green I and EvaGreen (Fischbach, Xander, Frohme & Glokler, 2015; Loo *et al.*, 2019; Mori, Nagamine, Tomita & Notomi, 2001). Other than a colour change, the result could also be observed by the change in turbidity due to the increase of magnesium pyrophosphate precipitate, which is the by-product of amplification (Li, Xiong, Liu, Liang & Zhou, 2016). As a highly sensitive and specific detection method, LAMP has been applied to identify *Hedyotis diffusa* (Li *et al.*, 2013), *Catharanthus roseus* (Chaudhary, Hemant & Ahmad, 2012), *Taraxacum formosanum* (Lai *et al.*, 2015), *Aristolochia manshuriensis* (Wu *et al.*, 2016), *Crocus sativus* (Zhao *et al.*, 2016), *Polygonum multiflorum* (Lee & Hxiao, 2019), and to differentiate *Curcuma longa* from *C. aromatica* (Sasaki & Nagumo, 2007), *P. ginseng* from *P. japonicus* (Sasaki, Komatsu & Nagumo, 2008), *Cordyceps sinensis* from its adulterants (Li *et al.*, 2011) and deer tendons from cattle tendons (Jiang, Liu, Wong, Nip & Shaw, 2015).

14.3 Materials and Methods

14.3.1 Materials

14.3.1.1 *Introduction of Materials*

Selachii, commonly called sharks, are characterised by their cartilaginous skeletons opening gill clefts and rigid dorsal fin (Nelson, Grande & Wilson, 2016). Under the group of Selachii, there are more than 500 species of sharks and they have existed for more than 420 million years (Nelson, Grande & Wilson, 2016). In Asian countries, shark fin has a long history of being consumed as a symbol of wealth and power, and also for its nutritional value as an ingredient of traditional food therapy (Cardenosa, Quinlan, Shea & Chapman 2018; Eriksson & Clarke, 2015; Vannuccini & Agriculture Organization of the United Nations, 1999). According to the Compendium of Materia Medica, consuming shark fin can help reinforce inner organs and restore normal functioning of stomach. Research have also shown shark fin having a positive effect on the immune system of immunosuppressed mice (Li *et al.*, 2011; Wang *et al.*, 2000).

The global shark fin market is estimated to be worth USD 400–550 million annually (Dulvy *et al.*, 2014). Shark fin in the Asian market are mostly in dried form, which is through sun drying, salting, or using processors to enhance the drying with extra flesh and cartilage removed for better preservation (Food and Agriculture Organisation [FAO], 2016a, 2016b; Musick, 2005; Vannuccini & Agriculture Organization of the United Nations, 1999). Since sharks grow slowly and reach sexual maturity late, and with a low fecundity and reproductive rate (Brautigam *et al.*, 2015; Cortes, 2002), overexploitation has led to serious decline in shark populations, and many populations are considered threatened or endangered (Baum *et al.*, 2003; Dulvy *et al.*, 2014; Barreto *et al.*, 2016; Jaiteh, Loneragan & Warren, 2017). According to the International Union for Conservation of Nature (IUCN) Red List of Threatened Species, more than 50% of the shark species are in the state of near extinction (Dulvy, Allen, Ralph & Walls, 2016).

As of October 2016, there are 12 shark species in the Appendix II of CITES, including, since 2000, the great white shark (*Carcharodon carcharias*), basking shark (*Cetorhinus maximus*) and whale shark (*Rhincodon typus*); since 2013, the oceanic whitetip shark (*Carcharhinus longimanus*), porbeagle shark (*Lamna nasus*) and three species of hammerhead sharks (*Sphyrna lewini, S. mokarran, S. zygaena*); and, since 2016, all three species of thresher sharks (*Alopias pelagicus, A. superciliosus, A. vulpinus*) and the silky shark (*Carcharhinus falciformis*). International trade of any part of the listed species must be accompanied by permits or licenses to certify that each specimen has been harvested sustainably and legally (CITES, 2019). Shark fins of these species are commercially valuable, especially for those that have been added to the list of CITES Appendix II since 2013, and they are traded in large volumes (Clarke, 2004; Clarke, Magnussen, Abercrombie, McAllister & Shivji, 2006; Fields *et al.*, 2018; Jabado *et al.*, 2015). Therefore, there is a need for an easy-to-use, rapid, and effective diagnostic method for species-level identification.

14.3.1.2 *Samples*

Total of 291 samples of 93 shark and shark-related species from seven orders and 26 families was collected from various sources (Table 14.1). For the 12 CITES-listed shark species, at least two samples were collected for each species. All samples, including

Table 14.1 Shark and Shark-related Samples for the Validation of Loop-Mediated Isothermal Amplification (LAMP) and Polymerase Chain Reaction (PCR) Assay

Order	Family	Species	Common name	Number of samples (unprocessed/processed)
Carcharhiniformes	Carcharhinidae	*Carcharhinus acronotus*	Blacknose shark	0/1
Carcharhiniformes	Carcharhinidae	*Carcharhinus albimarginatus*	Silvertip shark	7/1
Carcharhiniformes	Carcharhinidae	*Carcharhinus altimus*	Bignose shark	3/2
Carcharhiniformes	Carcharhinidae	*Carcharhinus amblyrhynchoides*	Graceful shark	0/1
Carcharhiniformes	Carcharhinidae	*Carcharhinus amblyrhynchos*	Grey reef shark	0/1
Carcharhiniformes	Carcharhinidae	*Carcharhinus amboinensis*	Pigeye shark	0/1
Carcharhiniformes	Carcharhinidae	*Carcharhinus brachyurus*	Copper shark	4/3
Carcharhiniformes	Carcharhinidae	*Carcharhinus brevipinna*	Spinner shark	3/3
Carcharhiniformes	Carcharhinidae	*Carcharhinus falciformis**	Silky shark	2/7
Carcharhiniformes	Carcharhinidae	*Carcharhinus galapagensis*	Galapagos shark	0/1
Carcharhiniformes	Carcharhinidae	*Carcharhinus isodon*	Finetooth shark	0/1
Carcharhiniformes	Carcharhinidae	*Carcharhinus leucas*	Bull shark	1/4
Carcharhiniformes	Carcharhinidae	*Carcharhinus limbatus*	Blacktip shark	5/2
Carcharhiniformes	Carcharhinidae	*Carcharhinus longimanus**	Oceanic whitetip shark	2/5
Carcharhiniformes	Carcharhinidae	*Carcharhinus macloti*	Hardnose shark	0/1
Carcharhiniformes	Carcharhinidae	*Carcharhinus melanopterus*	Blacktip reef shark	1/2

Carcharhiniformes	Carcharhinidae	*Carcharhinus obscurus*	Dusky shark	1/2
Carcharhiniformes	Carcharhinidae	*Carcharhinus perezi*	Caribbean reef shark	0/1
Carcharhiniformes	Carcharhinidae	*Carcharhinus plumbeus*	Sandbar shark	4/2
Carcharhiniformes	Carcharhinidae	*Carcharhinus porosus*	Smalltail shark	0/1
Carcharhiniformes	Carcharhinidae	*Carcharhinus sorrah*	Spottail shark	1/6
Carcharhiniformes	Carcharhinidae	*Galeocerdo cuvier*	Tiger shark	2/4
Carcharhiniformes	Carcharhinidae	*Lamiopsis temminckii*	Broadfin shark	0/1
Carcharhiniformes	Carcharhinidae	*Loxodon macrorhinus*	Sliteye shark	0/1
Carcharhiniformes	Carcharhinidae	*Negaprion acutiden*	Sharptooth lemon shark	0/2
Carcharhiniformes	Carcharhinidae	*Negaprion brevirostris*	Lemon shark	0/1
Carcharhiniformes	Carcharhinidae	*Prionace glauca*	Blue shark	2/4
Carcharhiniformes	Carcharhinidae	*Rhizoprionodon acutus*	Milk shark	0/1
Carcharhiniformes	Carcharhinidae	*Rhizoprionodon longurio*	Pacific sharpnose shark	0/1
Carcharhiniformes	Carcharhinidae	*Rhizoprionodon taylori*	Australian sharpnose shark	0/1
Carcharhiniformes	Carcharhinidae	*Scoliodon laticaudus*	Spadenose shark	0/1
Carcharhiniformes	Hemigaleidae	*Hemigaleus australiensis*	Australian weasel shark	0/1
Carcharhiniformes	Hemigaleidae	*Hemipristis elongata*	Snaggletooth shark	0/1
Carcharhiniformes	Hemigaleidae	*Hemitriakis japanica*	Japanese topeshark	7/0
Carcharhiniformes	Pentanchidae	*Apristurus macrorhynchus*	Flathead catshark	3/0
Carcharhiniformes	Proscylliidae	*Proscyllium habereri*	Graceful catshark	7/0

(Continued)

Table 14.1 (*Continued*)

Order	Family	Species	Common name	Number of samples (unprocessed/processed)
Carcharhiniformes	Scyliorhinidae	*Apristurus nakayai*	Milk-eye catshark	1/0
Carcharhiniformes	Scyliorhinidae	*Apristurus platyrhynchus*	Borneo catshark	1/0
Carcharhiniformes	Scyliorhinidae	*Atelomycterus marmoratus*	Coral catshark	6/0
Carcharhiniformes	Scyliorhinidae	*Cephaloscyllium umbratile*	Blotchy swell shark	4/0
Carcharhiniformes	Scyliorhinidae	*Galeus sauteri*	Blacktip sawtail catshark	7/0
Carcharhiniformes	Scyliorhinidae	*Parmaturus xaniurus*	Filetail catshark	1/0
Carcharhiniformes	Sphyrnidae	*Eusphyra blochii*	Winghead shark	0/1
Carcharhiniformes	Sphyrnidae	*Sphyrna lewini**	Scalloped hammerhead shark	1/6
Carcharhiniformes	Sphyrnidae	*Sphyrna mokarran**	Great hammerhead shark	0/9
Carcharhiniformes	Sphyrnidae	*Sphyrna tiburo*	Bonnethead shark	0/1
Carcharhiniformes	Sphyrnidae	*Sphyrna tudes*	Smalleye hammerhead shark	0/1
Carcharhiniformes	Sphyrnidae	*Sphyrna zygaena**	Smooth hammerhead shark	0/6
Carcharhiniformes	Triakidae	*Galeorhinus galeus*	Tope shark	0/1
Carcharhiniformes	Triakidae	*Mustelus californicus*	Gray smoothhound shark	0/1
Carcharhiniformes	Triakidae	*Mustelus canis*	Dusky smoothhound shark	0/1
Carcharhiniformes	Triakidae	*Mustelus griseus*	Spotless smoothhound shark	3/0
Carcharhiniformes	Triakidae	*Mustelus henlei*	Brown smoothhound shark	0/1
Carcharhiniformes	Triakidae	*Mustelus lunulatus*	Sicklefin smoothhound shark	0/1

Carcharhiniformes	Triakidae	*Mustelus manazo*	Starspotted smoothhound shark	9/0
Carcharhiniformes	Triakidae	*Mustelus mosis*	Arabian smoothhound shark	0/1
Carcharhiniformes	Triakidae	*Mustelus mustelus*	Common smoothhound shark	0/1
Carcharhiniformes	Triakidae	*Mustelus punctulatus*	Blackspotted smoothhound shark	0/1
Chimaeriformes	Callorhinchidae	*Callorhinchus callorynchus*	American elephantfish	0/1
Chimaeriformes	Chimaeridae	*Hydrolagus novaezealandiae*	Dark ghost shark	0/1
Hexanchiformes	Hexanchidae	*Heptranchias perlo*	Sharpnose sevengill shark	2/0
Hexanchiformes	Hexanchidae	*Hexanchus griseus*	Bluntnose sixgill shark	0/1
Lamniformes	Alopiidae	*Alopias pelagicus**	Pelagic thresher shark	4/6
Lamniformes	Alopiidae	*Alopias superciliosus**	Bigeye thresher shark	3/7
Lamniformes	Alopiidae	*Alopias vulpinus**	Common thresher shark	0/2
Lamniformes	Cetorhinidae	*Cetorhinus maximus**	Basking shark	0/5
Lamniformes	Lamnidae	*Carcharodon carcharias**	Great white shark	2/1
Lamniformes	Lamnidae	*Isurus oxyrinchus*	Shortfin mako	10/6
Lamniformes	Lamnidae	*Isurus paucus*	Longfin mako	1/2
Lamniformes	Lamnidae	*Lamna ditropis*	Salmon shark	5/0
Lamniformes	Lamnidae	*Lamna nasus**	Porbeagle	1/2
Lamniformes	Megachasmidae	*Megachasma pelagios*	Megamouth shark	4/0
Lamniformes	Mitsukurinidae	*Mitsukurina owstoni*	Goblin shark	1/0
Lamniformes	Odontaspididae	*Carcharias taurus*	Sand tiger shark	0/1

(*Continued*)

Table 14.1 (*Continued*)

Order	Family	Species	Common name	Number of samples (unprocessed/processed)
Orectolobiformes	Ginglymostomatidae	*Ginglymostoma cirratum*	Nurse shark	0/1
Orectolobiformes	Orectolobidae	*Orectolobus maculatus*	Spotted wobbegong	0/1
Orectolobiformes	Rhincodontidae	*Rhincodon typus**	Whale shark	1/2
Squaliformes	Centrophoridae	*Centrophorus acus*	Gulper shark	2/0
Squaliformes	Centrophoridae	*Deania profundorum*	Arrowhead dogfish	0/1
Squaliformes	Centrophoridae	*Deania quadrispinosa*	Longsnout dogfish	1/0
Squaliformes	Dalatiidae	*Dalatias licha*	Kitefin shark	0/1
Squaliformes	Echinorhinidae	*Echinorhinus cookei*	Prickly shark	2/0
Squaliformes	Echinorhinidae	*Etmopterus brachyurus*	Shorttail lanternshark	5/0
Squaliformes	Echinorhinidae	*Etmopterus decacuspidatus*	Combtoothed lanternshark	1/0
Squaliformes	Echinorhinidae	*Etmopterus fusus*	Pygmy lanternshark	2/0
Squaliformes	Echinorhinidae	*Etmopterus molleri*	Mollers lantern shark	2/0
Squaliformes	Echinorhinidae	*Etmopterus pusillus*	Smooth lanternshark	4/0
Squaliformes	Etmopteridae	*Centroscyllium fabricii*	Black dogfish	4/0
Squaliformes	Etmopteridae	*Trigonognathus kabeyai*	Viper dogfish	1/0
Squaliformes	Somniosidae	*Somniosus pacificus*	Pacific sleeper shark	2/0
Squaliformes	Squalidae	*Squalus brevirostris*	Japanese shortnose spurdog	4/0
Squaliformes	Squalidae	*Squalus japonicus*	Japanese spurdog	4/0
Squatiniformes	Squatinidae	*Squatina legnota*	Indonesian angel shark	1/0

*CITES-listed shark species.

dried processed fin samples, were stored at −80°C until DNA extraction and downstream experiments.

In order to confirm the species identity of the samples, the DNA of all samples were extracted using a Biomed Genomic DNA/Tissue Extraction Kit (Biomed, Beijing, China) according to the manufacturer's instructions (~60 min). PCR was performed to amplify the cytochrome c oxidase I (*COI*) gene using universal fish primers, FISHCOILBC_ts (5′-ACT TCY GGG TGR CCR AAR AAT CA-3′), FISHCOIHBC_ts (5′-TCA ACY AAT CAY AAA GAT ATY GGC AC-3′) (Handy *et al.*, 2011), FishF1 (5′-TCA ACC AAC CAC AAA GAC ATT GGC AC-3′) and FishR1 (5′-TAG ACT TCT GGG TGG CCA AAG AAT CA-3′) (Ward, Zemlak, Innes, Last & Hebert, 2005), for all the samples with an expected product size of ~700 bp. Sanger sequencing of PCR products purified with a gel extraction kit (Biomed, Beijing, China) was performed by Tech Dragon Ltd., Hong Kong. Samples were identified using the Basic Local Alignment Search Tool (BLAST) search against nucleotide sequences available on GenBank. The top-match results with a sequence similarity of at least 99% were used for species confirmation.

14.3.2 Methods

14.3.2.1 *Total Genomic Preparation*

To obtain DNA samples for species identification and testing of specific primers, spin column–based nucleic acid purification was used to remove potential PCR inhibitors, including polysaccharides, protein, salt residues, etc. DNA was extracted using a Biomed Genomic DNA/Tissue Extraction Kit (Biomed, Beijing, China) according to the manufacturer's instructions.

Equipment

- Centrifuge
- Heat block
- Scissors

Reagents

- Ethanol, 100%
- Isopropanol
- Proteinase K (20 mg/mL)
- BioMed Tissue DNA Extraction Kit:
    - Elution Buffer (EB)
    - Lysis Buffer (TL)
    - Binding Buffer (CB)
    - Washing Buffer (WB)

Procedures

1. Pre-warm the EB at 65°C before extraction starts.
2. Add 100% ethanol into WB according to the instructions on the bottle of WB.
3. Put 1 cm^2 of a shark sample and 180 μL of TL in a 1.5-mL micro-centrifuge tube. Cut the samples into small pieces using scissors.
4. Add 20 μL of Proteinase K, mix and incubate for 60 min at 55°C.
5. After incubation, add 200 μL of CB and mix well.
6. Incubate for 10 min at 70°C.
7. Add 100 μL of isopropanol into the supernatant, lightly vortex for about 5 s.
8. Fit a binding column into a 2-mL collection tube.
9. Transfer the mixture in the tube into the binding column and centrifuge at 12,100 × g for 1 min.

10. Pour off the liquid in the collection tube and place back the binding column to the collection tube.
11. Add 500 μL WB to the column and centrifuge at 12,100 × g for 30 s.
12. Pour off the liquid in the collection tube and refit the binding column to the collection tube.
13. Add 500 μL of WB and centrifuge at 12,100 × g for 30 s.
14. Pour off the liquid in the collection tube and place back the binding column to the collection tube.
15. Spin down at 12,100 × g for 2 min to completely remove the ethanol since residual WB left in the binding column will hinder the following steps.
16. Transfer the binding column to a new 1.5-mL Eppendorf tube.
17. Add 100 μL of pre-warmed EB and incubate for 5 min.
18. Elute the DNA by spinning down at 12,100 × g for 2 min.
19. DNA eluted is stored at −20°C.

14.3.2.2 *Genomic DNA Amplification*

Equipment

- Genie II (OptiGene, Horsham, UK)

Reagents

- Isothermal Mastermix (OptiGene, Horsham, UK)
- Forward outer primer F3 (5 μmol/L)
- Backward outer primer B3 (5 μmol/L)
- Forward inner primer FIP (50 μmol/L)
- Backward inner primer BIP (50 μmol/L)
- Forward loop primer LF (25 μmol/L)
- Backward loop primer LB (25 μmol/L)

Procedures

1. Prepare and mix well the LAMP reaction mixture as follows:

	Volume per reaction		
Ingredient	**Reaction without FIP and BIP**	**Reaction with either FIP or BIP**	**Reaction with both FIP and BIP**
Double-distilled water (ddH_2O)	2.0 μL	1.5 μL	1.0 μL
Isothermal Mastermix	7.5 μL	7.5 μL	7.5 μL
F3 (5 μmol/L)	0.5 μL	0.5 μL	0.5 μL
B3 (5 μmol/L)	0.5 μL	0.5 μL	0.5 μL
FIP (50 μmol/L)	0.5 μL	0.5 μL	0.5 μL
BIP (50 μmol/L)	0.5 μL	0.5 μL	0.5 μL
LF (25 μmol/L)	/	0.5 μL of either LF or LB	0.5 μL
LB (25 μmol/L)	/		0.5 μL
Template DNA (10.0 ng/μL)	1.0 μL	1.0 μL	1.0 μL
Total	12.5 μL	12.5 μL	12.5 μL

2. Perform LAMP reaction at the corresponding temperature and reaction time (Table 14.2).

14.3.2.3 *Fluorescence Detection and Data Analysis*

After LAMP, 2 μL 1000X SYBR Green I dye (Invitrogen, Waltham, MA) was added into the end-product of the LAMP reaction for naked-eye detection. End point assays were achieved by naked-eye visualisation under ambient white light. If there is positive LAMP reaction, colour would chang simultaneously with the addition of SYBR Green I dye. Positive LAMP results were shown in green colour, whereas negative results remained in orange colour.

Table 14.2 Loop-Mediated Isothermal Amplification (LAMP) and Polymerase Chain Reaction (PCR) Primers for CITES-Listed Shark Detection

Target	Region	Reaction	Primer type	Primer name	Sequence (5′ to 3′)	Reaction temperature and period	Amplicon size (bp)
Alopias pelagicus (Pelagic thresher shark)	*COI*	LAMP	F3	AP02A	TTA TAC CCG TGA TAA TTG GC	70°C for 60 min	296
			B3	AP03B	TGA TAG TTG TAA TAA AGT TG		
			FIP	AP2A3B FIPV2	GAG GGG GGA AGG AGT CAA AAG GAT TTG GAA ACT GAC TAG TGC		
			BIP	AP2A3B BIPV9	GGA GCC GGT ACT GGT TGA ACC CTG CTA AAT GGA GAG AGA A		
		PCR	LP	AP02A	TTA TAC CCG TGA TAA TTG GC	94°C for 5 min; 35 cycles of 94°C for 30 s, 58°C for 30 s, and 72°C for 1 min; 72°C for 5 min	
			RP	AP03B	TGA TAG TTG TAA TAA AGT TG		

(Continued)

Table 14.2 (*Continued*)

Target	Region	Reaction	Primer type	Primer name	Sequence (5′ to 3′)	Reaction temperature and period	Amplicon size (bp)
Alopias superciliosus (Bigeye thresher shark)	*COI*	LAMP	F3	AS10A	GTT GAC TTG GCC ATT TTC TCG	65°C for 60 min	211
			B3	AS11B	CGA TCA GTT AAT AAT ATT GTG		
			FIP	AS10A11B FIPV2	GTT GTA ATA AAG TTA ATT GAA GCT CTT CAT TTA GCA GGT ATC		
			BIP	AS10A11B BIPV2	TCA AAC ACC ATT ATT TGT ATG ATC ACT GGG AGG GAT AAG AGG A		
		PCR	LP	AS10A	GTT GAC TTG GCC ATT TTC TCG	94°C for 5 min; 35 cycles of 94°C for 30 s, 62°C for 30 s, and 72°C for 1 min; 72°C for 5 min	
			RP	AS11B	CGA TCA GTT AAT AAT ATT GTG		

Alopias vulpinus (Common thresher shark)	*NADH2*	LAMP	F3	AV02A	AAT TGG CCT AGC CCC ACT T	65°C for 60 min	179
			B3	AV03B	CCT ACT ATA GTT GAT AGT ACT CCT		
			FIP	AV2A3B FIPV2	TCT AAG CCT TGG AGA ACT TCC ACT TCT GAT TAC CCG AA		
			BIP	AV2A3B BIPV2	TAC TAC CGG CCT CAT TCT TTG TTT AGT GAA GGG TAA AGT TGT		
		PCR	LP	AV02A	AAT TGG CCT AGC CCC ACT T	94°C for 5 min; 35 cycles of 94°C for 30 s, 60°C for 30 s, and 72°C for 1 min; 72°C for 5 min	
			RP	AV03B	CCT ACT ATA GTT GAT AGT ACT CCT		
Carcharodon carcharias (Great white shark)	*COI*	LAMP	F3	CC05A	TCT TCA TGG TAA TGC CCA TC	70°C for 50 min	236
			B3	CC04B	CCA GGT CAA CGG ATG CTC CT		

(*Continued*)

Table 14.2 (***Continued***)

Target	Region	Reaction	Primer type	Primer name	Sequence (5′ to 3′)	Reaction temperature and period	Amplicon size (bp)
			FIP	CC5A4B FIPV1	TAT GTT ATT TAT TCG GGG GAA GGC GGG AAT TGA CTA ATC CCG TTA A		
			BIP	CC5A4B BIPV4	CTA GCT TCA GCC GGA GTT GAG TGC TAA ATT ACC GGC CAG		
			LF	CC5A4B F1B4 LF V1	TGT CCG GGG CAC CAA TTA		
			LB	CC5A4B F1B4 LBV1	GGA GCC GGC ACT GGT TGA A		
		PCR	LP	CC05A	TCT TCA TGG TAA TGC CCA TC	94°C for 5 min; 35 cycles of 94°C for 30 s, 66°C for 30 s, and 72°C for 1 min; 72°C for 5 min	
			RP	CC04B	CCA GGT CAA CGG ATG CTC CT		

Carcharhinus falciformis (Silky shark)	*NADH2*	LAMP	F3	CF04A	TCA CCA CAG GAC TTA TCT TG	70°C for 60 min	270
			B3	CF07B	GTA AGT GTT ATG ATA ATG TAC		
			FIP	CF4A7B FIPV5	TCC TCA TCC TCC AAT GAT TGT TGA GGC CCC ATT TGC TAT TTT GC		
	COI		BIP	CF4A7B BIPV5	TTC TAG CCT ACT CAT CAA TCG CAG GAT GAG GTT AAG TAG GGT C		
		PCR	LP	CF01A	TCT TCT AAT TCG AGC TGA G	94°C for 5 min; 35 cycles of 94°C for 30 s, 64°C for 30 s, and 72°C for 1 min; 72°C for 5 min	383
			RP	CF01B	ATT GAA GCT AGA ATA GAT GAC		
Carcharhinus longimanus (Oceanic whitetip shark)	*NADH2*	LAMP	F3	CL02A	CTC CTC TCC CTA GGA GGA TTG	70°C for 60 min	302
			B3	CL05B	TGG GAT GAG TGT AAA GAT TGC		

(Continued)

Table 14.2 (*Continued*)

Target	Region	Reaction	Primer type	Primer name	Sequence (5′ to 3′)	Reaction temperature and period	Amplicon size (bp)
			FIP	CL2A5B FIPV1	GAG GGC TAT AAT AGT AGC TGG AGT ACC TCC ACT CTC CGG ATT C		
			BIP	CL2A5B BIPV5	TGC TAC AAC ACT AAC TAT AAG CCC CAG GAG GAT AGA TAA GGT TGC		
		PCR	LP	CL02A	CTC CTC TCC CTA GGA GGA TTG	94°C for 5 min; 35 cycles of 94°C for 30 s, 68°C for 30 s, and 72°C for 1 min; 72°C for 5 min	
			RP	CL05B	TGG GAT GAG TGT AAA GAT TGC		
Cetorhinus maximus (Basking shark)	*COI*	LAMP	F3	CM01A	ACC CGG ATC ACT TCT TGG T	68°C for 60 min	530
			B3	CM02B	AAG AAT GTT GTG TTT AGG TTC		
			FIP	CM1A2B FIPV2	GTG GGA AGG CTA TGT CTG GCG GGG TTT TGG GAA CTG AT		

			BIP	CM1A2B BIPV8	ATA AGC TTT TGA CTC CTC CCT CCG GGC TAA AAG AAG AAG GAT G		
		PCR	LP	CM01A	ACC CGG ATC ACT TCT TGG T	94°C for 5 min; 35 cycles of 94°C for 30 s, 64°C for 30 s, and 72°C for 1 min; 72°C for 5 min	
			RP	CM02B	AAG AAT GTT GTG TTT AGG TTC		
Lamna nasus (Porbeagle shark)	*NADH2*	LAMP	F3	LN02A	CCT GAC AAA AAC TTG CCC CT	65°C for 60 min	444
			B3	LN07B	ATG GCT GGG ATA ACT AAG TTC		
			FIP	LN2A7B FIPV10	CTA CTA TGG TCG AGA GCA CAT TTA CCC CTC ATT AAA TCC CAA		
			BIP	LN2A7B BIPV9	ACT TTC CAT TAT TGC CCT CAT AAC CAA TAA GTC ATT TTG GTA TGA AGC		
			LF	LN2A7B F10B9 LFV1	CCA AGA AAG ATA AGA AGG		

(*Continued*)

Table 14.2 (*Continued*)

Target	Region	Reaction	Primer type	Primer name	Sequence (5′ to 3′)	Reaction temperature and period	Amplicon size (bp)
	COI	PCR	LP	LN06A	TGG CTC CCT CCT AGG CGA C	94°C for 5 min; 35 cycles of 94°C for 30 s, 66°C for 30 s, and 72°C for 1 min; 72°C for 5 min	488
			RP	LN06B	GAT CAC ACA AAT AGG GGT GTC		
Rhincodon typus (Whale shark)	*COI*	LAMP	F3	RT02A	ATT ACT TCC ACC TTC ATT CTT AT	70°C for 50 min	265
			B3	RT04BI	TAG TTA CAA GAA TAG ATC AGA CG		
			FIP	RT2A4BI FIPV3	GAT CAA CTG ATG CTC CCG CGC AGG AAC AGG CTG AAC TG		
			BIP	RT2A4BI BIPV7	CTC CTT ACA TCT AGC AGG AAT TTC ATG TTT GGT ATT GAG AGA TAG CT		
		PCR	LP	RT02A	ATT ACT TCC ACC TTC ATT CTT AT	94°C for 5 min; 35 cycles of 94°C for 30 s, 62°C for 30 s, and 72°C for 1 min; 72°C for 5 min	

			RP	RT04BI	TAG TTA CAA GAA TAG ATC AGA CG		
Sphyrna lewini (Scalloped hammerhead shark)	*COI*	LAMP	F3	SL04A	AGC TAT CTT TTC TCT CCA CC	68°C for 60 min	174
			B3	SL04B	TGC AAG AAC TGG AAG TGA TAG G		
			FIP	SL44A4B FIPV1	AGG TTT CAT GTT AAT GAT AGT AGC CGG TGT ATC ATC AAT T		
			BIP	SL44A4B BIPV1	CCA GCC ATT TCT CAA TAT CAA AGT AGG ATA GTA GTT ACA AGG		
		PCR	LP	SL04A	AGC TAT CTT TTC TCT CCA CC	94°C for 5 min; 35 cycles of 94°C for 30 s, 65°C for 30 s, and 72°C for 1 min; 72°C for 5 min	
			RP	SL04B	TGC AAG AAC TGG AAG TGA TAG G		
Sphyrna mokarran (Great hammerhead shark)	*COI*	LAMP	F3	SM03A	CTT TCG TAA TAA TCT TTT TTA TGG TA	70°C for 50 min	389

(*Continued*)

Table 14.2 (*Continued*)

Target	Region	Reaction	Primer type	Primer name	Sequence (5′ to 3′)	Reaction temperature and period	Amplicon size (bp)
			B3	SM04B	TAG TTA CAA GAA TAG ATC AG		
			FIP	SM3A4B FIPV1	TTC GTG GGA AAG CTA TAT CTG GTG GGT GGT TTT GGG AAT TGA CT		
			BIP	SM3A4B BIPV1	CCA CTT AGC TGG TAT CTC ATC AAT CTT GAG AAA TAG CTG GGG GT		
			LB	SM3A4B F1B1 LBV1	CTG GCC TCA ATT AAT TTC ATC ACA A		
		PCR	LP	SM03A	CTT TCG TAA TAA TCT TTT TTA TGG TA	94°C for 5 min; 35 cycles of 94°C for 30 s, 59°C for 30 s, and 72°C for 1 min; 72°C for 5 min	
			RP	SM04B	TAG TTA CAA GAA TAG ATC AG		

Sphyrna zygaena (Smooth hammerhead shark)	*COI*	LAMP	F3	SZ03A	CAT GAG CAG GTA TAG TTG GG	68°C for 60 min	299
			B3	SZ04B	TTC CTG CTC CAG CTT CTA CC		
			FIP	SZ3A4B FIPV5	TGG TCA TCT CCT AGA AGA GAT CCA GCC CTA AGT CTC TTA ATT CG		
			BIP	SZ3A4B BIPV2	AAT CAT AAT TGG TGG CTT CGG GGG AGG AGA AGA AAT GAT GGT G		
		PCR	LP	SZ03A	CAT GAG CAG GTA TAG TTG GG	94°C for 5 min; 35 cycles of 94°C for 30 s, 68°C for 30 s, and 72°C for 1 min; 72°C for 5 min	
			RP	SZ04B	TTC CTG CTC CAG CTT CTA CC		
Internal control	12S rRNA	LAMP	F3	UPCG01A	CCC CAA ACT AGG ATT AGA TA	55°C for 60 min	308
			B3	UPCG01B	ATG TAG CCC ATT TCT ATC CA		

(*Continued*)

Table 14.2 (*Continued*)

Target	Region	Reaction	Primer type	Primer name	Sequence (5′ to 3′)	Reaction temperature and period	Amplicon size (bp)
			FIP	UPCG1A1B FIPV4	CTA GGT GGG TTT GGG ACA CCC GCC AGA GTA CTA CAA GC		
			BIP	UPCG1A1B BIPV7	TAA ACC TCA CCA CTT CTG GCC TTT GCT ACA CCT CGA CCT		
			LF	UPCG1A1B F4B7 LFV1	CCA AGT CCT TTG GGT TTY AAG CTA G		
			LB	UPCG1A1B F4B7 LBV3	CGT CGT CAG CYH ACC YT		
	COI	PCR	LP	UP01A	YTT TGG TGC ATG AGC AGG	94°C for 5 min; 35 cycles of 94°C for 30 s, 40°C for 30 s, and 72°C for 1 min; 72°C for 5 min	148
			RP	UP01B	TAA CTA TAA AGA AGA TTA TTA C		

14.4 Result

14.4.1 Real-Time Amplification

The LAMP assays developed for the 12 CITES-listed shark species specifically amplified their target species only and non-target species were not detected (Figure 14.2). All reactions were able to give clear real-time amplification curves within 60 min. LAMP for internal control were able to amplify all 93 species within 60 min. Shown in Figure 14.3, the melting temperatures of LAMP products of the 12 LAMP assays were 81.1°C (bigeye thresher shark), 81.6°C (scalloped hammerhead shark), 82.9°C (oceanic whitetip shark), 83.1°C (silky shark and smooth hammerhead shark), 83.9°C (pelagic thresher shark and porbeagle shark), 84.1°C (basking shark), 84.8°C (common thresher shark), 85.4°C (great hammerhead shark and whale shark), 85.7°C (pelagic thresher shark) and 86.6°C (great white shark).

14.4.2 Visual Detection by Naked Eye and Gel Electrophoresis

Apart from the real-time amplification curve and melting curve obtained from Genie II, positive LAMP signals could be observed by the naked eye after the addition of SYBR Green I dye. As shown in Figure 14.4, under ambient white light, all positive LAMP reactions turned green in colour and negative reactions remained orange. Since the LAMP technique is mostly applied for rapid detection, gel electrophoresis is less used for result observation. Figure 14.5 shows the amplification result of samples of *C. longimanus*, *C. falciformis* and *S. lewini* with species-specific LAMP primers targeting the oceanic whitetip shark *C. longimanus*. Clear amplification was found only with the *C. longimanus* sample while no amplification was found with the *C. falciformis* and *S. lewini* samples.

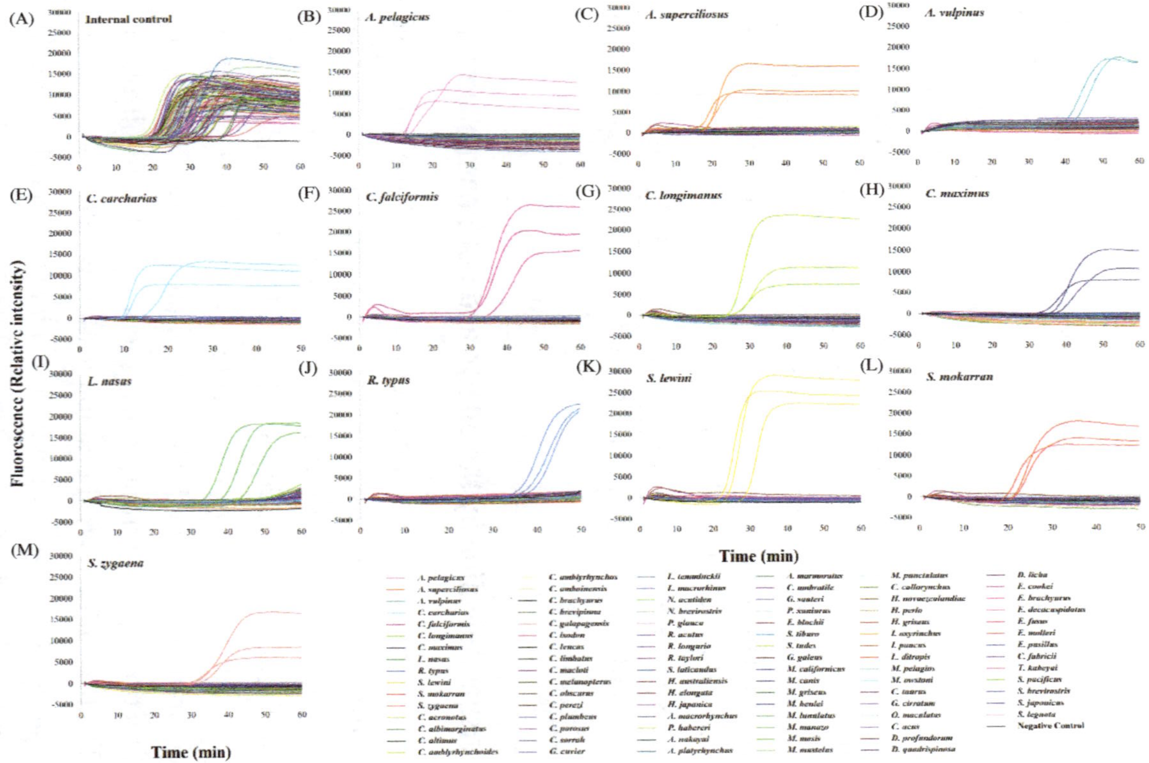

Fig. 14.2 Amplification curves of loop-mediated isothermal amplification (LAMP) assays for 93 species with species-specific primers targeting corresponding species. Rising fluorescence signals indicate positive amplification. Clear amplification was only found with the target species in three different samples.

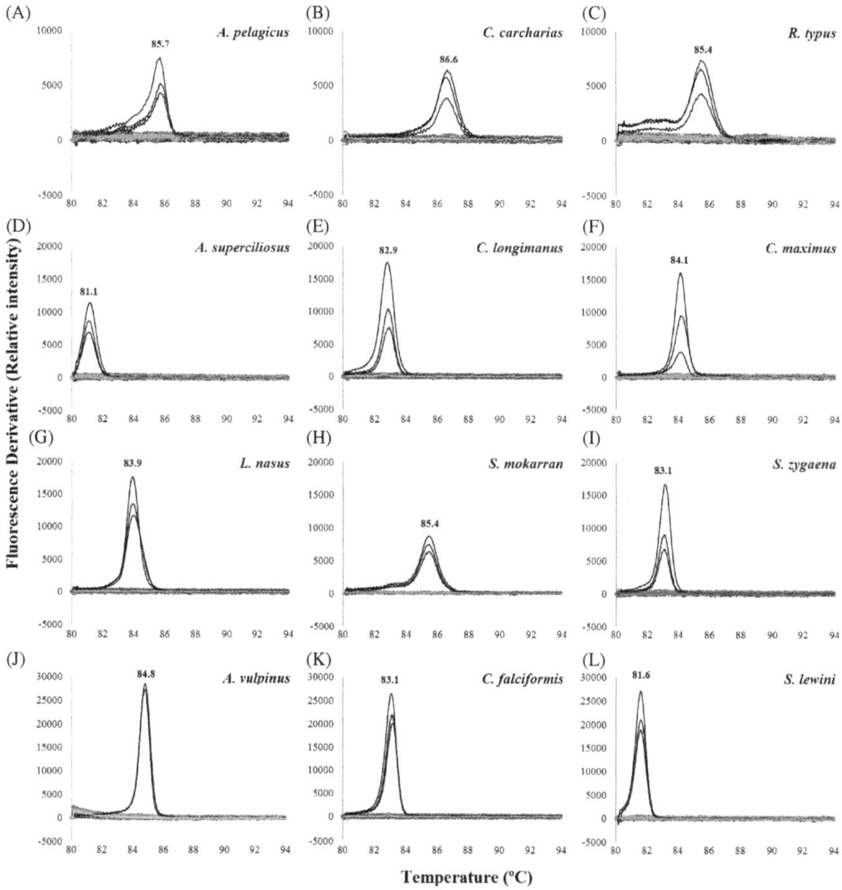

Fig. 14.3 Melting curves of the loop-mediated isothermal amplification (LAMP) products for the corresponding species. The melting temperature is shown as a peak.

14.5 Discussion

14.5.1 Design of LAMP Primer

The pair of outer primer — forward outer primer (F3) and backward outer primer (B3) — is designed based on the nucleotide difference between the target species and its closely-related species, which is similar to the design of species-specific conventional PCR primers (refer to Chapter 3). The size of the amplified product is suggested

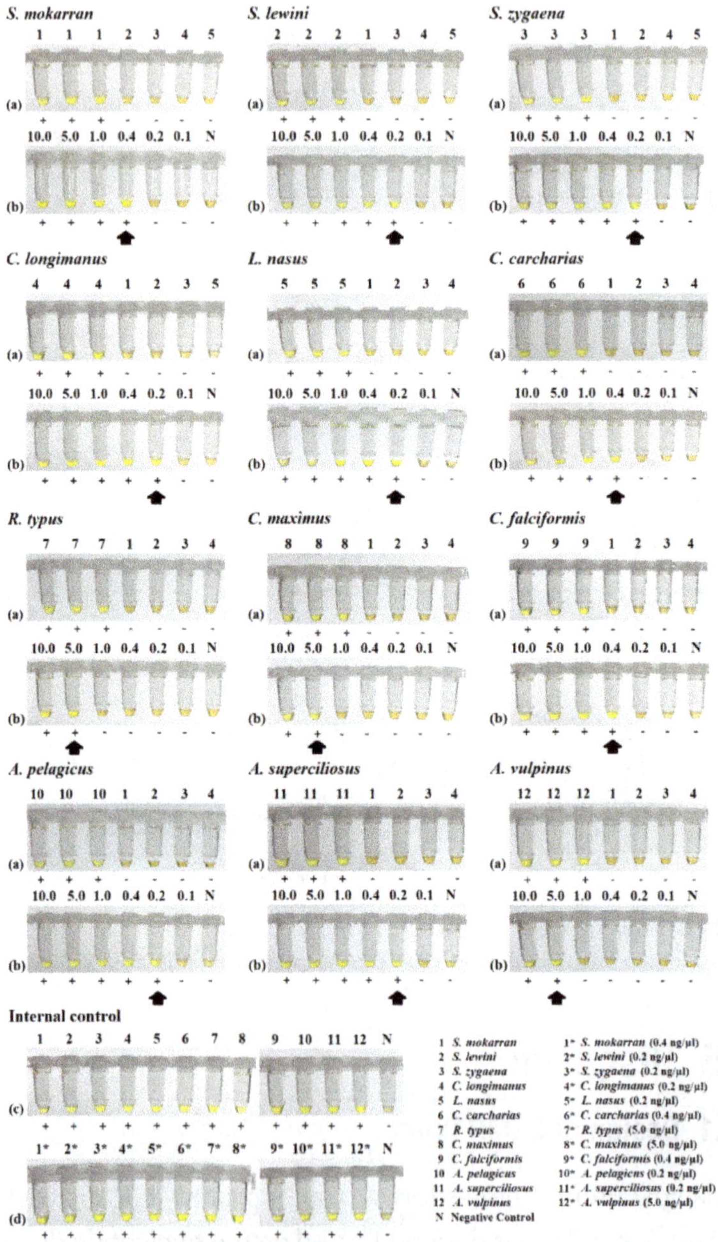

Fig. 14.4 Visual detection of loop-mediated isothermal amplification (LAMP) products of LAMP assays targeting corresponding shark species. End-point assays were achieved by naked-eye visualisation under ambient white light. Green colour represents positive LAMP results ('+' with arrow) while orange represents negative results ('–').

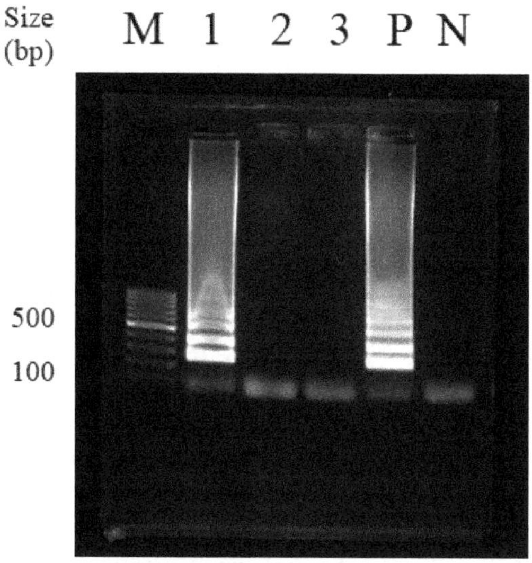

Fig. 14.5 Amplification result with species-specific loop-mediated isothermal amplification (LAMP) primers targeting the oceanic whitetip shark *Carcharhinus longimanus*. Lane M: 100 bp DNA size marker, 1: *Carcharhinus longimanus*, 2: *C. falciformis*, 3: *Sphyrna lewini*, P: positive control, N: negative control. Clear amplification was found with the *C. longimanus* sample while no amplification was found with the *C. falciformis* and *S. lewini* samples.

to be 150–300 bp. For the pair of inner primer, FIP and BIP, and loop primer, they are designed using the software PrimerExplorer V5 (Eiken Chemical Co. Ltd., Tokyo, Japan). All the LAMP primers designed are suggested to share similar T_m value and GC content. There are also several key points when designing LAMP primers:

1. Distance between 5′ end of F2 and B2 is suggested to be 120–180 bp, and that between F2 and F3 as well as B2 and B3 is suggested to be 0–20 bp.
2. A distance of 40–60 bp should also be considered for loop formation (5′ of F2 to 3′ of F1, 5′ of B2 to 3′ of B1).
3. For the T_m value and GC content for the primers, it is suggested to be about 60–65°C and 50–60% for the GC-rich primer and about 55–60°C for the AT-rich primer.

4. Primers should be designed to avoid the formation of secondary structures and the 3′ end sequence should not be rich in AT content or complementary to other primers.

The following sections will further discuss different approaches to increase the specificity and sensitivity of LAMP assays and choice of region for the primer design.

14.5.2 LAMP Amplification and Optimisation

LAMP allows rapid amplification of DNA using *Bst* polymerase with high strand displacement activity at isothermal temperature within an hour. This facilitates on-site diagnosis with limited equipment and provides species-level identification in a short period of time, thus increasing the efficiency of law enforcement. Although the optimal temperature for *Bst* polymerase is between 60°C and 65°C (Fukuta *et al.*, 2004), the optimal reaction temperatures for most of the LAMP assays developed were found to be 68°C or 70°C, except for those targeting the bigeye thresher shark, common thresher shark and porbeagle shark. Increase in LAMP reaction temperature allows better specificity, especially for eliminating congeneric species.

Apart from increasing the reaction temperature, another common approach of optimising LAMP reaction is the addition of loop primers, which can increase the sensitivity of LAMP reaction. The LAMP assays targeting the great white shark, porbeagle shark and great hammerhead shark and that for the internal control include loop primers in their primer sets. Loop primers are designed to bind to the additional sites that are not accessed by the internal primers and accelerate the rate of LAMP reaction and provide higher sensitivity (Nagamine, Hase & Notomi, 2002). This allows the LAMP assay for the internal control to amplify all shark species in Table 14.1 at a relatively low reaction temperature, which also favours primer annealing and amplification. The presence of loop primers also allows the LAMP assays developed to give amplification with a detectable threshold within 60 min, reducing the reaction time required for the assays. For LAMP and PCR assays amplifying the same region of a species, the species-specific LAMP assays generally have better sensitivity than species-specific PCR assays. Looped DNA product increases the sensitivity of the LAMP assay and hence facilitates detection with a limited sample amount from dried shark fin. In addition to better sensitivity, since LAMP produces more DNA product than the conventional PCR method, it allows easy visual detection with the naked eye to tell between positive and negative results without fluorescence detection equipment. On-site detection of CITES-listed shark species can be achieved.

14.5.3 Choice of Region for Primer Design

For the shark LAMP assays, the primers are designed based on *COI* and *NADH2* loci for the CITES-listed shark species and on the 12S ribosomal RNA (rRNA) locus for the internal control. Previous studies about species-specific primers on shark species identification are mostly focused on the ITS2 locus (Abercrombie, Clarke & Shivji, 2005; Chapman *et al.*, 2003; Magnussen *et al.*, 2007; Shivji *et al.*, 2002). The *COI* locus, a standard marker for fish and shark species DNA barcoding (Chang, Lin, Ren, Lin & Shao, 2016; Chang *et al.*, 2017; Handy *et al.*, 2011; Fields, Abercrombie, Eng, Feldheim & Chapman, 2015; Ward, Zemlak, Innes, Last & Hebert, 2005), is highly species specific and the number of nucleotide difference of congeneric species is sufficient for designing species-specific primers. For the common thresher shark, silky shark, oceanic whitetip shark and porbeagle shark, the *NADH2* locus is a better region for designing a species-specific primer, due to high nucleotide sequence differences between the target species and the corresponding congeneric species (Naylor *et al.*, 2012). High degree of nucleotide sequence difference allows the design of LAMP primers targeting four to six species-specific regions instead of only two for conventional PCR. The developed LAMP assays are highly specific, especially for species with many congeneric species such as the silky shark and the ocean whitetip shark.

Furthermore, care should be taken to avoid sites of known intraspecific variation among sharks from different regions or ocean basins during primer design, so that amplification success would not be affected by intraspecific nucleotide variation. 12S rRNA locus is a suitable target for designing primers for the internal control as it has high sequence homology among different shark species. This allows the design of six LAMP primers that can amplify all the shark species in this work.

14.5.4 Pros and Cons of LAMP Approach

In comparison to the conventional PCR approach, LAMP shows the advantages in the aspects of specificity and sensitivity. Furthermore, LAMP provides high amplification efficiency and allows simultaneous detection. LAMP approach does not require thermal cycler and special equipment. On the other hand, a LAMP approach needs more effort at the development stage, as primer design is more complicated. Since FIP and BIP are primers joined by two different primers without overlapping, to avoid failure of amplification or formation of primer dimers, rules mentioned in Section 14.5.1 must be followed strictly for the design of LAMP primers. Researchers can also use the software PrimerExplorer V5 to design the FIP, BIP, and loop primers. Many primer combinations can be generated but they must be screened and tested for optimal temperature and amplification time, in order to find out the best-match primers for amplifying the target species. Besides the complexity of primer design and workload of primer screening, the LAMP approach is more expensive than the conventional PCR method because of the use of commercial LAMP reagent. Furthermore, since the template is highly amplified, there may be a chance of cross contamination leading to false positive results. Therefore, it is important to clean the equipment before tests and keep good laboratory practice.

14.6 Conclusion

As a rapid authentication method, the LAMP technique has been widely applied on species differentiation of medicinal materials from their common adulterants and congeneric species. In this chapter, detection of shark fin products of CITES-listed shark species, as a kind of materials used in traditional Chinese medicine, has been demonstrated using LAMP and PCR techniques. LAMP and PCR primers designed based on *COI* or *NADH2* regions were able to differentiate target shark species from non-target species with a detection limit of 0.2–5.0 ng/μL DNA for LAMP assays and 0.2–10.0 ng/μL DNA for PCR assays. Target shark species were able to be differentiated from non-target species within an hour with the LAMP assays, thus providing a simple and robust solution with potential for on-site detection of CITES-listed shark species with shark fin products. Rapid and effective authentication and identification method can be carried using LAMP techniques. More investigation is needed for the application of LAMP techniques on the authentication of highly processed medicinal materials, along with the use of multiplex LAMP techniques.

Acknowledgements

We thank the Agriculture, Fisheries and Conservation Department of the Hong Kong SAR, Biodiversity Research Centre of Academia Sinica, Taiwan, Institute of Marine Biology of National Taiwan Ocean University, Kadoorie Farm & Botanic Garden Hong Kong, Ocean Park Hong Kong and Ocean Park Conservation Foundation Hong Kong for providing shark samples. This work was supported by Environment and Conservation Fund (ECF Project 80-2015) from the Hong Kong SAR.

References

Abercrombie, D. L., Clarke, S. C., & Shivji, M. S. (2005). Global-scale genetic identification of hammerhead sharks: Application to assessment of the international fin trade and law enforcement. *Conserv Genet, 6*, 775–788.

Barreto, R. F., Ferretti, J. M., Flemming, A., Amorim, H. A., Worm, B., & Lessa, R. P. T. (2016). Trends in the exploitation of South Atlantic shark populations. *Conserv Biol, 30*(4), 792–804.

Baum, J. K., Myers, R. A., Kehler, D. G., Worm, B., Harley, S. J., & Doherty, P. A. (2003). Collapse and conservation of shark populations in the Northwest Atlantic. *Science, 299*(5605), 389–392.

Brautigam, A., Callow, M., Campbell, I. R., Camhi, M. D., Cornish, A. S., Dulvy, N., S. V. Fordham, S. L. Fowler, A. R. Hood, C. McClennen, E. L. Reuter, G. Sant, C. A. Simpfendorfer, & Welch, D. J. (2015). *Global Priorities for Conserving Sharks and Rays: A 2015–2025 Strategy.* United Nations: The Global Sharks and Rays Initiative. http://www.iucnssg.org/uploads/5/4/1/2/54120303/grsi_report_21-12-15_websingles.pdf

Cardenosa, D., Quinlan, J., Shea, K. H., & Chapman, D. D. (2018). Multiplex real-time PCR assay to detect illegal trade of CITES-listed shark species. *Sci Rep, 8*, 16313.

Chang, C. H., Lin, H. Y., Ren, Q., Lin, Y. S., & Shao, K. T. (2016). DNA barcode identification of fish and fishery products in Taiwan: Government-commissioned authentication cases. *Food Control, 66*, 38–43.

Chang, C. H., Shao, K. T., Lin, H. Y., Chiu, Y. C., Lee, M. Y., Liu, S. H., & Lin, P. L. (2017). DNA barcodes of the native ray-finned fishes in Taiwan. *Mol Ecol Resour, 17*, 796–805.

Chapman, D. D., Abercrombie, D. L., Douady, C. J., Pikitch, E. K., Stanhopen, M. J., & Shivji, M. S. (2003). A streamlined, bi-organelle, multiplex PCR approach to species identification: Application to global conservation and trade monitoring of the great white shark, *Carcharodon carcharias*. *Conserv Genet, 4*, 415–425.

Chaudhary, A. A., Hemant, M. M., & Ahmad, A. (2012). Application of loop-mediated isothermal amplification (LAMP)-based technology for authentication of *Catharanthus roseus* (L.) G. Don. *Protoplasma, 249*(2), 417–422.

Clarke, S. C. (2004). *Shark Product Trade in Hong Kong and Mainland China and Implementation of the CITES Shark Listings*. China: TRAFFIC East Asia.

Clarke, S. C., Magnussen, J. E., Abercrombie, D. L., McAllister, M. K., & Shivji, M.S. (2006). Identification of shark species composition and proportion in the Hong Kong shark fin market based on molecular genetics and trade records. *Conserv Biol, 20*(1), 201–211.

Cortes, E. (2002). Incorporating uncertainty into demographic modeling: Application to shark populations and their conservation. *Conserv Biol, 16*(4), 1048–1062.

Dulvy, N. K., Allen, D. J., Ralph, G. M., & Walls, R. H. L. (2016). *The Conservation Status of Sharks, Rays and Chimaeras in the Mediterranean Sea* [Brochure]. Malaga, Spain: The International Union for Conservation of Nature.

Dulvy, N. K., Fowler, S. L., Musick, J. A., Cavanagh, R. D., Kyne, P. M., Harrison, L. R., Carlson, J. K., Davidson, L. N. K., Fordham, S. V., Francis, M. P., Pollock, C. M., Simpfendorfer, C. A., Burgess, G. H., Carpenter, K. E., Compagno, L. J. V., Ebert, D. A., Gibson, C., Heupel, M. R., Livingstone, S. R., Sanciangco, J. C., Stevens, J. D., Valenti, S., & White, W. T. (2014). Extinction risk and conservation of the world's sharks and rays. *eLife*, 3, e00590.

Eriksson, H., & Clarke, S. (2015). Chinese market responses to overexploitation of sharks and sea cucumbers. *Biol Conserv, 184*, 163–173.

Fields, A. T., Abercrombie, D. L., Eng, R., Feldheim, K., & Chapman, D. D. (2015). A novel mini-DNA barcoding assay to identify processed fins from internationally protected shark species. *PLoS One, 10*, e0114844.

Fields, A. T., Fischer, G. A., Shea, S. K. H., Zhang, H., Abercrombie, D. L., Feldheim, K. A., Elizabeth A. Babcock, & Chapman, D. D. (2018). Species composition of the international shark fin trade assessed through a retail-market survey in Hong Kong. *Conserv Biol, 32*(2), 376–389.

Fischbach, J., Xander, N. C., Frohme, M., & Glokler, J. F. (2015). Shining a light on LAMP assays — a comparison of LAMP visualization methods including the novel use of berberine. *BioTechniques, 58*(4), 189–194.

Food and Agriculture Organisation (FAO). (2016a). *FAO Fishery Commodities Global Production and Trade Database Updated to 2013*. Italy: Food and Agriculture Organization of the United Nations. Retrieved from http://www.fao.org/fishery/statistics/global-commodities-production/en (Accessed Mar 15, 2019).

Food and Agriculture Organisation (FAO). (2016b). *FAO Global Capture Production Database Updated to 2014*. Italy: Food and Agriculture Organization of the United Nations. Retrieved from http://www.fao.org/fishery/statistics/global-capture-production/en (Accessed Mar 15, 2019).

Fukuta, S., Mizukami, Y., Ishida, A., Ueda, J., Hasegawa, M., Hayashi, I., Hashimoto, M., & Kanbe, M. (2004). Real-time loop-mediated isothermal amplification for the CaMV-35S promoter as a screening method for genetically modified organisms. *Eur Food Res Technol, 218*, 496–505.

Handy, S. M., Deeds, J. R., Ivanova, N. V., Herber, P. D. N., Hanner, R., Ormos, A., Weigt, L. A., Moore, M. M., & Yancy, H. F. (2011). A single laboratory validated method for the generation of DNA barcodes for the identification of fish for regulatory compliance. *J AOAC Int, 94*, 201–210.

Jabado, R. W., Ghais, S. M. A., Hamza, W., Henderson, A. C., Spaet, J. L. Y., Shivji, M. S., & Hanner, R. H. (2015). The trade in sharks and their products in the United Arab Emirates. *Biol Conserv, 181*, 190–198.

Jaiteh, V. F., Loneragan, N. R., & Warren, C. (2017). The end of shark finning? Impacts of declining catches and fin demand for coastal community livelihoods. *Mar Policy, 82*, 224–233.

Jiang, L. L., Liu, C. L., Wong, Y. L., Nip, C. F., & Shaw, P. C. (2015). Differentiation of deer tendons from cattle tendons by a loop-mediated isothermal amplification (LAMP) test and bone remodeling bioassays. *Chin Med, 10*, 33.

Kim, Y., Jeong, S. M., Kim, B., Kim, D. P., & Cho, Y. K. (2015). Rapid and automated quantification of microalgal lipids on a spinning disc. *Anal Chem, 87*(15), 7865–7871.

Lai, G. H., Chao, J., Lin, M. K., Chang, W. T., Peng, W. H., Sun, F. C., Lee, M. S., & Lee, M. S. (2015). Rapid and sensitive identification of the herbal tea ingredient *Taraxacum formosanum* using loop-mediated isothermal amplification. *Int J Mol Sci, 16*(1), 1562–1575.

Lee, M. S., & Hxiao, H. J. (2019). Rapid and sensitive authentication of *Polygonum multiflorum* (He-Shou-Wu) of Chinese medicinal crop using specific isothermal nucleic acid amplification. *Ind Crops Prod, 29*, 281–289.

Li, J. J., Xiong, C., Liu, Y., Liang, J. S., & Zhou, X. W. (2016). Loop-mediated isothermal amplification (LAMP): Emergence as an alternative technology for herbal medicine identification. *Front Plant Sci, 7*, 1956.

Li, K., Li, Q., Yuan, Y., Chen, J. Y., Huang, L. Q., & Liu, Z. G. (2011). Identification and detection of *Cordyceps sinensis* with LAMP. *Chin Tradit Herbal Drugs, 42*(8),1605–1608.

Li, M., Wong, Y. L., Jiang, L. L., Wong, K. L., Wong, Y. T., Lau, C. B., & Shaw, P. C. (2013). Application of novel loop-mediated isothermal amplification (LAMP) for rapid authentication of the herbal tea ingredient *Hedyotis diffusa* Willd. *Food Chem, 141*(3), 2522–2525.

Liu, Y., Wang, X. Y., Wei, X. M., Gao, Z. T., & Han, J. P. (2018). Rapid authentication of Ginkgo biloba herbal products using the recombinase polymerase amplification assay. *Sci Rep, 8*, 8002.

Loo, J. F., But, G. W. C., Kwok, H. C., Lau, P. M., Kong, S. K., Ho, H. P., & Shaw, P. C. (2019). A rapid sample-to-answer analytical detection of genetically modified papaya using loop-mediated isothermal amplification assay on lab-on-a-disc for field use. *Food Chem, 274*, 822–830.

Magnussen, J. E., Pikitch, E. K., Clarke, S. C., Nicholson, C., Hoelzel, A. R., & Shivji, M. S. (2007). Genetic tracking of basking shark products in international trade. *Anim Conserv, 10*, 199–207.

Mori, Y., Nagamine, K., Tomita, N., & Notomi, T. (2001). Detection of loop-mediated isothermal amplification reaction by turbidity derived from magnesium pyrophosphate formation. *Biochem Biophys Res Commun, 289*(1), 150–154.

Musick, J. A. (2005). *Shark Utilization. Management Techniques for Elasmobranch Fisheries.* Italy: Food and Agriculture Organization of the United Nations.

Nagamine, K., Hase, T., & Notomi, T. (2002). Accelerated reaction by loop-mediated isothermal amplification using loop primers. *Mol Cell Probes, 16*, 223–229.

Naylor, G. J. P., Caira, J. N., Jensen, K., Rosana, K. A. M., White, W. T., & Last, P. R. (2012). A DNA sequence-based approach to the identification of shark and ray species and its implications for global elasmobranch diversity and parasitology. *Bull Am Mus Nat Hist, 367*, 1–262.

Nelson, J. S., Grande, T. C., & Wilson, M. V. H. (2016). *Fishes of the World.* New Jersey, USA: John Wiley & Sons, Inc.

Notomi, T., Okayama, H., Masubuchi, H., Yonekawa, T., Watanabe, K., Amino, N., & Hase, T. (2000). Loop-mediated isothermal amplification of DNA. *Nucleic Acids Res, 28*(12), E63.

Sasaki, Y., Komatsu, K., & Nagumo, S. (2008). Rapid detection of *Panax ginseng* by loop-mediated isothermal amplification and its application to authentication of Ginseng. *Biol Pharm Bull, 31*(9), 1806–1808.

Sasaki, Y., & Nagumo, S. (2007). Rapid identification of *Curcuma longa* and *C. aromatica* by LAMP. *Biol Pharm Bull, 30*(11), 2229–2230.

Shivji, M., Clarke, S., Pank, M., Natanson, L., Kohler, N., & Stanhope, M. (2002). Genetic identification of pelagic shark body parts for conservation and trade monitoring. *Conserv Biol, 16*, 1036–1047.

Tian, E., Liu, Q., Ye, H., Li, F., & Chao, Z. (2017). A DNA barcode-based RPA assay (BAR-RPA) for rapid identification of the dry root of *Ficus hirta* (Wuzhimaotao). *Molecules, 22*(12), E2261.

Tomita, N., Mori, Y., Kanda, H., & Notomi, T. (2008). Loop-mediated isothermal amplification (LAMP) of gene sequences and simple visual detection of products. *Nat Protoc, 3*(5), 877–882.

Vannuccini, S. F., & Agriculture Organization of the United Nations. (1999). *Shark Utilization, Marketing, and Trade.* Italy: Food and Agriculture Organization of the United Nations.

Wang, G., Ding, X., Hu, J., Wu, W., Sun, J., & Mu, Y. (2017). Unusual isothermal multimerization and amplification by the strand-displacing DNA polymerases with reverse transcription activities. *Sci Rep, 7*, 13928.

Wang, J., Yang, F., Zhang, J., Shen, X., Dai, G., & Zhou, Z. (2000). The research on anticarcinogenosis and immunologic regulation of shark chondric powder. *Chin J Mar Drugs, 74*, 14–17.

Ward, R. D., Zemlak, T. S., Innes, B. H., Last, P. R., & Hebert, P. D. (2005). DNA barcoding Australia's fish species. *Philos Trans R Soc Lond, B, Biol Sci, 360*, 1847–1857.

Yang, Z., McLendon, C., Hutter, D., Bradley, K. M., Hoshika, S., Frye, C. B., & Benner, S. A. (2015). Helicase-dependent isothermal amplification of DNA and RNA by using self-avoiding molecular recognition systems. *Chembiochem, 16*(9), 1365–1370.

Zhao, M., Shi, Y., Wu, L., Guo, L., Liu, W., Xiong, C., Yan, S., Sun, W., & Chen, S. (2016). Rapid authentication of the precious herb saffron by loop-mediated isothermal amplification (LAMP) based on internal transcribed spacer 2 (ITS2) sequence. *Sci Rep, 6*, 25370.

Chapter 15

Rapid Identification of Medicinal Materials by Lateral Flow Dipstick Diagnosis

Grace Wing-Chiu But, Ka-Lok Wong & Pang-Chui Shaw

15.1 Introduction

Lateral flow dipstick (LFD) is a simple diagnostic device for detecting the presence of a target substance. LFD diagnostic tests have been widely used for testing different target analyte for clinical analysis, e.g., microbial in human or animals, and ingredients or contaminants in food and environments (Lee *et al.*, 2015; Tang *et al.*, 2009; Weng, Gaur & Neethirajan, 2016).

Generally, there are four major parts on LFD, which include the sample application part, the conjugate release part, the testing part and the absorbent part (Figure 15.1). For a non-competitive assay (sandwich assay), when a liquid sample, such as a polymerase chain reaction (PCR) product diluted with reaction buffer, is placed on the sample application part, the liquid sample will run along the dipstick due to capillary action. At the conjugate release part, there are dried detection labels conjugated with molecular markers (antibody). When the liquid sample passes through the conjugate release part, the sample rehydrates the detection labels, and the PCR product binds with specific detection labels. At the testing part, there are test and control sites, which are fabricated

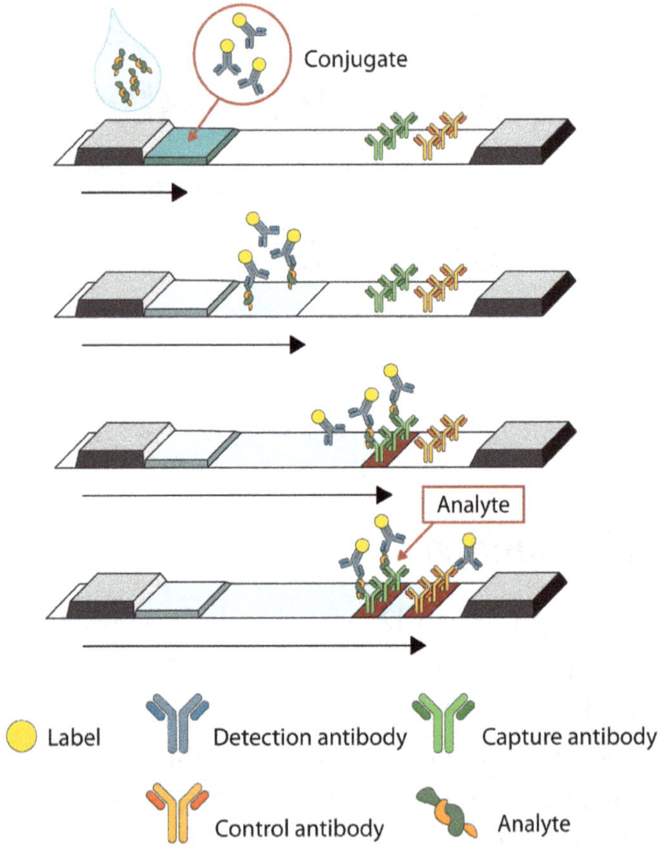

Fig. 15.1 Schematic diagram on lateral flow dipstick (LFD).

with capture reagents (anti-antibody or biotin ligand). When the sample bound with specific detection labels are captured by the capture reagents, they accumulate at that site. Those free, non-bound molecular markers continue to flow through the testing sites and are captured at the control site. When there is enough accumulation of samples on the test site or non-bound molecular markers on the control site, the accumulation captured will be visible and form a coloured line, which can be observed by the naked eye. After the testing part, the liquid flows to the absorbent part where liquid is soaked up.

As a device for the analysis of nucleic acid amplification, LFD also has advantages: low cost, short preparation and result analysis time, and high stability and portability. LFD is also simple to perform, and its result is easy to be analysed by the general public. For detection and authentication, LFD has been applied to differentiate toxic mushroom *Amanita phalloides* from 18 closely related edible and toxic mushroom species (Vaagt, Hasse & Fischer, 2013), differentiate between Arabian coffee (*Coffea arabica* L.) and robusta coffee (*Coffea canephora* Pierre) (Trantakis *et al.*, 2012), and detect components in Lonicerae Japonicae Flos (*Lonicera japonica* Thumnb.) (Zhang *et al.*, 2019).

In this chapter, Cordyceps is differentiated from its common adulterants by the HybriDetect 2T dipstick system. HybriDetect 2T dipstick system allows multiplexed lateral flow assay, with more than one target being detected simultaneously. Other than time and cost savings and being less labour intensive, multiplexed lateral flow assay also has the advantages of low sample volume requirement.

15.2 Materials and Methods

15.2.1 Materials

15.2.1.1 *Introduction of Materials*

Cordyceps (Dongchongxiacao) is a precious traditional Chinese medicinal materials. Cordyceps is composed of the fruiting body of *Ophiocordyceps sinensis* (syn. *Cordyceps sinensis*) parasitic on the caterpillar of a ghost-moth species (Family: Hepialidae). In Asian countries, Cordyceps has a long history of being consumed for its pharmacological value in replenishing the kidney and soothing the lung. Previous pharmacological studies have also shown that Cordyceps is beneficial to the circulatory, immune, respiratory and male reproductive systems (Fung *et al.*, 2011; Jiang *et al.*, 2011; Lee, Wong, Kong, Leung & Lam, 2006; Panda & Swain, 2011; Sirisidthi, Kosai & Jiraungkoorskul, 2015; Wang, Lee, Chen, Yu & Duh, 2012). The growth of demand of Cordyceps results in a dramatic rise in the price of Cordyceps. The Cordyceps industry in China was estimated to be worth USD 1.5 billion in 2004 (Dong, Guo, Wang & Liu, 2015). Owing to the high price, *Cordyceps gunnii* and *C. militaris* have been found in the market to adulterate *O. sinensis* from time to time, resulting in potential threat to public health in consumption of adulterants or substitutes, thus reducing public confidence in traditional medicinal materials. Traditionally, Cordyceps is identified by its morphological characteristics, which is highly relied on by experienced experts (Shrestha, Zhang, Zhang & Liu, 2010). There are also various authentication methods to differentiate *O. sinensis* from its commonly found adulterants, including chemical methods (Hu *et al.*, 2015; Zhang *et al.*, 2015) and molecular methods, e.g., DNA barcoding (Chen, Wang, Zhou & Qu, 2002; Xiang *et al.*, 2013) and species-specific amplification with PCR-based methods (Lam *et al.*, 2015; Li *et al.*, 2011; Liu, Wang, Gao, Han & Xiang, 2017). In this study, a species-specific PCR assay cum multiplex LFD detection for the differentiation of *O. sinensis* from its adulterants *C. gunnii* and *C. militaris* is described.

15.2.1.2 *Samples*

Nine Cordyceps products and related samples of three species, *O. sinensis*, *C. gunnii* and *C. militaris*, were collected from various locations in China (Table 15.1). The samples were identified based on the morphological characteristics and sequencing of the translation elongation factor 1-alpha (EF-1α) region. Samples were stored at room temperature in the Institute of Chinese Medicine, The Chinese University of Hong Kong.

Table 15.1 Samples of Cordyceps and Related Species Studied

Genus	Species	Collection place	Voucher
Ophiocordyceps	*Ophiocordyceps sinensis*	Hong Kong, China	T2973
		Hong Kong, China	T3399
		Hong Kong, China	T3400
Cordyceps	*Cordyceps gunnii*	Hong Kong, China	T2984
		Hong Kong, China	T3454
		Hong Kong, China	T3455
	Cordyceps militaris	Hong Kong, China	T3004
		Shenzhen, China	T3155
		Guangdong, China	T3181

15.2.2 Methods

15.2.2.1 *Total Genomic Preparation*

Spin column-based nucleic acid purification was used to obtain DNA samples and remove potential PCR inhibitors, including polysaccharides, protein, salt residues, etc. DNA was extracted using the Biomed Plant Genomic DNA/Tissue Extraction Kit (Biomed, Beijing, China) according to the manufacturer's instructions.

Equipment

- Centrifuge
- Heat block
- Scissors

Reagents

- Ethanol, 100%
- BioMed Tissue DNA Extraction Kit (Biomed, Beijing, China)
    - Lysis Buffer (AP1)
    - RNase A (100 mg/mL)

- Precipitation Buffer (AP2)
- Binding Buffer (AP3/E)
- Washing Buffer (WB)
- Elution Buffer (EB)

Procedures

1. Pre-warm the EB at 65°C before extraction starts.
2. Add 100% ethanol into AP3/E and WB according to the instructions on the bottles of AP3/E and WB, respectively.
3. Put 20 mg of sample and 400 μL of AP1 in a 1.5-mL micro-centrifuge tube. Cut the samples into small pieces using scissors.
4. Add 4 μL of RNase A (100 mg/mL), mix and incubate for 1 h at 65°C.
5. After incubation, add 130 μL of AP2 and mix well.
6. Incubate for 10 min on ice.
7. After incubation, centrifuge at 12,100 × g for 10 min.
8. Transfer the supernatant to a new 1.5-mL micro-centrifuge tube.
9. Add 1.5-fold volume of AP3/E and mix well.
10. Fit a binding column into a 2-mL collection tube.
11. Transfer the mixture in the tube into the binding column and centrifuge at 12,100 × g for 1 min.
12. Pour off the liquid in the collection tube and place back the binding column to the collection tube.
13. Add 500 μL of WB to the column and centrifuge at 12,100 × g for 30 s.
14. Pour off the liquid in the collection tube and place back the binding column to the collection tube.
15. Add 500 μL of WB and centrifuge at 12,100 × g for 30 s.
16. Pour off the liquid in the collection tube and place back the binding column to the collection tube.

17. Spin down at 12,100 × g for 2 min to completely remove the ethanol since residual WB left in the binding column will hinder the following steps.
18. Transfer the binding column to a new 1.5-mL Eppendorf tube.
19. Add 100 μL of pre-warmed EB and incubate for 5 min.
20. Elute the DNA by spinning down at 12,100 × g for 2 min.
21. DNA eluted is stored at –20°C.

15.2.2.2 *Primer Design*

As shown in Table 15.2, nucleotide sequences of the EF-1α region of *O. sinensis* and adulterants derived from *C. gunnii* and *C. militaris* were retrieved from GenBank, National Centre for Biotechnology Information (GenBank, NCBI) and the Medicinal Materials DNA Barcode Database (MMDBD) (Wong *et al.*, 2018). Nucleotide sequences obtained were aligned using biological sequence alignment software BioEdit (Ibis Therapeutics, Florida). Primers were designed targeting the EF-1α region for both internal control and species-specific primers using the OligoAnalyzer 3.1 (Integrated DNA technologies, Iowa). Sequences of primers are shown in Table 15.3 and Figure 15.2.

Table 15.2 DNA Sequence of EF-1α Region of Cordyceps and Related Species Retrieved from NCBI GenBank and MMDBD (Wong *et al.*, 2018)

Species	Accession number of NCBI			Sequence retrieved from MMDBD	
Ophiocordyceps sinensis	KJ364496.1	KJ364497.1	HM595936.1		
Cordyceps gunnii	AY489616.1	HM140636.1		T2984	T3454
Cordyceps militaris	XM 006665968.1	HM595940.1	DQ070019.1		

Table 15.3 Polymerase Chain Reaction (PCR) Primers Targeting EF-1α Region for Differentiation between Cordyceps and Related Species

Target	Primer name	Sequence (5′ to 3′)	Amplicon size (bp)
Internal control	EF-F1-b-DIG	CAA CTT CAT CAA GAA GGT CGG CT	246
	EF-R1-FITC	TTG TAC ACA TCC TGG AGG GG	
Ophiocordyceps sinensis	EF-CS-F1-Biotin	CGA CAA CAT GAT TGA TTC CTC CC	177
	EF-R1-FITC	TTG TAC ACA TCC TGG AGG GG	
Cordyceps gunnii	EF-CG-F1-Biotin	AAC ATG TTG GCC GCT TCC A	173
	EF-R1-FITC	TTG TAC ACA TCC TGG AGG GG	
Cordyceps militaris	EF-CM-F1-Biotin	ATG GTT CTG CCC ACC GAG	170
	EF-R1-FITC	TTG TAC ACA TCC TGG AGG GG	

15.2.2.3 *PCR Amplification*

Equipment

- Thermocycler

Reagents

- dNTPs, 2.5 mmol/L
- PCR buffer, 10×
  - 750 mM Tris-HCl, pH 8.8
  - 200 mM $(NH_4)_2SO_4$
  - 0.1% Tween 20
  - 15 mM $MgCl_2$
- *Taq* DNA polymerase, 5 U/μL
- Internal control forward primer (EF-F1-b-DIG), 10 μmol/L
- Internal control reverse primer (EF-R1-FITC), 10 μmol/L
- Species-specific forward primer, 10 μmol/L

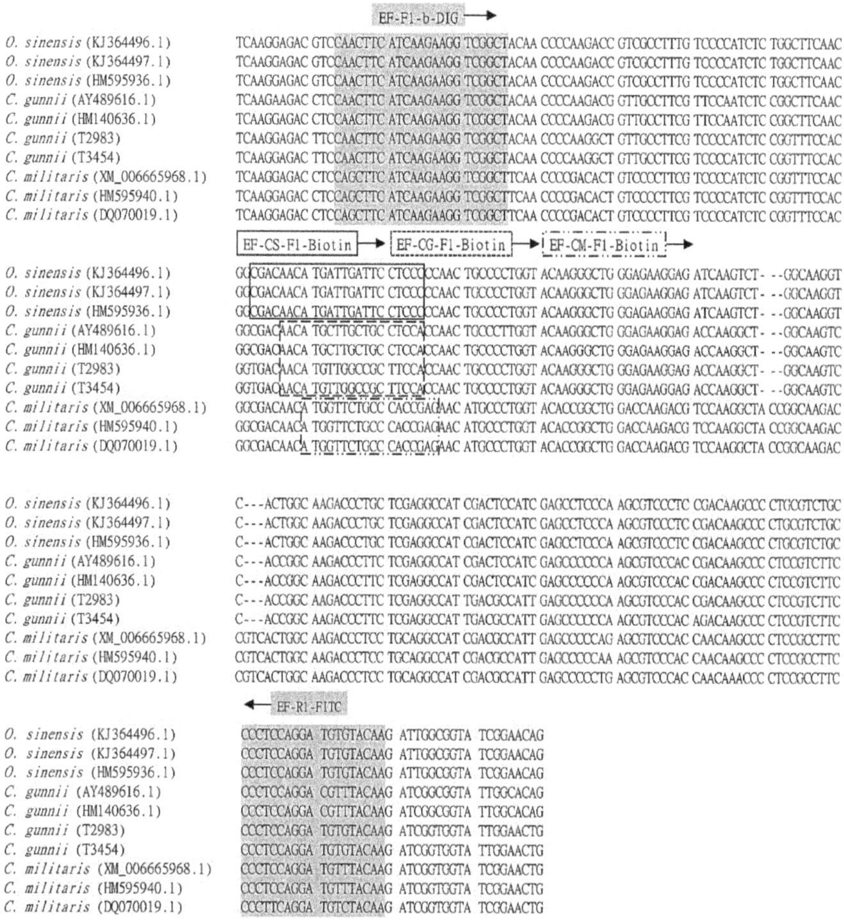

Fig. 15.2 Primer design based on sequence alignment of EF-1α region of *Ophiocordyceps sinensis*, *Cordyceps gunnii* and *C. militaris* for internal control and species-specific polymerase chain reaction (PCR) assays. The loci for internal control (EF-F1-b-DIG and EF-R1-FITC) are highlighted in grey. Species-specific primers (EF-CS-F1-Biotin, EF-CG-F1-Biotin and EF-CM-F1-Biotin) were designed and labelled, respectively. Arrows represent the direction of amplification.

Procedures

1. Prepare and mix the PCR reaction mixture on ice as follow:

Ingredient	Final volume per reaction	Final concentration
Taq buffer	2.5 μL	1×
dNTPs	2 μL	0.2 μM
Internal control forward primer (EF-F1-b-DIG)	0.5 μL	0.2 μM
Internal control reverse primer (EF-R1-FITC)	0.5 μL	0.2 μM
Species-specific forward primer	0.5 μL	0.2 μM
Template DNA	2 μL	
ddH_2O	16.6 μL	
Total	24.6 μL	

2. Perform a hot-start PCR reaction in a T-100 Thermo Cycler with an initial denaturation at 95°C for 5 min; then, add 0.4 μL of *Taq* polymerase into the reaction mixtures and perform the PCR reaction with PCR cycles consisting of 30 cycles of 15 s at 95°C, 15 s at 56°C and 30 s at 72°C, followed by a final extension at 72°C for 7 min.
3. PCR products are visualised in 3% agarose gel.

15.2.2.4 *LFD Testing*

Dual-labelled amplicons were detected with Milenia® HybriDetect 2T Dipstick from Milenia Biotec (Giessen, Hesse, Germany) according to the manufacturer's instructions.

Reagents

- HybriDetect 2T tool
  - HybriDetect 2T Dipsticks
  - HybriDetect 2T Assay Buffer

Procedures

1. Dilute 5 μL of PCR product with 95 μL of HybriDetect Assay Buffer in a new 1.5-mL micro-centrifuge tube.
2. Immerse the sample application area of the dipstick in the diluted PCR product.
3. Incubated the dipstick in an upright position for 5–15 min until a line is visible at the Dipstick-control site.

15.3 Result

15.3.1 PCR Amplification

As shown in Figure 15.3, clear amplification was shown with all nine samples representing the three species, *O. sinensis*, *C. gunnii* and *C. militaris*, in expected sizes (246 bp) using internal control primers EF-F1-b-DIG and EF-R1-FITC (Table 15.3). On the other hand, for species-specific amplification, only samples of target species were specifically amplified by their corresponding species-specific primers in expected sizes (Table 15.3)

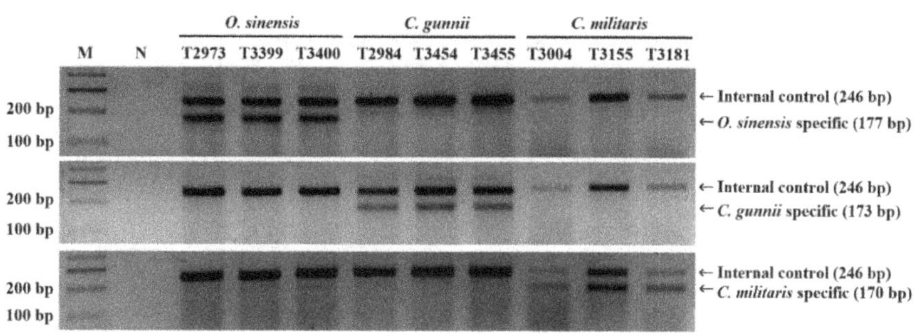

Fig. 15.3 Differentiation of Cordyceps by polymerase chain reaction (PCR) using a biotin-labelled species-specific primer. All samples from *Ophiocordyceps sinensis*, *Cordyceps gunnii* and *C. militaris* were detected in internal control (246 bp), while only corresponding species were detected in specific reactions (170–177 bp), respectively. PCR products were visualised by 3% agarose gel electrophoresis. PCR without DNA template was applied as the negative control (N). M represents 100 bp DNA size marker.

and no amplification was found for non-target species showing the specificity of each of the PCR assays.

15.3.2 Lateral Flow Dipstick

Apart from the gel electrophoresis, the result of the PCR amplification could also be observed visually using LFD. As shown in Figure 15.4, after immersion of the diluted PCR product and incubation, all dipsticks, including negative control, showed a signal at the Dipstick-control site. This represents the reaction was performed correctly. For the PCR-control site, all samples showed a signal at that position. This acts as an internal control for the reaction. For each of the species-specific reaction, only target species showed a signal at the species-specific site, showing the specificity of the PCR assay and the sensitivity of the LFD testing.

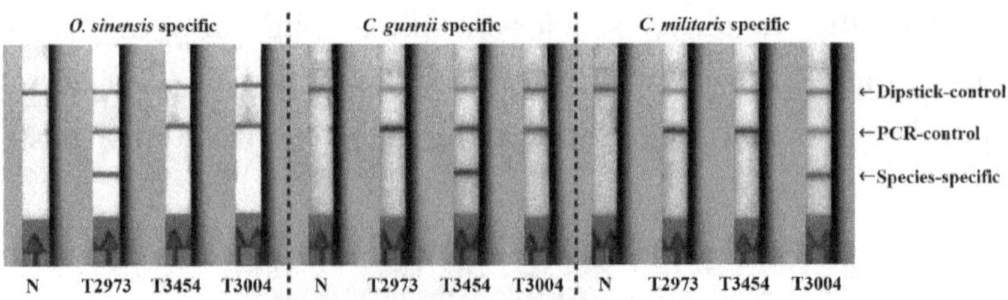

Fig. 15.4 Differentiation of Cordyceps by polymerase chain reaction (PCR) in combination with lateral flow dipstick (LFD). Labelled PCR products were detected using a HybriDetect 2T Dipstick. Primers for internal control: EF-F1-b-DIG and EF-R1-FITC; primers for specific reaction: biotin-labelled species-specific primers and FITC-labelled primer (EF-R1-FITC). PCR without DNA template was applied as the negative control (N).

15.4 Discussion

In this study, a species-specific PCR assay in combination with a LFD detection system was employed to differentiate *O. sinensis* from its common adulterant *C. gunnii* and *C. militaris*. Internal control was also included to avoid a false negative result due to DNA degradation or presence of PCR inhibitors. To our knowledge, this is the first developed LFD for the authentication of Chinese medicinal materials.

15.4.1 PCR Amplification

In this study, a PCR-based detection in combination of LFD was developed for rapid differentiation of *O. sinensis* and two common adulterants, *C. gunnii* and *C. militaris*. Species-specific primers targeting each of these three species and internal control primers were designed based on the EF-1α region (Table 15.3). As shown in Figure 15.2, internal control primers (EF-F1-b-DIG and EF-R1-FITC) were designed on section containing a minimum number of polymorphic sites, in which sequences of all three species have no nucleotide difference. This enables samples of all three species to be amplified by the internal control primers, to avoid a false negative result due to DNA amplifiability or the absence of DNA. On the other hand, for species-specific primers, all three forward primers (*O. sinensis*: EF-CS-F1-Biotin; *C. gunnii*: EF-CG-F1-Biotin; *C. militaris*: EF-CM-F1-Biotin) were designed to include the most polymorphic sites at the 3′ end (Figure 15.2). Only target species can bind with the corresponding forward primer, increasing the specificity of the PCR assay and allowing the differentiation of the concerned Cordyceps species. Furthermore, the PCR product of the species-specific amplification is designed to be ~70 bp smaller than that of the internal control amplification. This allows simple result analysis by the sizes of the PCR products.

15.4.2 Lateral Flow Dipstick

In this study, a HybriDetect 2T LFD system was employed for performing LFD testing. HybriDetect 2T LFD system has more than one testing site, allowing multiplexed lateral flow assay. Simultaneous detection of both internal control and species-specific reactions can be performed within the same dipstick in a single run. The presence of a PCR-control site (Figure 15.4) allows one to assess the DNA quality, avoiding the false negative result obtained in a species-specific reaction due to DNA template problems. On each dipstick, there are three testing sites, including (i) Dipstick-control site, (ii) PCR-control site and (iii) Species-specific site, which are fabricated with anti-rabbit antibody, anti-DIG antibody and biotin ligand, respectively. Each primer designed in this study has also been labelled. The forward internal control (EF-F1-b-DIG) was labelled with DIG and all three forward species-specific primers (*O. sinensis*: EF-CS-F1-Biotin; *C. gunnii*: EF-CG-F1-Biotin; *C. militaris*: EF-CM-F1-Biotin) were labelled with biotin. For the reverse primer (EF-R1-FITC), it was labelled with FITC. After successful PCR amplification, the internal control PCR product formed was tagged with both DIG and FITC while for species-specific PCR products, they were tagged with biotin and FITC.

As explained in Section 15.1, after being diluted by the HybriDetect 2T Assay Buffer, the PCR product placed on the sample application region of the dipstick ran along the dipstick due to capillary force. At the conjugate release region, the dried gold-labelled FITC-specific antibody was rehydrated and bound with the FITC-tag on the PCR product. As a result, complex gold particles were formed (internal control PCR product: gold particle-FITC-PCR product-DIG; species-specific PCR product:

gold particle-FITC-PCR product-biotin). When the liquid sample reached the testing region, fabricated with anti-DIG antibody, the PCR-control site only captured the complex gold particles of the internal control PCR product (gold particle-FITC-PCR product-DIG). On the other hand, fabricated with biotin ligand, the species-specific region only captured the complex gold particles of the species-specific PCR product (gold particle-FITC-PCR product-biotin). For a negative reaction with no products, non-bound complexed gold particles flowed through the other sites and were captured by the anti-rabbit antibody at the Dipstick-control site. When there was enough accumulation of complex gold particles, a signal would be developed and became visible at each region (Figure 15.4). Comparing to traditional gel electrophoresis, LFD testing, along with its result analysis, is comparatively simple and does not need specific equipment.

15.4.3 Differentiation of Cordyceps

The PCR assay developed in this study is able to differentiate Cordyceps from its adulterants and result present in both the simple and easy LFD method, and traditional gel electrophoresis also shows the specificity of the PCR assay. Other than *C. gunnii* and *C. militaris*, *Metacordyceps liangshanensis*, *C. cicadae* and *O. nutans* are other commonly found adulterants of Cordyceps (Liu, Wang, Gao, Han & Xiang, 2017). By examining their nucleotide sequences of the EF-1α region (Table 15.4), high nucleotide sequence similarity was found among sequences of internal control primers (EF-F1-b-DIG and EF-R1-FITC) and those of the Cordyceps, while several nucleotide differences were found between the sequence of the species-specific primer (EF-CS-F1-Biotin) targeting *O. sinensis* and those of the common adulterants. This shows that the PCR

Table 15.4 Sequence Alignment of the Primers Used and the Binding Sites of the Targeted Species

Primer	NCBI accession number	Species	Sequence alignment
EF-F1-b-DIG	—	—	CAACTTCATCAAGAAGGTCGGCT
(Internal control)	HM595936.1	*O. sinensis*	....
	HM140636.1	*C. gunnii*	....
	HM595940.1	*C. militaris*	..G....................
	EF468756.1	*M. liangshanensis*	....
	EF468755.1	*M. liangshanensis*	....
	HQ881017.1.	*C. cicadae*	....
	AB968589.1	*O. nutans*	G........T...........G.
	DQ522333.1	*O. nutans*	G......................
EF-R1-FITC	—	—	CCCCTCCAGGATGTGTACAA
(Internal control)	HM595936.1	*O. sinensis*	....
	HM140636.1	*C. gunnii*	...........C..T.....
	HM595940.1	*C. militaris*	..............T.....
	EF468756.1	*M. liangshanensis*	..............C.....
	EF468755.1	*M. liangshanensis*	..............C.....
	HQ881017.1.	*C. cicadae*	.....T........C.....
	AB968589.1	*O. nutans*	..............T.....
	DQ522333.1	*O. nutans*	..............C.....
EF-CS-F1-Biotin (Target: *O. sinensis*)	—	—	CGACAACATGATTGATTCCTCCC
	HM595936.1	*O. sinensis*	....
	HM140636.1	*C. gunnii*	..........C...C.G.....A
	HM595940.1	*C. militaris*	..........G..CTGC..A..G
	EF468756.1	*M. liangshanensis*	T.........C...CCG.....A
	EF468755.1	*M. liangshanensis*	T.........C...CCG.....A
	HQ881017.1.	*C. cicadae*	..........C..ACGG.....A
	AB968589.1	*O. nutans*	...T......C.C.CCC.....A
	DQ522333.1	*O. nutans*	...T......C..ACCG.....A

assay, in combination of LFD, is likely able to differentiate *O. sinensis* from *M. liangshanensis*, *C. cicadae* and *O. nutans* as well.

15.4.4 Pros and Cons of LFD Approach

Comparing to traditional gel electrophoresis or hybridisation-based detection like fluorescent probe, LFD is more time-saving, which only needs 5–15 min and is less labour intensive, mostly a one-step procedure, for the analysis of the nucleic acid amplification product. LFD approach does not require equipment such as gel electrophoresis power supply and a gel tank. It is portable and can be carried easily outside the laboratory. Moreover, the result analysis of LFD testing is simple, which can be interpreted by a layman. On the other hand, more effort is required for the design and optimisation of primers to avoid a possible false positive. Therefore, the PCR assay, in combination of LFD, is more appropriate for on-site application and rapid screening.

15.5 Conclusion

As a rapid authentication method, LFD has been widely applied on clinic, food and environmental safety. In this chapter, we demonstrate that PCR, coupled with the LFD system, can differentiate Cordyceps (*O. sinensis*), its common adulterants, *C. gunnii* and *C. militaris*. Together with the control reaction, authentication can be achieved with high accuracy.

Acknowledgement

We thank Dr. Yuk-Lau Wong for the technical assistance and valuable suggestions.

References

Chen, Y., Wang, N., Zhou, H., & Qu, L. (2002). Differentiation of medicinal Cordyceps species by rDNA ITS sequence analysis. *Planta Med, 68*, 635–639.

Dong, C., Guo, S., Wang, W., & Liu, X. (2015). Cordyceps industry in China. *Mycology, 6*, 121–129.

Fung, J. C., Yue, G. G., Fung, K. P., Ma, X., Yao, X. Q., & Ko, W. H. (2011). *Cordyceps militaris* extract stimulates Cl(-) secretion across human bronchial epithelia by both Ca(2+)(-) and cAMP-dependent pathways. *J Ethnopharmacol, 138*, 201–211.

Hu, H., Xiao, L., Zheng, B., Wei, X., Ellis, A., & Liu, Y. M. (2015). Identification of chemical markers in *Cordyceps sinensis* by HPLC-MS/MS. *Anal Bioanal Chem, 407*, 8059–8066.

Jiang, Y., Wong, J. H., Fu, M., Ng, T. B., Liu, Z. K., Wang, C. R., N. Li, W. T. Qiao, T. Y. Wen, & Liu, F. (2011). Isolation of adenosine, iso-sinensetin and dimethylguanosine with antioxidant and HIV-1 protease inhibiting activities from fruiting bodies of *Cordyceps militaris*. *Phytomedicine, 18*, 189–193.

Lam, K. Y., Chan, G. K., Xin, G. Z., Xu, H., Ku, C. F., Chen, J. P., Yao, P., Lin, H. Q., Dong, T. T. X., & Tsim, K. W. (2015). Authentication of *Cordyceps sinensis* by DNA analyses: Comparison of ITS sequence analysis and RAPD-derived molecular markers. *Molecules, 20*, 22454–22462.

Lee, J. H., Seo, H. S., Kwon, J. H., Kim, H. T., Kwon, K. C., Sim, S. J., Cha, Y. J., & Lee, J. (2015). Multiplex diagnosis of viral infectious diseases (AIDS, hepatitis C, and hepatitis A) based on point of care lateral flow assay using engineered proteinticles. *Biosens Bioelectron, 69*, 213–225.

Lee, K. W. L., Wong, C. K., Kong, S. K., Leung, K. N., & Lam, C. W. K. (2006). Immunomodulatory activities of HERBSnSENSES Cordyceps — in vitro and in vivo studies. *Immunopharmacol Immunotoxicol, 28*, 341–360.

Li, K., Li, Q., Yuan, Y., Chen, J. Y., Huang, L. Q., & Liu, Z. G. (2011). Identification and detection of *Cordyceps sinensis* with LAMP. *Chin Tradit Herbal Drugs, 42*(8), 1605–1608.

Liu, Y., Wang, X., Gao, Z., Han, J., & Xiang, L. (2017). Detection of *Ophiocordyceps sinensis* and its common adulterates using species-specific primers. *Front Microbiol, 8*, 1179.

Panda, A. K., & Swain, K. C. (2011). Traditional uses and medicinal potential of *Cordyceps sinensis* of Sikkim. *J Ayurveda Integr Med, 2*, 9–13.

Shrestha, B., Zhang, W., Zhang, Y., & Liu, X. (2010). What is the Chinese caterpillar fungus *Ophiocordyceps sinensis* (Ophiocordycipitaceae)? *Mycology, 1*, 228–236.

Sirisidthi, K., Kosai, P., & Jiraungkoorskul, W. (2015). Antihyperglycemic activity of *Ophiocordyceps sinensis*: A review. *Indian J Agric Res, 49*, 400–406.

Tang, D., Sauceda, J. C., Lin, Z., Ott, S., Basova, E., Goryacheva, I., Lin, J., Niessner, R., & Knopp, D. (2009). Magnetic nanogold microspheres-based lateral-flow immunodipstick for rapid detection of aflatoxin B2 in food. *Biosens Bioelectron, 25*, 514–518.

Trantakis, I. A., Spaniolas, S., Kalaitzis, P., Ioannou, P. C., Tucker, G. A., & Christopoulos, T. K. (2012). Dipstick test for DNA-based food authentication. Application to coffee authenticity assessment. *J Agric Food Chem, 60*, 713–717.

Vaagt, F., Hasse, I., & Fischer, M. (2013). Loop-mediated isothermal amplification (LAMP)-based method for rapid mushroom species identification. *J Agric Food Chem, 61*, 1833–1840.

Wang, B., Lee, C. P., Chen, Z., Yu, H. M., & Duh, P. (2012). Comparison of the hepatoprotective activity between cultured *Cordyceps militaris* and natural *Cordyceps sinensis*. *J Funct Foods, 4*, 489–495.

Weng, X., Gaur, G., & Neethirajan, S. (2016). Rapid detection of food allergens by microfluidics ELISA-based optical sensor. *Biosensors, 6*, 24.

Wong, T. H., But, G. W., Wu, H. Y., Tsang, S. S., Lau, D. T., & Shaw, P. C. (2018). Medicinal Materials DNA Barcode Database (MMDBD) version 1.5-one-stop solution for storage, BLAST, alignment and primer design. *Database, 2018*, bay112.

Xiang, L., Song, J., Xin, T., Zhu, Y., Shi, L., Xu, X., Pang, X., Yao, H., Li, W., & Chen, S. (2013). DNA barcoding the commercial Chinese caterpillar fungus. *FEMS Microbiol Lett, 347*, 156–162.

Zhang, B., Nan, T. G., Xin, J., Zhan, Z. L., Kang, L. P., Yuan, Y., Wang, B. M., & Huang, L. Q. (2019). Development of a colloidal gold-based lateral flow dipstick immunoassay for rapid detection of chlorogenic acid and luteoloside in Flos Lonicerae Japonicae. *J Pharm Biomed Anal, 170*, 83–88.

Zhang, J., Wang, P., Wei, X, Li, L., Cheng, H., Wu, Y., Zeng, W., Yu, H., & Chen, Y. (2015). A metabolomics approach for authentication of *Ophiocordyceps sinensis* by liquid chromatography coupled with quadrupole time-of-flight mass spectrometry. *Food Res Int, 76*, 489–497.

Chapter 16

Barcoding High-Resolutions Melting Analysis

Suchada Sukrong, Kannika Thongkhao,
Chayapol Tungphatthong & Thatree Phadungcharoen

16.1 Introduction

DNA barcoding involves sequencing a short region of DNA as a tool for species identification. It is useful in plant identification, biodiversity assessment and conservation, adulteration detection and medicinal materials authentication. The DNA barcoding technique was first described in 2003 by Herbert and collaborators for the identification of animals (Hebert, Cywinska, Ball & Dewaard, 2003). Subsequently, the technique has been widely used and applied to many natural materials including plants. Maturase K (*mat*K), the large subunit of the ribulose-1,5-bisphosphate carboxylase/oxygenase (*rbc*L), the *psb*A-*trn*H intergenic spacer and the nuclear internal transcribed spacer (ITS) are the most commonly used DNA barcodes in plants (Mishra, Kumar, Nagireddy, Shukla & Sundaresan, 2017). These loci have also proved valuable to distinguish closely related species.

However, although the DNA barcoding technique is proven to be very useful for species identification, it has limitations, such as being time consuming and costly because of the requirements for sequencing equipment, for use in routine work. This leads us to search for a fast, reliable and inexpensive method. Recently, the DNA barcoding technique has been applied in combination with a high-resolution melting analysis called Barcoding High-Resolutions Melting (Bar-HRM) (Thongkhao, Tungphatthong, Phadungcharoen & Sukrong, 2020; Tungphatthong *et al.*, 2018).

The Bar-HRM is a sequencing free method using fluorescent dye for the detection of double-stranded DNA (dsDNA) dissociation in real-time polymerase chain reaction (PCR). Increasing temperature during the process leads to the dissociation of dsDNA into single-stranded DNA (ssDNA), and the melting temperature (T_m) is measured. The direct T_m can discriminate small sequence differences in PCR-amplified amplicons according to their composition, length and GC content. The recent advancement of the technique includes the precision of the instruments and development of saturating DNA dyes, which increase the resolution and permit the use of high-resolutions melting (HRM) for genotyping (Ganopoulos & Tsaftaris, 2011) and for quantification of adulterants (Mader, Ruzicka, Schmiderer & Novak, 2011).

HRM analysis begins after PCR amplification. The amplicon is gradually heated from around 60°C to approximately 90°C; the gradual denaturation resulting from incremental heating that produces a characteristic melting profile. When the dsDNA dissociates into ssDNA, the intercalating dye is released and fluoresces at a low level. The change in fluorescence is plotted against the temperature, generating a melting curve characteristic of the amplicon. Figure 16.1 shows the melting curves obtained for the assayed species, namely A, B and C. The melting curve analysis revealed peaks with very close T_m, though three groups can be seen: (i) at 74.3°C for species A; (ii) at 75.0°C for species B and (iii) at 75.8°C for species C. However, because of the close melting temperatures and similarity of profiles, it is not possible to clearly differentiate them by the conventional melting curve analysis.

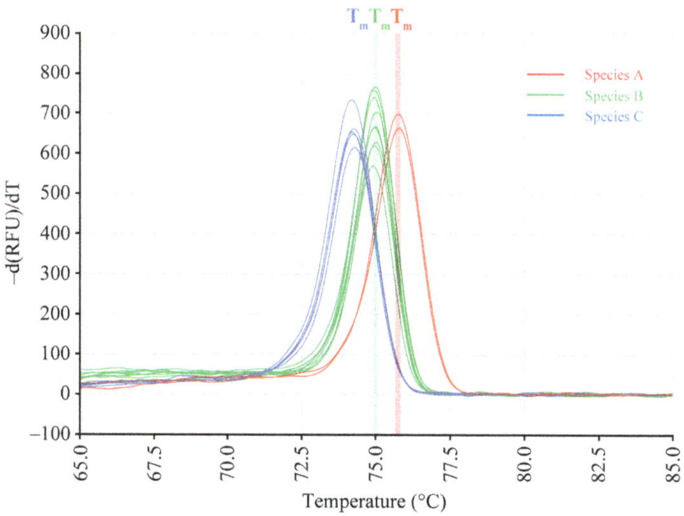

Fig. 16.1 The conventional melting curves of the amplicons from species A, B and C.

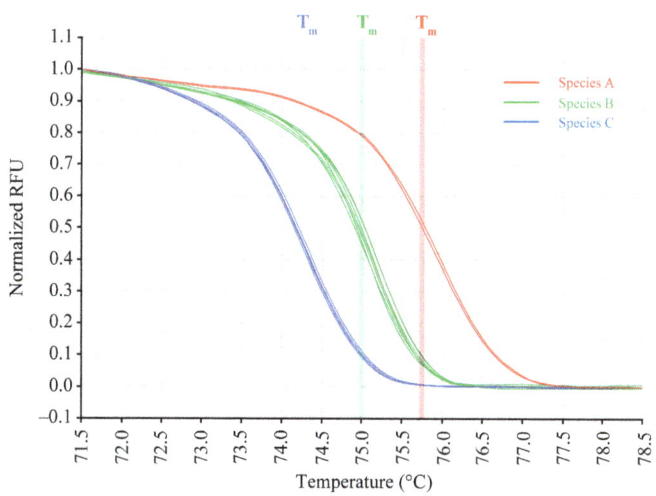

Fig. 16.2 The normalised high-resolutions melting (HRM) curves.

HRM was applied as a tool to discriminate closely related taxa and is displayed as normalised melt and difference curves in Figures 16.2 and 16.3, respectively. As can be seen, the specimens were divided into three distinct clusters in good agreement with the results of conventional melting curve analysis. HRM is sensi-

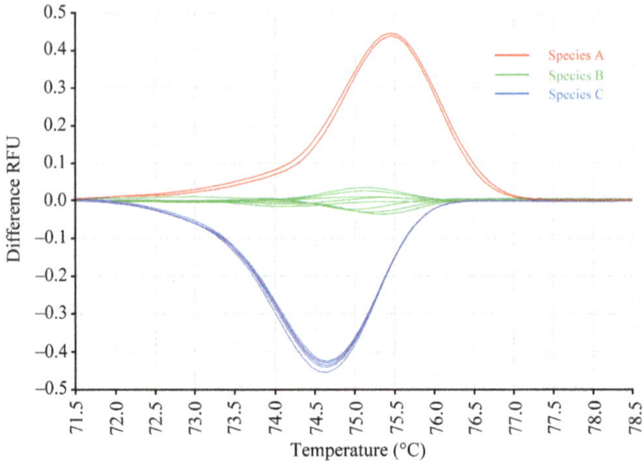

Fig. 16.3 Difference in high-resolutions melting (HRM) curves derived from the normalisation data.

tive enough to allow the detection of a single base change between otherwise identical nucleotide sequences (Tungphatthong *et al*., 2018).

16.2 Materials and Methods

16.2.1 Introduction to Plant Materials

Melientha suavis Pierre (Pak Wan Pa), *Sauropus androgynus* (L.) Merr (Pak Wan Baan) and *Urobotrya siamensis* Hiepko (Pak Wan Mao) share the vernacular name in Thai — 'Phak Wan'. *M. suavis* and *S. androgynus* are edible plants, whereas *U. siamensis* is a poisonous species (Figure 16.4). Shoots and young leaves of *M. suavis* and *S. androgynus* have a sweet taste and high nutrient value (Julapak, Mankeb, Mekhora & Chulilung, 2016). Presently, demand for *M. suavis* and *S. androgynus* is increasing, and their price is continuously rising. This results in increasing farming areas for the production of both valuable vegetables.

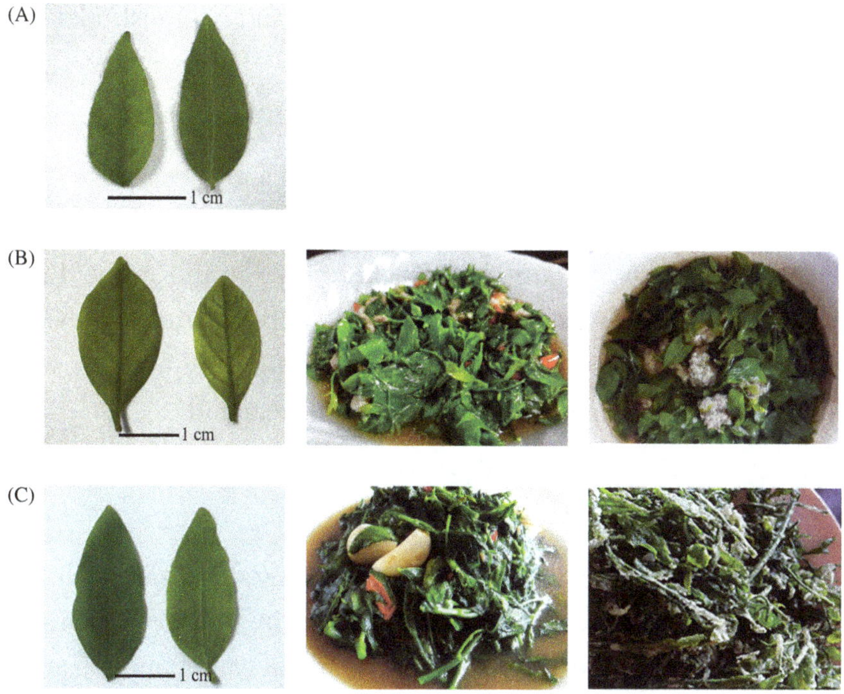

Fig. 16.4 Plants used in this study and dishes made from their leaves. (A) *Urobotrya siamensis*, (B) *Melientha suavis* and (C) *Sauropus androgynus*.

Confusion between *M. suavis* and the poisonous *U. siamensis* species caused an outbreak of *U. siamensis*–related death in 2005 (Tourdjman *et al.*, 2009). Deaths were also reported in 2007 in the rural areas of Thailand where people gathered *U. siamensis* shoots and consumed them due to misidentification (http://webdb.dmsc.moph.go.th/ifc_toxic/, accessed on 24 January 2021). Contamination of the poisonous species of *U. siamensis* in crop fields is possible because of similar appearances, and the poisonous species is commonly found in the same habitat as that of the edible species (Hiepko, 1979). Therefore, it is difficult for consumers, including farmers, who lack experience in species identification to differentiate them. Unintentional spread of poisonous plants to crop fields or markets would have detrimental effects and we must take this safety concern seriously.

16.2.2 Plant Samples

Twenty-two authenticated samples, *U. siamensis* ($n = 8$), *M. suavis* ($n = 7$) and *S. androgynus* ($n = 7$), were used in the study (Table 16.1). All voucher specimens were stored at the Museum of Natural Medicine, Chulalongkorn University. Thirteen unknown samples were received from local nurseries in Thailand.

16.2.3 Genomic DNA Extraction

Young leaves of the specimens were collected, frozen with liquid nitrogen and ground into fine powder by mortar and pestle. Genomic DNA was extracted from 100 mg of each sample using a DNeasy™ Plant Mini Kit (Qiagen, Germany) following the manufacturer's instructions.

After DNA extraction, genomic DNA was purified using a GENECLEAN® Kit (MP Biomedicals, Irvine, CA, USA). DNA quality and quantity were determined by agarose gel electrophoresis. All DNA samples were kept at –20°C for further analysis.

Equipment

- Microcentrifuge
- Heating block
- Vortex mixer

Reagents

- Ethanol (100%)
- Deionised water
- GENECLEAN® II KIT
- 6 M NaI solutions

Table 16.1 Authentic Plants and Tested Samples

Plant species	Voucher No.	Place of collection (province)	Accession No.			
			*rbc*L	*mat*K	ITS2	*psb*A-*trn*H
Authentic species						
Urobotrya siamensis Hiepko	SS568	Bangkok	LC467714	LC467717	LC471213	LC473134
	SS569	Saraburi	—	—	—	—
	SS606	Loei	—	—	—	—
	SS607	Prachinburi	—	—	—	—
	SS608	Buriram	—	—	—	—
	SS609	Bangkok	—	—	—	—
	SS610	Saraburi	—	—	—	—
	SS615	Loei	—	—	—	—
Melientha suavis Pierre	SS558	Bangkok	LC467713	LC467716	LC471212	LC473133
	SS559	Saraburi	—	—	—	—
	SS560	Prachinburi	—	—	—	—
	SS561	Nakhon Ratchasima	—	—	—	—
	SS562	Buriram	—	—	—	—
	SS611	Bangkok	—	—	—	—
	SS612	Loei	—	—	—	—
Sauropus androgynus (L.) Merr.	SS553	Bangkok	LC466956	LC467715	LC471211	LC473132
	SS554	Prachinburi	—	—	—	—

(*Continued*)

Table 16.1 (*Continued*)

Plant species	Voucher No.	Place of collection (province)	Accession No.			
			*rbc*L	*mat*K	ITS2	*psb*A-*trn*H
	SS555	Bangkok	—	—	—	—
	SS556	Nonthaburi	—	—	—	—
	SS557	Loei	—	—	—	—
	SS613	Nakhon Si Thammarat	—	—	—	—
	SS614	Songkla	—	—	—	—
Unknown samples			—	—	—	—
Phak-Wan 1	TS1	Bangkok	—	—	—	—
Phak-Wan 2	TS2	Prachinburi	—	—	—	—
Phak-Wan 3	TS3	Bangkok	—	—	—	—
Phak-Wan 4	TS4	Loei	—	—	—	—
Phak-Wan 5	TS5	Bangkok	—	—	—	—
Phak-Wan 6	TS6	Prachinburi	—	—	—	—
Phak-Wan 7	TS7	Prachinburi	—	—	—	—
Phak-Wan 8	TS8	Prachinburi	—	—	—	—
Phak-Wan 9	TS9	Buriram	—	—	—	—
Phak-Wan 10	TS10	Nakhon Ratchasima	—	—	—	—
Phak-Wan 11	TS11	Nakhon Ratchasima	—	—	—	—
Phak-Wan 12	TS12	Tak	—	—	—	—
Phak-Wan 13	TS13	Buriram	—	—	—	—

- GLASSMILK® beads
- NEW Wash concentrate solution
- TBE Modifier solution

Procedures

1. Measure the volume of the extracted genomic DNA.
2. Add a threefold volume of NaI solution to the DNA and mix well by pipetting.
3. Calculate the amount of GLASSMILK® needed according to the manufacturer's instructions.
4. Resuspend GLASSMILK® by vortexing for 1 min and mix with DNA/NaI solution.
5. Incubate at room temperature for 5 min and mix well.
6. Pellet the GLASSMILK® with the bound DNA and discard the supernatant.
7. Add 500 μL prepared NEW Wash and resuspend.
8. Centrifuge at 12,100 ×g for 5 s and discard supernatant.
9. Repeat Steps 7 and 8.
10. Dry the pellet to remove residual ethanol.
11. Add onefold volume of TE or water equal to the amount of GLASSMILK® added.
12. Resuspend pellet to mix and elute DNA.
13. Centrifuge at 12,100 ×g for 30 s and remove supernatant containing DNA.
14. Store the purified genomic DNA at –20°C for further analysis.

16.2.4 Amplification of DNA Barcoding Regions and Sequence Analysis

Four core DNA barcode regions, *rbc*L, *mat*K, ITS2 and *psb*A-*trn*H, were assessed by PCR. The DNA barcode regions were amplified by universal primers (Table 16.2).

Table 16.2 Primers Used for DNA Barcode Generation, Sequencing and Barcoding High-Resolutions Melting Analysis

Barcode region	Primer name	Primer sequence (5′ to 3′)	Reference
*rbc*L	*rbc*L_aF	ATGTCACCACAAACAGAGACTAAAGC	Levin *et al*., 2003
	*rbc*L_aR	GTAAAATCAAGTCCACCR(G/A)CG	Kress *et al*., 2009
*mat*K	*mat*K_xF	TAATTTACGATCAATTCATTC	Ford *et al*., 2009
	*mat*K-MALPR1	ACAAGAAAGTCGAAGTAT	Dunning & Savolainen, 2010
	UroF	CTTCGCATTTACGATCAACAT	This study
	UroR	CTAACATAATGCATGAAAGGATC	This study
*trn*H-*psb*A	*psb*A-*trn*HF	GTTATGCATGAACGTAATGCTC	Sang, Crawford & Stuessy, 1997
	*psb*A-*trn*HR	CGCGCATGGTGGATTCACAAATC	Sang *et al*., 1994
ITS	ITS1	TCCGTAGGTGAACCTGCGG	White, Bruns, Lee & Taylor, 1990
	ITS4	TCCTCCGCTTATTGATATGC	White *et al*., 1990
ITS2	ITS_S2F	ATGCGATACTTGGTGTGAAT	Chen *et al*., 2010
	ITS_S3R	GACGCTTCTCCAGACTACAAT	Chen *et al*., 2010

Equipment

- PCR Thermocycler (T100 Thermal Cycler, Bio-Rad Hercules, CA, USA)

Reagents

- *Taq* polymerase (Platinum, Invitrogen, Waltham, MA, USA)
- dNTPs, 10 mM
- $MgCl_2$, 50 mM
- Forward and reverse primer, 10 mM each
- PCR buffer, 10×
- Deionised water

Procedures

PCR amplification was performed in 25 μL of reaction mixture consisting of 1× PCR buffer with 1.5 mM $MgCl_2$, 0.2 mM dNTPs mix, 0.2 mM each of the forward and reverse primer, 0.5 U of *Taq* polymerase and 30 ng of genomic DNA. PCR was carried out in a T100 Thermal Cycler (Bio-Rad) using cycling conditions of 94°C for 4 min; followed by 30 cycles of 94°C for 30 s, 57°C for 30 s and 72°C for 1 min (for *mat*K and *rbc*L) or 45 s (for ITS2 and *psb*A-*trn*H); and a final extension at 72°C for 10 min. PCR amplification was observed by agarose gel electrophoresis. PCR amplicons were subsequently sequenced bidirectionally by Sanger sequencing. Nucleotide sequences were edited by BioEdit software version 7.2.6. The corrected sequences were deposited to GenBank (Table 16.1), National Centre for Biotechnology Information (NCBI).

16.2.5 Bar-HRM Analysis by Real-Time PCR

16.2.5.1 *Bar-HRM Primer Design*

The chloroplast *mat*K gene was selected as a target for the Bar-HRM assay to distinguish the three plant species. The forward and reverse primers were located on the conserved regions of *M. suavis*, *S. androgynus* and *U. siamensis* flanking a 145 bp amplicon from the *mat*K gene (Figure 16.5).

16.2.5.2 *Bar-HRM Assay*

Equipment

- Real-time PCR Thermocycler, CFX96™ Real-time System (Bio-Rad)

Reagents

- Forward and reverse primer, 10 μM each
- SsoFast™ EvaGreen® Supermix (Bio-Rad), 2×
- Deionised water

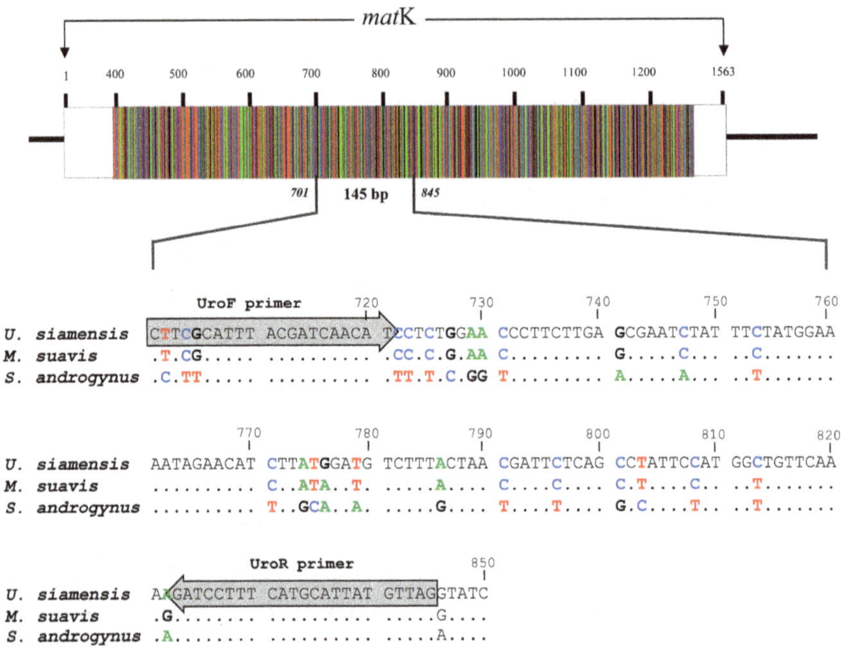

Fig. 16.5 The alignment of the *mat*K target region of the three plant species for barcoding high-resolutions melting (Bar-HRM) analysis. Grey arrows show the directions of annealing sites for forward (UroF) and reverse (UroR) primers. The amplification target is 145 bp. Nucleotide variable sites are indicated. The numbers indicate the positions according to the *mat*K gene.

Procedures

Real-time PCR was performed on a CFX96™ real-time PCR machine. The amplification reaction was carried out in 10 μL containing 1× SsoFast™ EvaGreen® Supermix (Bio-Rad), 0.5 μM forward primer (UroF: 5′-CTT CGC ATT TAC GAT CAA CAT-3′) and reverse primer (UroR: 5′-CTA ACA TAA TGC ATG AAA GGA TC-3′) and 10 ng of genomic DNA. The real-time PCR conditions consisted of an initial denaturing step at 95°C for 1 min, followed by 39 cycles of 95°C for 15 s (denaturation), 63°C for 20 s (annealing) and 72°C for 20 s (extension). Fluorescence data were collected during the extension step. Subsequently, the

PCR amplicons were denatured for HRM analysis at 95°C for 1 min and reannealed at 60°C for 1 min to form random DNA duplexes. Temperature was then increased from 60°C to 95°C at 0.1°C increments, and the fluorescence intensity from each individual increasing step was measured to generate the melting curves. Melting curves were analysed using CFX Manager™ software (version 3.1 upgrade) and Precision Melt Analysis™ software (version 3.1 upgrade). Normalised and differential melting curves were plotted. *M. suavis* was set as the reference species. All reactions were performed in triplicate. Bar-HRM analysis sensitivity was analysed by using a *U. siamensis* genomic DNA template with different amounts at 10, 1, 0.1 and 0.01 ng.

16.2.6 Detection of Plant Samples

To test the unknown species from local nurseries, genomic DNA of 13 unknown plants was extracted. Genomic DNA of all samples was subsequently examined by Bar-HRM analysis. Real-time PCR amplification and HRM analysis were applied as described earlier to identify the characteristic T_m. All real-time PCR was performed in triplicate. Melting, normalised and differential melting curves were analysed and plotted against temperature using CFX Manager™ software (version 3.1 upgrade) and Precision Melt Analysis™ software (version 3.1 upgrade). *M. suavis* was set as the reference species.

16.3 Results

16.3.1 Generation of Core DNA Barcodes

Core DNA barcodes, *rbc*L, *mat*K, ITS2 and *psb*A-*trn*H, were established from 22 specimens representing the three

Table 16.3 Sequence Characteristics of the Four DNA Barcodes from *Melienthasuavis, Sauropus androgynus* and *Urobotrya siamensis*

	*rbc*L	*mat*K	ITS2	*psb*A-*trn*H
Length (bp)	542–554	830–920	470–478	337–394
Number of variations (bp)	42	189	129	141
Nucleotide variation (%)	7.58	20.54	25.39	27.81

authentic species, namely, *M. suavis*, *S. androgynus* and *U. siamensis*. DNA barcode regions of each species were aligned, and the result revealed differences in the length of the amplicons. The amplicons of the *rbc*L, *mat*K, ITS2 and *psb*A-*trn*H regions were 542–554, 830–920, 470–478 and 337–394 bp, respectively (Table 16.3). Nucleotide variation and insertion–deletions (indels) were found in all barcode regions. *rbc*L showed the lowest sequence variation, followed by *mat*K, ITS2 and *psb*A-*trn*H. Identical nucleotide sequences were observed from the same species. Therefore, a DNA sequence from each DNA barcode was submitted to GenBank (refer to accession numbers in Table 16.1).

16.3.2 Differentiation of Edible Plants from Poisonous Plants

The plastidial *mat*K gene was selected as the DNA-targeted region for the differentiation of edible plants, *M. suavis* and *S. androgynus,* from the poisonous plant *U. siamensis*. Positive amplification of the *mat*K primer pair produced an amplicon of 145 bp in length with 26 variable sites (Figure 16.5). The melting profiles of the three plant species were clearly separated into three different categories, as illustrated by melting, normalised and difference plots (Figure 16.6). The T_m values for *M. suavis, S. androgynus*

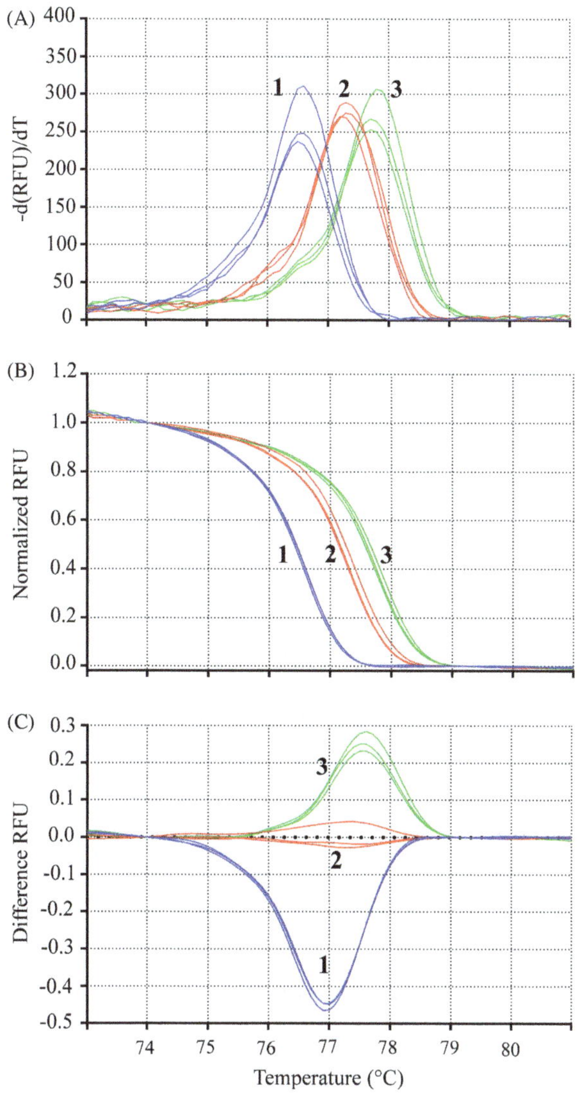

Fig. 16.6 (A) Conventional melting, (B) normalised curves and (C) difference curves obtained by high-resolutions melting (HRM) analysis targeting the *mat*K gene of (1) *Sauropus androgynus*, (2) *Melientha suavis* and (3) *Urobotrya siamensis*.

and *U. siamensis* were 77.47 ± 0.00°C, 76.80 ± 0.06°C and 77.94 ± 0.06°C, respectively, with a confidence level of >99% confidence level (Table 16.4).

Table 16.4 Bar-HRM Analysis of *Sauropus androgynus*, *Melientha suavis* and *Urobotrya siamensis*

		HRM analysis		
Species	**C_t value ± SD**	**T_m (°C) ± SD**	**Cluster**	**Level of confidence (%) ± SD**
S. androgynus	19.44 ± 0.15	76.80 ± 0.00	1	99.13 ± 0.15
M. suavis	13.67 ± 0.24	77.47 ± 0.06	2	99.23 ± 0.15
U. siamensis	16.43 ± 0.58	77.94 ± 0.06	3	99.73 ± 0.06

16.3.3 Specificity and Sensitivity

This primer for amplifying a small *mat*K region of 145 bp was specifically designed to differentiate *U. siamensis* from the other two species. Bar-HRM analysis sensitivity was analysed by using a *U. siamensis* genomic DNA template at different amounts with 10, 1, 0.1 and 0.01 ng (Figure 16.7). Similar melting profiles were found in conditions with different amounts of template DNA (Figure 16.7A). The lowest concentration of the DNA template that the Bar-HRM method was capable to amplify was 0.01 ng. Conventional PCR was performed to compare the sensitivity of PCR and Bar-HRM methods using the same primers. From the result, the PCR product was detected at 0.1 ng of the DNA template, which is 10 times lower than that of the Bar-HRM method (Figure 16.7B).

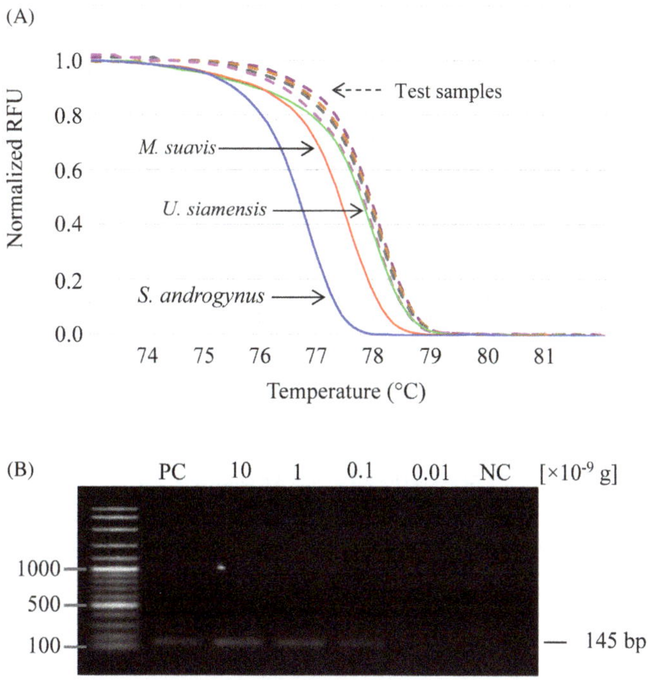

Fig. 16.7 Sensitivity of barcoding high-resolutions melting (Bar-HRM) analysis for the detection of *Urobotrya siamensis*. (A) Normalised curves of *U. siamensis* DNA at various amounts at 10, 1, 0.1 and 0.01 ng (dash lines) compared to authentic samples and (B) 2% agarose gel electrophoresis revealed 145 bp amplicon from different DNA template concentrations. PC and NC represent positive and negative control, respectively. Lane M: 100 bp DNA size marker.

16.3.4 Detection of Unknown Samples

Thirteen unknown samples were obtained from local nurseries, and the expected species as claimed by farmers were recorded (Table 16.5). Three distinct plant groups were separated by Bar-HRM analysis (Figure 16.8). Four samples (TS1, TS2, TS3 and TS4) exhibited T_m values of 76.80°C, and the species were

Table 16.5 List of Plant Samples from Local Nurseries in Thailand Tested by Bar-HRM Analysis

Tested samples	T_m (°C) ± SD	Claimed species	Detected species
TS 1	76.80 ± 0.00	*S. androgynus*	*S. androgynus*
TS 2	76.80 ± 0.00	*S. androgynus*	*S. androgynus*
TS 3	76.80 ± 0.00	*S. androgynus*	*S. androgynus*
TS 4	76.80 ± 0.00	*S. androgynus*	*S. androgynus*
TS 5	77.50 ± 0.05	*M. suavis*	*M. suavis*
TS 6	77.50 ± 0.06	*M. suavis*	*M. suavis*
TS 7	77.50 ± 0.00	*M. suavis*	*M. suavis*
TS 8	77.50 ± 0.00	*M. suavis*	*M. suavis*
TS 9	77.50 ± 0.05	*M. suavis*	*M. suavis*
TS 10	77.60 ± 0.05	*M. suavis*	*M. suavis*
TS 11	77.50 ± 0.00	*M. suavis*	*M. suavis*
TS 12	77.50 ± 0.05	*M. suavis*	*M. suavis*
TS 13	77.50 ± 0.01	*U. siamensis*	*M. suavis*

identified to be *S. androgynus*. T_m values of 77.5°C–77.6°C were observed in nine samples (TS5, TS6, TS7, TS8, TS9, TS10, TS11, TS12 and TS13), and the samples were identified as *M. suavis* species. A claimed *U. siamensis* species (TS13) was clustered into the *M. suavis* group by Bar-HRM analysis, and the findings agreed with the sequencing results.

16.4 Discussion

16.4.1 Necessity of Plant Authentication

M. suavis and *S. androgynus* are popular vegetables because their young leaves can be cooked in many favourite menu items.

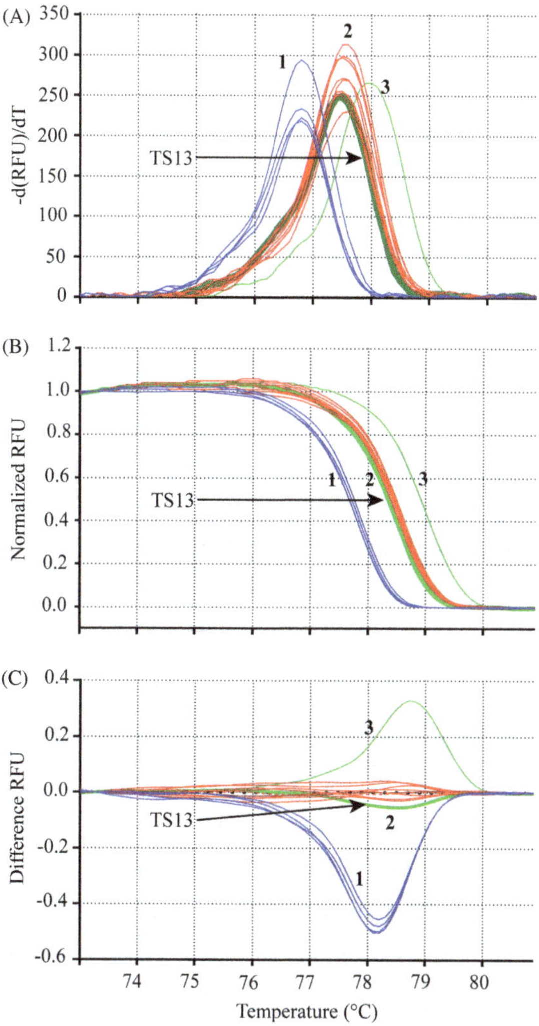

Fig. 16.8 Application of barcoding high-resolutions melting (Bar-HRM) analysis for differentiation of unknown samples from local nurseries. (A) Conventional melting curves, (B) normalised curves and (C) difference curves obtained by HRM analysis targeting the *mat*K gene of (1) *Sauropus androgynus*, (2) *Melientha suavis* and (3) *Urobotrya siamensis*. TS13 was clustered into the *M. suavis* group by Bar-HRM analysis.

However, misidentification with the poisonous *U. siamensis* caused deaths in the last decade. Thus, the authenticity of edible *M. suavis* and *S. androgynus* is a crucial issue for food safety concerns.

16.4.2 Choice of Barcode Regions for Plant Species Differentiation

The *mat*K gene has been proposed as a universal DNA barcode for flowering plants (Lahaye *et al.*, 2008). The gene has a high evolutionary rate, suitable length, interspecies divergence and low transition/transversion rate (Li *et al.*, 2015). Many reports have successfully used *mat*K as a DNA barcode for the differentiation of related plant species, such as *Crocus sativus* (Villa, Costa, Oliveira & Mafra, 2017), *Mitragyna speciosa* (Jaipaew, Padungchareon & Sukrong, 2018) and *Vitex glabrata* (Phoolcharoen & Sukrong, 2013). *MatK* is easy to be amplified and has a high discrimination value for the detection of various poisonous plant DNA sequences (Bruni *et al.*, 2010). Although the ITS2 and *psb*A-*trn*H regions revealed a higher percentage variation than the *mat*K region, the wide spread of variation sites across the targeted amplicons caused a lack of suitable places to position the Bar-HRM primers. *rbcL* has been used as a land-plant DNA barcode (Hollingsworth, Li, van der Bank & Twyford, 2016), and the application of an HRM primer set targeting this gene has been successfully performed in many plant species. However, *M. suavis*, *S. androgynus* and *U. siamensis* sequences exhibited low nucleotide variation rates, and Bar-HRM analysis might not be able to distinguish among the three species. Taken together, the *mat*K region was selected for its specific amplification in this study.

16.4.3 Application of Bar-HRM to Differentiate Poisonous Plants from Edible Plants

Testing on 13 unknown species from local nurseries by Bar-HRM analysis revealed that the species had been cultured. One of the samples, TS13, was suspected to be *U. siamensis* because their leaves looked alike. After testing by Bar-HRM analysis, TS13 was clustered into the *M. suavis* group with a high degree of confidence (>99%), showing that it was not *U. siamensis*, which was consistent with direct sequencing results. The similarity of leaves TS13 to *U. siamensis* may be due to genetic variation within the population, as stated in a previous report (Prathepha, 2000). In addition, leaf morphology is also affected by environmental factors such as local climate (Cetin, Sevik & Yigit, 2018).

16.4.4 Potential and Limitation of Bar-HRM Approach

This study showed that the primers designed for HRM analysis resulted in extremely high sensitivity and could be applied to a limited amount of the sample. As shown previously, Bar-HRM analysis exhibited high sensitivity of detection over conventional PCR when the same primer set was used (Figure 16.7). In addition, Bar-HRM has been proven to be an efficient and reliable method to identify processed or finished products such as tablets and capsules (Tungphatthong *et al.*, 2018).

However, for a successful analysis, many factors such as genomic DNA quality, amplicon length, primer design, dye selection, PCR reagents and cycling conditions should be considered to ensure the experiment is optimised for HRM. They will all affect the melting behaviour (Montgomery, Wittwer, Palais & Zhou, 2007). Achieving amplicon-specific amplification is critical to the success of the assay since any non-specific amplification will impair the melting curve analysis. Another important factor is the choice of intercalating dye. Several different HRM dyes should be tested to determine which functions best in each experimental system. One factor affecting dye functionality is the instrument itself, since different instruments use different detection methods.

16.5 Conclusion

DNA Bar-HRM analysis based on the chloroplast *mat*K gene was shown to be an effective method for species differentiation. The melting profiles can differentiate edible *M. suavis* and S. *androgynus* from poisonous *U. siamensis*. This strategy could be extended to other plants to avoid misidentification problems. Bar-HRM analysis would benefit agricultural and industrial quality control during the crop production phase through to the food process phase before releasing agricultural products to the markets.

Acknowledgements

We are grateful to the Center of Excellence in DNA Barcoding of Thai Medicinal Plants, Faculty of Pharmaceutical Sciences, Chulalongkorn University, for providing facilities.

Reprinted from "The use of plant DNA barcoding coupled with HRM analysis to differentiate edible vegetables from poisonous plants for food safety" in *Food Control*, 109, 106896 by Thongkhao, K., Tungphatthong, C., Phadungcharoen, T., & Sukrong, S. (2020), with permission from Elsevier. Readers may refer to these papers for further information.

References

Bruni, I., De Mattia, F., Galimberti, A., Galasso, G., Banfi, E., Casiraghi, M., & Labra, M. (2010). Identification of poisonous plants by DNA barcoding approach. *Int J Legal Med, 124*(6), 595–603.

Cetin, M., Sevik, H., & Yigit, N. (2018). Climate type-related changes in the leaf micromorphological characters of certain landscape plants. *Environ Monit Assess, 190*(7), 404.

Chen, S. L., Yao, H., Han, J. P., Liu, C., Song, J. Y., Shi, L. C., Zhu, Y. J., Ma, X. Y., Gao, T., Pang, X. H., Luo, K., Li, Y., Li, X. W., Jia, X. C., Lin, Y. L., & Leon, C. (2010). Validation of the ITS2 region as a novel DNA barcode for identifying medicinal plant species. *PLoS One, 5*(1), e8613. doi:10.1371/journal.pone.0008613.

Dunning, L. T., & Savolainen, V. (2010). Broad-scale amplification of *mat*K for DNA barcoding plants, a technical note. *Bot J Linn Soc, 164*(1), 1–9.

Ford, C. S., Ayres, K. L., Toomey, N., Haider, N., Stahl, J. V., Kelly, L. J., Wikstrom, N., Hollingsworth, P. M., Duff, R. J., Hoot, S. B., Cowan, R. S., Chase, M. W., & Wilkinson, M. J. (2009). Selection of candidate coding DNA barcoding regions for use on land plants. *Bot J Linn Soc, 159*(1), 1–11.

Ganopoulos, A., & Tsaftaris, A. (2011). Microsatellite high resolution melting (SSR-HRM) analysis for authenticity testing of protected designation of origin (PDO) sweet cherry products. *Food Control, 22*(3–4), 532–541.

Hebert, P., Cywinska, A., Ball, S. L., & Dewaard, J. (2003). Biological identification through DNA barcodes. *Proc Royal Soc Lond B, 270*, 313–321.

Hiepko, P. (1979). A revision of opiliaceae I. Genera of the eastern old world, excluding *Opilia*. *Willdenowia, 9*, 13–56.

Hollingsworth, P. M., Li, D. Z., van der Bank, M., & Twyford, A. D. (2016). Telling plant species apart with DNA: From barcodes to genomes. *Philos Trans R Soc Lond, B, Biol Sci, 371*(1702), 20150338.

Jaipaew, J., Padungchareon, T., & Sukrong, S. (2018). PCR-reverse dot blot of the nucleotide signature sequences of *mat*K for the identification of *Mitragyna speciosa*, a narcotic species. *Plant Gene, 14*, 46–54.

Julapak, P., Mankeb, P., Mekhora, T. S. S., & Chulilung, P. (2016). Financial cost and benefit analysis of Pak-wan Pa (Melientha sauvis Pierre) farming in Ban Mo District, Saraburi Province,Thailand. *Int J Agric Technol, 12*(7.2), 1845–1856.

Kress, W. J., Erickson, D. L., Jones, F. A., Swenson, N. G., Perez, R., Sanjur, O., & Bermingham, E. (2009). Plant DNA barcodes and a community phylogeny of a tropical forest dynamics plot in Panama. *Proc Nat Acad Sci USA, 106*(44), 18621–18626.

Lahaye, R., van der Bank, M., Bogarin, D., Warner, J., Pupulin, F., Gigot, G., Maurin, O., Duthoit, S., Barraclough, T. G., & Savolainen, V. (2008). DNA barcoding the floras of biodiversity hotspots. *Proc Nat Acad Sci USA, 105*(8), 2923–2928.

Levin, R. A., Wagner, W. L., Hoch, P. C., Nepokroeff, M., Pires, J. C., Zimmer, E. A., & Sytsma, K. J. (2003). Family-level relationships of Onagraceae based on chloroplast *rbc*L and *ndh*F data. *Am J Bot, 90*(1), 107–115.

Li, X., Yang, Y., Henry, R. J., Rossetto, M., Wang, Y., & Chen, S. (2015). Plant DNA barcoding: From gene to genome. *Biol Rev Camb Philos Soc, 90*(1), 157–166.

Mader, E., Ruzicka, J., Schmiderer, C., & Novak, J. (2011). Quantitative high-resolution melting analysis for detecting adulterations. *Anal Biochem, 409*(1), 153–155.

Mishra, P., Kumar, A., Nagireddy, A., Shukla, A. K., & Sundaresan, V. (2017). Evaluation of single and multilocus DNA barcodes towards species delineation in complex tree genus *Terminalia*. *PLoS One*, *12*(8), e0182836. doi:10.1371/journal.pone.0182836

Montgomery, J., Wittwer, C. T., Palais, R., & Zhou, L. (2007). Simultaneous mutation scanning and genotyping by high-resolution DNA melting analysis. *Nat Protoc, 2*(1), 59–66. doi:10.1038/nprot.2007.10

Phoolcharoen, W., & Sukrong, S. (2013). Molecular analysis of *Vitex* species using candidate DNA barcoding and PCR-RFLP of the *mat*K gene for authentication of *Vitex glabrata*. *Nat Prod Commun, 8*(1), 125–128.

Prathepha, P. (2000). Detection of RAPD variation in a forest tree species, *Melientha suavis* Pierre (Opiliaceae) from Thailand. *Sci, 26*, 213–218.

Sang, T., Crawford, D., & Stuessy, T. (1997). Chloroplast DNA phylogeny, reticulate evolution, and biogeography of Paeonia (Paeoniaceae). *Am J Bot, 84*(8), 1120.

Thongkhao, K., Tungphatthong, C., Phadungcharoen, T., & Sukrong, S. (2020). The use of plant DNA barcoding coupled with HRM analysis to differentiate edible vegetables from poisonous plants for food safety. *Food Control, 109*, 106896. doi:10.1016/j.foodcont.2019.106896

Tourdjman, M., Srihawong, R., Soy, T. K., Touch, S., Hul, S., Janssens, B., Galliot-Guilley, M., & Vong, S. (2009). Plant poisoning outbreak in the western area of Cambodia, 2005. *Trans R Soc Trop Med Hyg, 103*(9), 949–951.

Tungphatthong, C., Somnuek, J., Phadungcharoen, T., Ingkaninan, K., Denduangboripant, J., & Sukrong, S. (2018). DNA barcoding of *Bacopa* species coupled with high-resolution melting analysis. *Genome, 61*(12), 867–877. doi:10.1139/gen-2018-0059

Villa, C., Costa, J., Oliveira, M. B., & Mafra, I. (2017). Novel quantitative real-time PCR approach to determine safflower (*Carthamus tinctorius*) adulteration in saffron (*Crocus sativus*). *Food Chem, 229*, 680–687.

White, T. J., Bruns, T., Lee, S., & Taylor, J. (1990). Amplification and direct sequencing of fungal ribosomal RNA genes for phylogenetics. In Innis, M. A., Gelfand, D. H., Sninsky, J. J. & White, T. J. (Eds.), *PCR Protocols: A Guide to Methods and Applications* (pp. 315–322). New York, NY: Academic Press.

Chapter 17

Setting Up a DNA Laboratory for Molecular Authentication

Ka-Lok Wong & Wai-Yan Ha

17.1 Introduction

Decisions on many areas of our daily life, such as food ingredient analysis, healthcare safety, radiofrequency radiation measurement, oil exploration and air pollution monitoring, heavily rely on laboratory test results. The quality of these tests are undoubtedly critical as wrong decisions can be made based on misleading information. To maintain consistent quality for the operation and validity of test results, organisations can adopt a quality assurance system to set up quality requirements to find out and correct the defects in their processes and products. For a testing laboratory, quality management ensures that most test and calibration results are trustworthy, whereas invalid ones can be detected and corrected in a timely manner. Global quality standards for test and calibration developed by several organisations, namely, International Organization for Standardization (ISO), International Electrotechnical Commission (IEC) and US Food and Drug Administration (FDA), are valuable references for laboratories to design their own quality management systems.

To achieve internationally recognised quality standard and pursuing of accreditation, *ISO/IEC 17025 General requirements for the competence of testing and calibration laboratories* is world-wide adopted (ISO/IEC 17025[2017]). ISO/IEC 17025:2017, which is published by ISO and IEC, is a conformity assessment standard that defines the requirements for testing and calibration laboratories, including general requirements, structural requirements, resource requirements, process requirements and management system requirements. The general requirements relate to impartiality and confidentiality of laboratory activities. The structural requirements cover matters of the organisation and management structure of the laboratory and personnel responsible for the range of laboratory activities. Resource requirements describe the personnel, facilities and environmental conditions, equipment, metrological traceability, externally provided products and services necessary to manage and perform the laboratory activities. Process requirements relate to more technical matters such as review of requests, verification and validation of methods, sampling, handling of test or calibration items, technical records, evaluation of measurement uncertainty, ensuring the validity of results, reporting of results, nonconforming work, control of data and information management. Management system requirements focus on establishing, documentation, implementation and maintaining a management system that is capable of supporting and demonstrating the consistent achievement of requirements of the ISO document and assuring the quality of the laboratory results.

In general, the requirements of establishing laboratories undertaking different categories of analysis are nearly the same, but special precautionary measures should be considered according to the particular needs of each category. For example, if the test aims at trace level analysis, measures should be taken to minimise cross-contamination. DNA testing, which employs the polymerase chain reaction (PCR) technique, is highly sensitive but prone to cross-contamination as nucleic acids can be amplified up to a billion time of their original concentration.

Contamination, for a DNA laboratory, is the introduction of unwanted nucleic acids into test items. Typically, there are three types of contaminations: (1) starting material contamination caused by an invasion of bacteria, fungi or other microorganisms into test items because of the poor sample storage condition prior to or after receipt by the laboratory; (2) sample-to-sample contamination caused by sample materials/genomic DNA from one source to one or more other samples during sample pre-treatment or preparation; and (3) amplified product-to-sample contamination caused by an amplified product from one PCR amplification to another sample or even to the working environment prior to its amplification step.

For a DNA laboratory, the workflow may involve (1) sample pre-process; (2) nucleic acid extraction; (3) nucleic acid amplification and (4) post amplification. In order to minimise the risk of co-amplification of target DNA with contaminants, two major principles should be followed when setting up a DNA laboratory: (1) separation of time and space and (2) forward flow of sample movement. In the first principle, physical separation of incompatible experimental steps is the most effective way to prevent contamination. The second principle is that the flow of test items should be unidirectional. Therefore, the laboratory space arrangement can be simply divided into two zones: pre-PCR and post-PCR as depicted in Figure 17.1. More specifically, the movement of the test item and its derivatives should start from the pre-PCR area to post-PCR zone, and the reverse must be restricted. These

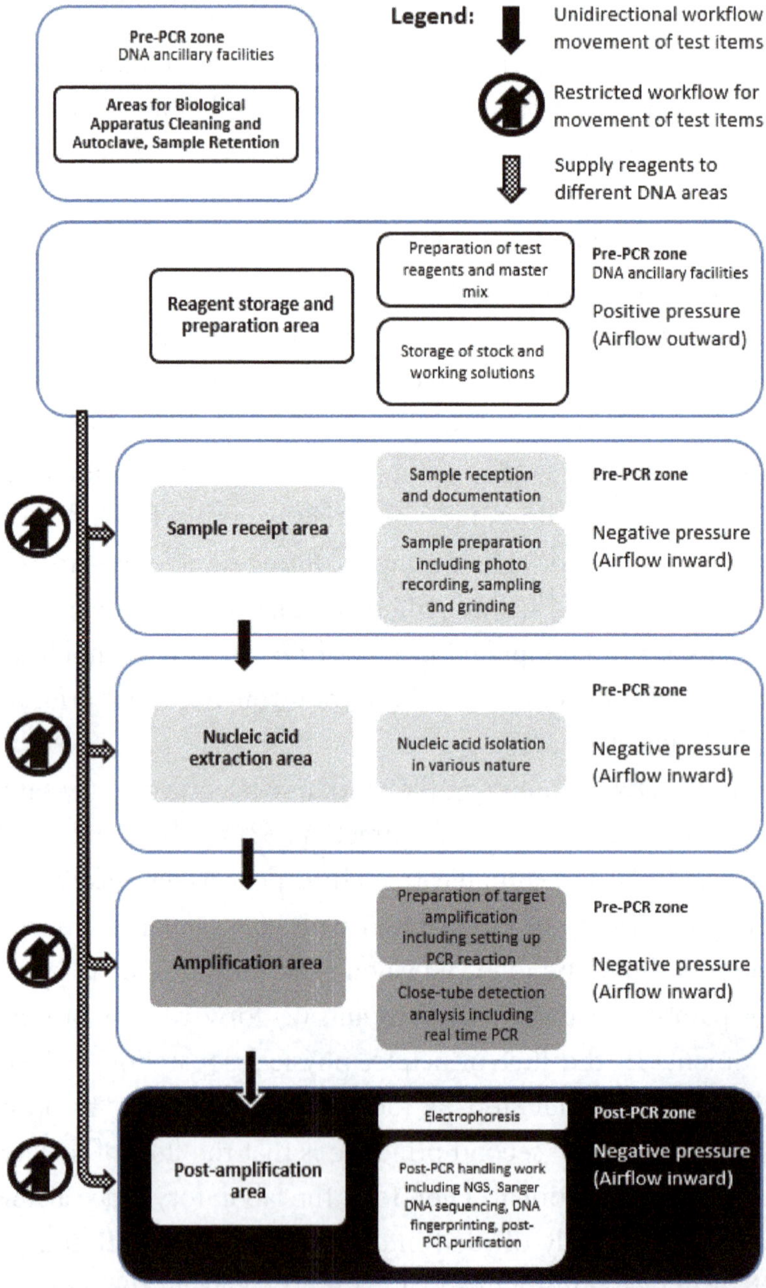

Fig. 17.1 A sketch depicting the model layout for a DNA laboratory.

two principles must be implemented concurrently. Think about the following scenarios: (1) Laboratory A has designated rooms for pre-PCR and post-PCR process, but there is no restriction of the movement of amplification products from post-PCR to pre-PCR zones; (2) Laboratory B literally obeys the second principle, but the pre-PCR and post-PCR steps are actually conducted on the same bench without effective physical separation. Obviously, the anti-contamination measurements by neither Laboratory A nor Laboratory B are effective, which may lead to invalid or incorrect results.

In the following sections, requirements and implementations related to setting up and operating a DNA laboratory for molecular authentication of Chinese Materia Medica (CMM) will be exhaustively discussed in respect to some requirements under the resource and process requirements of ISO17025 and the Hong Kong Laboratory Accreditation Scheme (HOKLAS) supplementary criteria published by the local accreditation body, Hong Kong Accreditation Service (HKAS) (HOKLAS 003:2015; HOKLAS Supplementary Criteria No. 43). It is essential to mention that the contents are not a replacement of the aforementioned standards or supplementary criteria as they will not cover all stipulated requirements. Instead, the discussion will focus on the implementation and practice connected with DNA analysis in the opinions and experience of the authors. Readers should always refer to the standard to have a complete view for particular applications.

17.2 Resource Requirements

17.2.1 Facilities and Environmental Conditions

The facilities and environmental conditions should be suitable for the laboratory activities and should not adversely affect the validity of test results. With the concept of separating the working environment into pre-PCR and post-PCR zones, the laboratory area can be further subdivided based on the major steps of most DNA analytical processes (European Network of Forensic Science Institute; Scientific Working Group on DNA Analysis Methods) as depicted in Figure 17.1. Depending on the DNA techniques to be employed and the commitment to the international standard for the DNA test, five separate areas should be clearly designated for conducting activities related to (i) sample receipt and processing, (ii) DNA extraction, (iii) amplification of target DNA, (iv) manipulation of post-PCR product and (v) ancillary facilities for reagent preparation. The following sections will introduce the functions and major activities in each area. Besides, DNA analysis-related environmental conditions and facilities will be discussed.

17.2.1.1 *Sample Receipt Area*

This area belongs to the pre-PCR zone. This area is designed for receipt, recording, storage and grinding of test items for subsequent nucleic acid extraction process. Physically, separate space is allocated solely for test item handling. Grinding of test items is conducted in a biosafety cabinet (BSC) to prevent spreading of powders over other areas to cause environmental and sample-to-sample contamination. Extracted DNA and PCR products are not allowed to enter into this room. Tools or glassware should be sterilised or decontaminated before use.

17.2.1.2 *Nucleic Acid Extraction Area*

This area belongs to the pre-PCR zone, in which extraction of nucleic acids from the test item is conducted. Other major activities involve the yield determination and storage of DNA extracts. If organic solvents, such as phenol and chloroform, are required in extraction steps, all steps involving these chemicals must be performed inside the designated fume hood. After DNA extraction, the operator has to keep the extracts in the designated low-temperature cabinets.

17.2.1.3 *Amplification Area*

This area is the watershed moment in the DNA analytical process and belongs to pre-PCR zone where the amplification of nucleic acids takes place. The function of this area is to (1) set up PCR reaction and (2) carry out nucleic acid amplification using a thermal cycler or close-tube detection such as real-time PCR. If the preparation of PCR master mix and addition of genomic DNA have to be performed in the same room, the best way is to conduct these two activities in two designated PCR hoods individually to ensure that the preparation of the master mix is in a DNA-free environment. Usage of barrier-tips are highly recommended to prevent aerosol spreading over the thermal cycler and facilities. No PCR tube containing amplified products can be opened in this room in order to prevent aerosol accumulation. The amplification products should be transferred and stored in the post-amplification area immediately.

17.2.1.4 *Post-Amplification Area*

This area is designated for post-PCR analysis. Major activities include the analysis of amplified PCR products by electrophoresis, purification of amplification product, determination of concentration of amplification product, sequencing and storage of amplification products. The mixing of reagent, such as the thermal cycling reagent and restriction enzyme digestion, should be performed in a designated hood. Glassware and other consumables cannot be taken out of this area without prior decontamination.

17.2.1.5 *Ancillary Facilities Located in Pre-PCR Zone*

Reagent storage and preparation area

The supply of clean and proper test reagents is of paramount importance to the validity of the test result. The major activities conducted in this area are the preparation of stock reagents, aliquoting of working solutions and setting up a master mix for applications. It should house storage appliance and dedicated equipment and apparatus for master mix preparation, such as the designated PCR hood for the sole purpose of handling reagents. Test items, DNA extracts or amplification products cannot be brought or stored in this area.

Other areas for biological apparatus cleaning and autoclave, sample retention

Depending on the need and nature of individual laboratory, additional area may be considered for the storage of special test items or reference materials at dedicated conditions. Such an area may be equipped with a temperature monitoring system, temperature-controlled desiccator and/or cold storage. One may also consider defining an area for biological apparatus cleaning and autoclaving in order to decontaminate and sterilise all used items for reuse.

17.2.1.6 *Other Environmental Conditions and Facilities to be Considered*

Relative room pressure differentials

Air pressure differential can alter the flow direction of air particles between a room and its surroundings (Lstiburek, 2008). A negative-pressure room prevents air particles from escaping whereas a positive one keeps air from getting into the room. Except for the reagent preparation area, slight negative pressure differential should generally be built in all areas in order to trap and prevent the spreading of contaminants. Slight positive pressure in the reagent preparation area ensures no contaminant presents during the preparation of reagents. It is important that the windows are well-sealed, and doors are closed at all time; otherwise, a stable pressure differential cannot be built up or maintained. Air pressure monitoring systems with a pressure deviation alarm should be fitted in each area to alert the operator.

Physical separation

If, because of environmental constraints, all steps have to be performed in a single room, the boundary of each work area needs to be clearly defined and the layout is in accordance with the forward flow principle. Appropriate protection and separation facilities should be housed to prevent cross-contamination among areas. It is highly recommended that the operator conduct analytical steps vulnerable to the contamination in a dead air box with ultraviolet (UV) light or PCR hood to minimise the chance of amplification of unwanted nucleic acids. In some circumstances, appropriate decontaminants such as bleach or commercial reagent for the removal of nucleic acid may also be used for decontamination.

Monitoring the environment

It is essential to demarcate high-risk places in the laboratory, like the working bench, PCR hood, BSC and fume hood. Appropriate measures, such as a surface swab test or open tube test, should be taken regularly to detect the presence of nucleic acids in working areas (Wu, Wu, Zhang & Cheng, 2018). Corrective actions have to be taken if contamination is found.

17.2.2 Equipment

The laboratory should have access to equipment including, but not limited to, measuring instruments, software, measurement standards, reference materials, reference data, reagents, consumables or auxiliary apparatus. It is recommended that the functionality and quality of equipment, reagent and apparatus should be monitored by an assigned officer. The precaution on some critical aspects related to DNA laboratory are discussed as follows:

17.2.2.1 *Performance and Maintenance*

Operator should ensure the performance and precision of commonly used equipment such as balances, micropipette and spectrophotometer meeting the specification of the tests. Critical analytical equipment like the thermal cycler and DNA sequencer must be verified regularly to ensure that its performance is within the tolerance of the tests. One example is the temperature accuracy of the thermal cycler, which exerts a great impact on the validity of the DNA test. Procedures and records of performance checks, maintenance activities and calibration should be available.

17.2.2.2 *Location and Placement of Equipment*

Each area should have designated sets of equipment and apparatus. When the equipment and apparatus are moved to other areas or relocated after repair, the operator needs to clean and decontaminate them accordingly.

17.2.2.3 *Pipette*

Repeated amplification of nucleic acids may lead to the accumulation of amplification products dramatically in the laboratory environment if improperly controlled. Therefore, each area should have at least one set of designated pipettes, and transferring them to other areas for use without a decontamination procedure is prohibited. It is highly recommended to use barrier filter pipette tips, especially for steps involving the manipulation of DNA templates and amplification products to prevent carryover.

17.2.2.4 *BSC and PCR Hood*

BSC or PCR hood can provide a confined area for critical steps in the analytical process, such as the preparation of reagents, addition of DNA templates into the master mix and preparation of cycle sequencing reagents. In particular, it is of utmost importance for laboratories without separate rooms. To diminish the risk of contamination, designated equipment and apparatus to be used within the BSC or PCR hood, such as pipetting for the preparation of the master mix, should not be removed for other purposes. The work-surface and equipment inside can be decontaminated by UV irradiation using the built-in UV germicidal lamps.

17.2.2.5 *Sterilisation*

Reagents, buffers, apparatus and consumables should be sterilised by autoclaving with the aim of breaking down residual DNA molecules and denaturing DNase/RNase. Sterile syringe filters with a pore size of 0.22 microns can be used for sterilising heat-sensitive reagents by removing microorganisms. UV irradiation can cross-link the strands of DNA to make them un-amplifiable, and it is particularly useful for treating the water, plasticwares and racks in a UV cross-linker before preparing master mixes.

17.2.2.6 *Reagents*

The laboratory needs to identify critical reagents for the tests. The preparation step, precautions and person responsible should be documented.

Operator should always aliquot and take the required amount of reagents from the stock. Repeated freeze-thaw cycles of easily degraded reagents such as primers, nucleotides and fluorescent reagents are not recommended. Expired reagents should not be used for testing as it may affect the testing performance and result in incorrect findings.

The service, materials and supplies provided by third parties must meet the requirements for DNA tests. Generally, chemicals and reagents used are at a molecular biology grade or equivalent, certified with including but not limited to 'PCR grade', 'DNase free' or 'DNA free'. Verification procedure, criteria for acceptance, shelf life and special storage conditions should be documented and traceable in the test records.

There should be documentation stipulating and recording the procedures for the purchasing, handling, storage, verification, preservation, maintenance and the use of reference materials and stocks. For method validation and quality control of the test method, reference material should be obtained mainly from reputable national institutes or authorities. If the original form of reference material is not available, genomic or plasmid DNA of known provenance is also acceptable for the use of DNA analysis.

17.2.3 Personnel

Personnel who have impact on the quality of test should be adequately qualified. The laboratory needs to provide training to newly recruited staff members, who will carry out tests and maintain full records of training and competent assessment.

17.3 Process Requirements

17.3.1 Sampling

There should be documentation stipulating the minimum sample size, sampling procedures and chain-of-custody. The sampling method should address the factors to be controlled to ensure the validity of subsequent testing results. Operator should possess the knowledge to select a DNA technique that is fitted for identifying target species from a single source or mixed sources of the test item. For example, direct sequencing by the Sanger method is applicable to a single species of medicinal material. Individual items in the sample should not be mixed and homogenised.

17.3.2 Handling of Test Items

Laboratory should document the procedure and precaution for the handling, transportation, storage, retention and disposal of test item as follows:

17.3.2.1 *Record of Test Item*

Once the test items arrive, it is necessary to register them into the record system of the laboratory, preferably with a unique laboratory identification number. The physical appearance and condition of test item and its container should be examined and recorded carefully. If a photo record is needed, the laboratory may consider placing a colour correction card as a reference when taking the photos. The work area should be decontaminated before processing the next test item. Operator has to handle one test item at a time to prevent sample-to-sample contamination.

17.3.2.2 *Storage of Test Items*

The storage location for test items has to be kept away from the analytical areas. Storage conditions for test items should be documented and fulfil the requirements of test standards to prevent deterioration, loss or damage of test items.

Fresh test items should be kept in a refrigerator or freezer to minimise the degradation. The temperature of the low-temperature storage cabinet must be monitored to ensure that it is within the acceptable range. No consumables and reagents should be placed in the cabinets reserved for fresh test items.

Dried test items, such as plant voucher specimens, should be deposited in an area protected from bacterial contamination, cross-contamination, heat and sunlight. There should be appropriate utilities, such as uninterrupted electricity power supply, air conditioning and a dehumidifier, to ensure the storage condition fulfilling the requirement of the test.

17.3.2.3 *Transferring Materials among Areas*

The movement of test items should be in accordance with the forward flow principle. Designated containers are used for transporting the test items, DNA extracts and amplification products across areas. Before and after transferring the materials to the next area or bringing them back to the storage location, the operator has to clean the container with the appropriate decontaminating reagent, such as 10% bleach or 70% ethanol or by UV irradiation.

The movement of test items and materials from the post-PCR zone to pre-PCR zone should be minimised. When it is unavoidable, it can only be allowed after thorough decontamination of the container for test items and changes of protective clothing for the pre-PCR zone.

17.3.3 Test Method and Method Validation

It is recommended to use the national, regional or international standard method. For the in-house method, it should be fully validated before use. However, method validation is highly correlated to the type of DNA test to be employed. As special considerations are required, appropriate standards or guidelines should be referred to.

17.3.4 Ensuring the Validity of Results

To ensure the validity of test results, the laboratory should have a procedure for monitoring the test outcomes. The monitoring should be planned and reviewed, which may include, where appropriate, but not be limited to the following:

17.3.4.1 *Quality Control Plan*

Quality control plan should be established and implemented. Use of reference materials or quality control materials have to be included for every test run, including (1) Extraction negative control; (2) Extraction positive control; (3) PCR/Sequencing negative control; and (4) PCR/sequencing positive control. Operator needs to process test items and all kinds of positive and negative controls in parallel throughout the analytical process, from sample handling to data analysis. Duplicate measurement of each test item or random sample duplicate, depending on the choice of DNA technique, should be applied. It is essential to state the frequencies and acceptance criteria of these controls and actions to be taken when results are out of the control limits.

17.3.4.2 *Interlaboratory Comparison or Proficiency Testing*

The laboratory should participate in proficiency testing activities or interlaboratory comparison at regular time intervals to demonstrate its competence. If unsatisfactory results are obtained from the proficiency testing program, the laboratory needs to investigate and rectify the problem, and all findings should be recorded.

17.3.5 Other Related Practices

1. Wearing gloves while handling test items can provide two-way protection: (i) against hazards associated with test items to the operator; and (ii) avoiding transfer of proteolytic enzymes and nucleases from the operator to test items. To avoid sample-to-sample contamination, the operator should always change into new gloves before touching the next test item. After the test has been completed, discard the used gloves into the waste bin to prevent the spread of the test items outside the laboratory areas.
2. Operator must change protective clothing when moving between pre-PCR and post-PCR zones. It is desirable to have designated colours of laboratory coats for each area for easy identification. Whenever there is a suspicion that a laboratory coat might have been contaminated, it must be discarded at once.
3. The laboratory should have and follow a written procedure for monitoring, cleaning and decontaminating the working space, with designated cleaning utensils for each area. In case of a contamination event, the laboratory should implement corrective actions.
4. Visitors working in the laboratory, e.g., service engineer and maintenance worker, must be under supervision at all the time. Decontamination procedures should be taken after the service or visit.

17.4 Conclusion

In this chapter, we have covered and discussed the requirements and practices for setting up and operating a DNA laboratory for the molecular authentication of CMM with reference to the standards. It is worth noting that a number of management requirements in the standards have not been mentioned as they are indeed applied to various kinds of test and calibration services, but not specific to DNA tests. Besides, the laboratory should also recognise that different types of DNA tests have their unique requirements, and the laboratory needs to examine these carefully during the design phase and take corresponding measures. It is always necessary to refer to the standards to obtain a complete view.

References

European Network of Forensic Science Institute. DNA contamination prevention guidelines. Retrieved from https://enfsi.eu/wp-content/uploads/2017/09/DNA-contamination-prevention-guidelines-v2.pdf (Accessed Dec 1, 2020).

HOKLAS 003:2015. *Technical Criteria for Laboratory Accreditation*. Hong Kong: Hong Kong Accreditation Service.

HOKLAS Supplementary Criteria No. 43. *'Chinese Medicine' and 'Food' — Species Identification by DNA Sequencing for Authentication Purpose*. Hong Kong: Hong Kong Accreditation Service.

ISO/IEC 17025(2017). *General Requirements for the Competence of Testing and Calibration Laboratories*. Geneva: Organization for Standardization (ISO).

Lstiburek, J. (2008). *Air Pressure and Building Envelopes*. Building Science Press.

Scientific Working Group on DNA Analysis Methods. *Contamination Prevention and Detection Guidelines for Forensic DNA Laboratories*. Retrieved from https://media.wix.com/ugd/4344b0_c4d4dbba84f1400a98eaa2e48f2bf291.pdf (Accessed Dec 1, 2020).

Wu, Y. P., Wu, J. Y., Zhang, Z. H., & Cheng, C. (2018). DNA decontamination methods for internal quality management in clinical PCR laboratories. *J Clin Lab Anal, 32*(3), e22290.

Chapter 18 Concluding Remarks

Molecular authentication utilises various DNA techniques to examine genetic information in order to reveal the species identity of the target material. These techniques were originally for analysing the evolutionary and phylogenetic relationships of plant and animal materials. The use of molecular technology to authenticate Chinese medicinal materials was initiated in the mid-1990's and we were among the first research groups in this field. Since the publication of the first paper in 1994 (Cheung, Kwan, But & Shaw, 1994), rapid progress has been made and more than 2,000 papers and over 30 Chinese and US patents using molecular techniques are now available (Shaw, Wong, Chan, Wong & But, 2009). In addition, molecular authentication standards have been officially recorded in several pharmacopoeias.

18.1 The Pros and Cons of Molecular Authentication

There are several advantages of using molecular tools in authentication: (1) Unlike organoleptic examination, the techniques do not depend on the physical form of the material. (2) Small quantity of sample, usually a few milligrams, is sufficient for the analysis, as DNA can be amplified by polymerase chain reaction (PCR). (3) Differentiation can be done at different phylogenetic levels by selectively examining different regions of the genome. As discussed in Chapter 11, DNA sequences such as cytochrome c oxidase subunit I (*COI*), *rbcL* genes, internal transcribed spacer (ITS) and *psbA-trnH* intergenic spacer regions are served as standard DNA barcodes for authentication. In addition to studying individual DNA sequences, it is possible to generate fingerprints using random amplified polymorphic DNA (RAPD: Chapter 5), amplified fragment length polymorphism (AFLP: Chapter 6) and other related techniques that scan the polymorphism of the whole genome. (4) DNA sequences are the most basic signature of an organism, which is relatively conserved for a species. On the other hand, proteins and chemical compounds are phenotypic products of DNA. Their expression and composition are more significantly affected by growing conditions, collection time and age of the organism. (5) Every nucleotide in the DNA may be regarded as an individual marker. A DNA fragment of several hundred base pairs therefore constitutes a substantial amount of information. The ability to obtain this information is valuable for tracing the geographical source of a material ('Daodi' material in Chinese). (6) Molecular authentication may be used to identify medicinal materials in a mixture. For example, our previous study showed that ingredients in multi-ingredient decoctions can be identified using specific diagnostic PCR (Lo, Li & Shaw, 2015). (7) Equipment such as thermocyclers for DNA amplification, electrophoresis tanks for separating DNA fragments and DNA sequencing machine are easy to access and are affordable to many laboratories. (8) The development of next generation DNA sequencing may facilitate high-throughput identification of ingredients in medicinal products.

There are, however, limitations in applying molecular techniques: (1) The quality of DNA may directly affect the accuracy and reproducibility of the DNA profile. Obtaining high molecular weight DNA, free from contaminants, is the prerequisite to the success of many molecular techniques. For example, high molecular weight DNA is required for good AFLP fingerprints and the generation of some DNA barcode sequences. In our experience, some of the dried medicinal materials, including *Panax quinquefolius* (American ginseng), *Codonopsis pilosula* (Dangshen) and *Lycium barbarum* (Gouqi) produced DNA of good quality. However, in some other cases, DNA extracted from the material is degraded, owing to harsh processing procedures or adverse storage conditions. For example, DNA for some red ginseng and Dendrobii Caulis (Shihu) samples are too degraded for generating DNA fingerprints because they have been steamed or boiled. (2) The existence of secondary metabolites in some medicinal materials may hinder the extraction of DNA. Sometimes, it is necessary to develop an extraction protocol for a particular medicinal material and this slows down the authentication process. (3) Medicinal materials not stored properly are often contaminated by fungi and they may generate inaccurate fingerprints and cause false positive identification results. To tackle this problem, before extracting the DNA, it is necessary to wash the surface of the sample thoroughly with sterile water and ethanol. Nevertheless, direct sequencing of the PCR product of a sample contaminated by fungi may generate ambiguous data. If this is the case, one should first clone the PCR product into a vector and then extract the DNA from a few independent clones to find the correct sequence. A more efficient method is to sequence the PCR product by Next Generation Sequencing. In addition, it is imperative to check the data generated from a reliable reference. (4) Techniques such as

RAPD and arbitrarily primed PCR (AP-PCR) are widely used in molecular authentication because they are relatively simple and no prior knowledge about the template sequence is needed. However, because of the low stringency of the annealing step, these techniques are particularly sensitive to contaminants in the DNA preparation and even slight alternation in experimental conditions. To ensure the consistency of DNA fingerprints and to find the frequency of intraspecific variation, it is essential to examine many samples in the same batch of material.

18.2 Priority Issues in Molecular Authentication

We have identified areas for further development in molecular authentication. (1) Generation of standard DNA fingerprint and sequence database. At present, there is no consensus on the techniques or sequences used. The availability of reference techniques and sequences will reduce the ambiguity and aid data comparison across different laboratories. It is worth to develop a standard DNA fingerprint and sequence library for authentication, especially for those easily confused and expensive medicinal materials. This library should be inter-laboratories validated. The database should also include information of related species and common adulterant to increase the accuracy in data comparison. Many regulatory authorities including Government Chinese Medicines Testing Institute of Hong Kong SAR are actively generating DNA barcode sequences from authenticated herbal samples (https://www.cmro.gov.hk/html/eng/useful_information/gcmti/research/btc/DNA_sequences.html). A Global Pharmacopoeia Genome Database (GPGD) has been established to provide a uniform genomic data format for herb species across various pharmacopoeias (http://www.gpgenome.com, Liao *et al.*, 2022). (2) Development of locality-based ('Daodi') DNA markers and find their relationship with active ingredients. It is well known that medicinal materials grown in different localities may show different pharmacological efficacies. The use of different cultivars or the effect of environmental factors trigger the variation of gene expression. The origin of medicinal materials from different geographic locations may be identified by analysing the unique single nucleotide polymorphism (SNP) or epigenetic markers. There are a number of successful cases in locality authentication at species-, strain- and locality-levels by DNA markers (Chen, Duan, Zhou, Chen & Fu, 2011; Kumar & Roy, 2018; Tochika-Komatsu, Asaka & Ii, 2001; Wang, Hao, Chen & Li, 2016; Zhang *et al*., 2012; Zhang, Zhang, Huang, Yang & Cao, 2006). (3) Identification of constituents in commercial medicinal products. In recent years, Chinese medicinal products and health-enhancing natural products have become popular and well accepted by the public. For the benefit of consumers and the healthy development of the industry, standard methods should be developed to characterise the content of these products. Our successful cases in the authentication of ingredients in decoctions, traditional Chinese medicine (TCM) granules and highly processed materials indicate the feasibility of the molecular approach (Jiang, Lo, Chen & Shaw, 2016; Lo *et al.*, 2015; Lo & Shaw, 2018). Refinement of next-generation sequencing techniques and having more herbal species included in a designated genomic or chloroplast database will facilitate this area of work. (4) Using DNA techniques for the quantification of medicinal materials. Our previous study demonstrated the amount of individual component in concentrated Chinese medicine granules and their mixtures could be determined using quantitative PCR (qPCR) (Lo & Shaw, 2017), showing that the DNA technique is applicable for quantification under certain circumstances. (5) Automation of instruments for molecular authentication such as isolating, amplifying, separating, purifying and detecting DNA fragments. For example, a robot and automatic DNA extraction machine may help these processes. The advantages of using the automated method are to reduce the procedure time and manual labour, which leads to the decrease in costs and human errors. To use molecular authentication methods routinely, procedures in DNA extraction, amplification, sequencing and data analysis should also be simplified.

18.3 Other Uses of Molecular Markers

Apart from the use in authentication, molecular markers can also aid selection for breeding purposes. For example, ginseng is susceptible to pathogens including *Alternaria panax*, *Phytophthora cactorum*, *Rhizoctonia solani*, *Ramularia* spp. and *Fusarium* spp. The major solution for disease control nowadays is pesticide spraying that may be harmful to consumers if excessive residues remain in the medicinal materials. DNA technology can be used to locate marker genes that protect the medicinal materials from pathogens and help to develop a quick assay for breeders to ascertain individuals carry the pest resistance markers. In addition, DNA technology helps to identify genetically modified (GM) genes in medicinal materials. GM detection has already been applied for various food products that also have medicinal values, such as maize, soybean (Tengel, Schussler, Setzke, Balles & Sprenger-Haussels, 2001), potato (Watanabe *et al.*, 2004) and papaya (Loo et al., 2019). As organic products are usually sold at higher prices, DNA techniques can help to ensure the product is non-transgenic.

18.4 Conclusion

Although DNA techniques can be used alone for authentication, combining it with other methods such as organoleptic and chemical analyses will increase the accuracy of authentication. With the advancement of DNA sequencing and DNA fingerprinting, we foresee that more regulatory agencies and testing laboratories will use DNA authentication as a routine method in their authentication and quality control activities.

References

Chen, C., Duan, L. N., Zhou, X. L., Chen, B. L., & Fu, C. X. (2011). Molecular authentication of geo-authentic *Scrophularia ningpoensis*. *J Zhejiang Univ Sci B*, 12(5), 393-398. doi:10.1631/jzus.B1000179

Cheung, K. S., Kwan, H. S., But, P. P., & Shaw, P. C. (1994). Pharmacognostical identification of American and Oriental ginseng roots by genomic fingerprinting using arbitrarily primed polymerase chain reaction (AP-PCR). *J Ethnopharmacol, 42*(1), 67–69. doi:10.1016/0378-8741(94)90025-6

Jiang, L. L., Lo, Y. T., Chen, W. T., & Shaw, P. C. (2016). DNA authentication of animal-derived concentrated Chinese medicine granules. *J Pharm Biomed Anal, 129*, 398–404. doi:10.1016/j.jpba.2016.07.030

Kumar, V., & Roy, B. K. (2018). Population authentication of the traditional medicinal plant *Cassia tora* L. based on ISSR markers and FTIR analysis. *Sci Rep*, *8*(1), 10714. doi:10.1038/s41598-018-29114-1

Liao, B. S., Hu, H. Y., Xiao, S. M., Zhou, G. R., Sun, W., Chu, Y., Meng, X. X., Wei, J. H., Zhang, H., Xu, J., & Chen, S. L. (2022). Global Pharmacopoeia Genome Database is an integrated and mineable genomic database for traditional medicines derived from eight international pharmacopoeias. *Sci China Life Sci*, *65*(4), 809-817. doi:10.1007/s11427-021-1968-7

Lo, Y. T., Li, M., & Shaw, P. C. (2015). Identification of constituent herbs in ginseng decoctions by DNA markers. *Chin Med, 10*(1), 1. doi:10.1186/s13020-015-0029-x

Lo, Y. T., & Shaw, P. C. (2017). Quantification of concentrated Chinese medicine granules by quantitative polymerase chain reaction. *J Pharm Biomed Anal, 145*, 661–665. doi:10.1016/j.jpba.2017.07.047

Lo, Y. T., & Shaw, P. C. (2018). DNA barcoding in concentrated Chinese medicine granules using adaptor ligation-mediated polymerase chain reaction. *J Pharm Biomed Anal, 149*, 512–516. doi:10.1016/j.jpba.2017.11.048

Loo, J. F. C., But, G. W. C., Kwok, H. C., Lau, P. M., Kong, S. K., Ho, H. P., & Shaw, P. C. (2019). A rapid sample-to-answer analytical detection of genetically modified papaya using loop-mediated isothermal amplification assay on lab-on-a-disc for field use. *Food Chem, 15*(274), 822–830. doi: 10.1016/j.foodchem.2018.09.049

Shaw, P. C., Wong, K. L., Chan, A. W., Wong, W. C., & But, P. P. (2009). Patent applications for using DNA technologies to authenticate medicinal herbal material. *Chin Med, 4*, 21. doi:10.1186/1749-8546-4-21

Tengel, C., Schussler, P., Setzke, E., Balles, J., & Sprenger-Haussels, M. (2001). PCR-based detection of genetically modified soybean and maize in raw and highly processed foodstuffs. *BioTechniques, 31*(2), 426–429. doi:10.2144/01312pf01

Tochika-Komatsu, Y., Asaka, I., & Ii, I. (2001). A random amplified polymorphic DNA (RAPD) primer to assist the identification of a selected strain, aizu K-111 of Panax ginseng and the sequence amplified. *Biol Pharm Bull, 24*(10), 1210–1213. doi:10.1248/bpb.24.1210

Wang, H., Hao, N., Chen, L., & Li, G. (2016). Development of intron polymorphism markers in major latex-like protein gene for locality-level and cultivar identification of *Salvia miltiorrhiza*. *Springerplus*, *5*(1), 1919. doi:10.1186/s40064-016-3611-5

Watanabe, T., Kuribara, H., Mishima, T., Kikuchi, H., Kodama, T., Futo, S., Kasama, K., Toyota, A., Nouno, M., Saita, A., Takahashi, K., Hino, A., Akiyama, H., Maitani, T., & Kubo, M. (2004). New qualitative detection methods of genetically modified potatoes. *Biol Pharm Bull, 27*(9), 1333-1339. doi:10.1248/bpb.27.1333

Zhang, B., Yuan, Q., Huang, L., Liu, X., Li, X., Lin, S., Chen, M., & Ge, X. (2012). Locality identification of Chinese medicinal plant Scutellaria baicalensis (Lamiaceae) population-level DNA barcoding. *Zhongguo Zhong Yao Za Zhi, 37*(8), 1100–1106.

Zhang, Y., Zhang, J. C., Huang, M. H., Yang, M. S., & Cao, H. (2006). Detection of genetic homogeneity of Panax notoginseng cultivars by sequencing nuclear 18S rRNA and plastid matK genes. *Planta Med, 72*(9), 860–862. doi:10.1055/s-2006-946685

Index

adaptor ligation-mediated polymerase chain reaction, authentication of medicinal products by, 333–337, 341–342
- adaptor, design of, 354–355
- adaptor trimming, 352
- bioinformatics analysis, 344–349, 356–357
- database construction, 351–352
- data quality after, 351
- DNA extraction, 337–340
- DNA sample, adaptor assembly and pre-treatment of, 340–341
- *Hedyotis* samples, 337
- materials and methods, 337–351
- next generation sequencing and, 343–344
- NGS data, validation of identified species from, 353
- read counting, 352–353
- read mapping, 352
- validation, 349–351

adaptor short strand (AS1), 355

AFLP. *See* amplified fragment length polymorphism (AFLP)

agarose gel electrophoresis, 68, 77–79, 223
- DNA extraction, for medicinal materials, 52–53

amplification, 68

amplified fragment length polymorphism (AFLP), 503
- authentication of medicinal materials, 153–156
  - advantage of, 168
  - choice of primers and radiolabelling, 157
  - conversion of, 159–160
  - DAMD analysis, 162, 165
  - materials and methods, 156–160
  - minisatellite sequence, of *P. ginseng* polymorphic band, 164
  - of *P. ginseng*, 160–162
  - process, 157–158
  - reamplification and cloning of polymorphic DNA fragments, 159
  - samples studied and DNA extraction, 156
  - similarity index analysis of, 159

SI value of *P. ginseng*, 163
three steps of, 154
animal-derived CMMs, 29
DNA extraction from
equipment, apparatus and accessories, 46
modified CCDB spin column-based DNA extraction protocol, 48–50
modified DNA extraction protocol using DNeasy Mericon food kit, 50–52
reagents, 46–47
sample preparation, 47–48
animal medicines, of DNA barcoding, 326–329
antibodies, 8–9
AP-PCR. *See* arbitrarily primed PCR (AP-PCR)
arbitrarily primed PCR (AP-PCR), 130, 137–139, 504
authentication of medicinal materials
by adaptor ligation-mediated polymerase chain reaction and metabarcoding, 333–337, 341–342
adaptor, design of, 354–355
adaptor trimming, 352
bioinformatics analysis, 344–349, 356–357
database construction, 351–352
data quality after, 351
DNA extraction, 337–340
DNA sample, adaptor assembly and pre-treatment of, 340–341
Hedyotis samples, 337
materials and methods, 337–351
next generation sequencing and, 343–344
NGS data, validation of identified species from, 353
read counting, 352–353
read mapping, 352
validation, 349–351
amplified fragment length polymorphism, 153–156
advantage of, 168
choice of primers and radiolabelling, 157
conversion of, 159–160
DAMD analysis, 162, 165
materials and methods, 156–160

minisatellite sequence, of
P. ginseng polymorphic band, 164
of *P. ginseng*, 160–162
process, 157–158
reamplification and cloning of polymorphic DNA fragments, 159
samples studied and DNA extraction, 156
similarity index analysis of, 159
SI value of *P. ginseng*, 163
by multiplex polymerase chain reaction, 219–221
adulteration detection, 249
application of, 248–250
ARMS-PCR for *P. ginseng* identification, 245–246
built-in internal control, 222–223
close species discrimination, 248
cost-effective tool, 222
cultivar identification, 250
definition of targets, 241
DNA-intercalating dyes, 236, 239
as fit-for-purpose, 221–225
genomic DNA extraction, 246–247
homologous sequence-based primer design, 241–243
limitations, 250–253
multi-component medicinal materials verification, 249–250
multiplex end-point PCR-fragment size multiplexing, 223–235
multiplex real-time PCR, 235–238
number of analytes per multiplex assay, limit on, 252–253
PCR product, visualisation of, 247–248
for *P. ginseng* identification and its adulteration detection, 245–248
precise species identification, 221
probes-fluorophore colour multiplexing, 239–240
random amplification sequence characterised amplification region marker-based primer design, 243–244

screening of candidate primers, optimisation and pooling, 244–245
types of, 223–235
uneven detection limit, 251–252
unknown targets remain unidentified, 250–251
workflow, 241–245
polymerase chain reaction-restriction fragment length polymorphism, 171–172
Beimu, 172, 174, 181–182, 192–193
choice of primers, 175, 181
Daihuang, 172, 175–179
total genomic DNA preparation, 175
randomly primed polymerase chain reaction
arbitrarily primed PCR, 137–139
data analysis, 140–141
ginseng, 134, 141–145
guanghuoxiang, 134–136, 145–146
Kudidan, 133–134, 141–143
materials and methods, 133–137
random amplified polymorphic DNA, 139–140
total genomic DNA preparation, 137
Yu-Ping-Feng San, 137, 146–148
by sequence characterised amplified region, 199–202
materials, 202–203
non-stringent amplification conditions, 210
of *Panax ginseng* and *Panax quinquefolius*, 207
primer SCAR.F1 and SCAR.R1, 210
primers SCAR.F1 and SCAR.R1, 209
primers SCAR.F2 and SCAR.R2, 208
procedures, 204–207
pros and cons of, 211–212
RAPD markers and, 211
RAPD reaction, 203–204
total genomic DNA preparation, 203
autoradiography, 68

backward inner primer (BIP), 395, 428

Barcode of Life Data System (BOLD), 91–93
barcoding gap, 96, 98
Barcoding High-Resolutions Melting (Bar-HRM), 457–460
  application of, 477
  DNA barcodes, generation of, 469–470
  edible plants, differentiation of, 470–472
  materials and methods
    amplification of, 465–467
    detection of unknown samples, 473–474
    genomic DNA extraction, 462–465
    plant materials, 460–462
    plant samples, 462
    plant samples, detection of, 469
    real-time PCR, bar-HRM analysis by, 467–469
    specificity and sensitivity, 472, 473
  plant authentication, necessity of, 474–476
  plant species differentiation, choice of barcode regions, 476
  potential and limitation of, 477–478
  by real-time PCR, 467–469
barcoding targets, genome information for, 364–366
Basic Local Alignment Search Tool (BLAST), 95, 103–108, 243, 349
  alignments, 106
  descriptions, 104–105
  graphic summary, 105–106
  taxonomy, 106
Bayesian (BA) model, 116
BcaBEST polymerase, 395
Beimu, 172, 174, 181–182, 184–185, 192–193
BioEdit, 101
bioinformatics, 89
  adaptor ligation-mediated polymerase chain reaction and metabarcoding, 344, 356–357
    preparation of computational environment, 344–345
    reference database construction, 346
    reference database, read mapping to, 348–349
    reference sequences, read counting to, 349
    sequencing read data, quality control of, 346–347

setting up conda environment and installing required bioinformatics software, 345
databases, for bioinformatics analysis, 90
Barcode of Life Data System, 91–93
Medicinal Materials DNA Barcode Database, 93–94
medicinal materials, monographs of, 90–91
National Centre for Biotechnology Information, 94–95
taxonomy and DNA sequence databases, 91–95
taxonomic identification, 114–120
tools, for species identification
BOLD identification engine, 108–109
global alignment, 101–102
local alignment, 102–107
MMDBD, a one-stop solution, 109–114
raw data sequence pre-editing, 97–101
species identification, principle of, 95–97
biosafety cabinet (BSC), 488, 493
BIP. *See* backward inner primer (BIP)
BOLD identification engine, 108–109
Bsm polymerase, 395
Bst polymerase, 395

capillary electrophoresis (CE), 6
celery *(Apium graveolens)*, 240
central processing unit (CPU), 93
cetyl trimethyl ammonium bromide (CTAB), 30–33, 60–61, 277
Chinese Materia Medica (CMM), 29
decoction slices of, 29
Chinese medicinal materials, 501
Chinese Pharmacopoeia (ChP), 90
CITES-listed shark species, using loop-mediated isothermal amplification, 393–394
fluorescence detection and data analysis, 408
genomic DNA amplification, 407–420
LAMP amplification and optimisation, 426–427

LAMP approach, pros and cons of, 428–429
LAMP primer, design of, 423–426
LAMP, principles of, 395–397
materials, 398–399
naked eye and gel electrophoresis, visual detection by, 421, 423
primer design, choice of region for, 427–428
real-time amplification, 421, 422
samples, 399–405
total genomic preparation, 405–407
cleaved amplified polymorphic sequence (CAPS), 171
ClustalW function, 101
Cluster Database at High Identity with Tolerance (CD-HIT), 346
CMM. *See* Chinese Materia Medica (CMM)
codominant polymorphism, 200
complementary DNA (cDNA), 14
concentrated Chinese medicine granules (CCMG), 333
contaminations, types of, 485
Cordyceps (Dongchongxiacao), 201, 439–440, 451–453
core sequence (CORE), 154
CTAB. *See* cetyl trimethyl ammonium bromide (CTAB)
Cynanchum species, 377
cytochrome c oxidase subunit 1 *(COI)*, 278

Daihuang, 172, 175–179, 182–183, 185–195
denaturing PAGE, 79–82
de novo assembly using low-coverage whole genome shotgun sequence (dnaLCW), 366–371
false gaps, 371
false SNPs, 371
procedures, 368–371
TR copy number error, 371–372
directed amplification of the minisatellite-region DNA (DAMD), 160, 161, 165, 167
dispersed repeats, 15
DNA amplification, forensically informative nucleotide sequencing, 286–287
DNA authentication, 120
DNA barcoding, 17, 89, 270, 305–306, 457
animal medicines, authentication of, 326–329
data analysis, 317–318

fungal medicines,
authentication of, 324–326
genomic DNA amplification,
315–317
materials, 307–313
plant medicines,
authentication of,
318–324
total genomic DNA
preparation, 307, 315
DNA barcoding paradox,
376–379
DNA-based marker, 10
DNA concentration, and purity
measurement
NanoDrop™
spectrophotometer, 69–70
Qubit® fluorometer, 70–72
UV spectrophotometer, 69
DNA Data Bank of Japan
(DDBJ), 94
DNA extraction, 29–31
CTAB extraction, 31–33
DNA yield and purity, 53–55
forensically informative
nucleotide sequencing,
283–286
materials and methods
animal-derived CMMs,
46–52
nucleic acid
quantification,
52
PCR amplification
and agarose gel
electrophoresis, 52–53
plant-derived CMMs,
40–46
sample information and
storage, 36–40
PCR success rate, 55–60
potassium acetate/SDS
precipitation method,
33–35
RNase A digestion, 35–36
DNA fingerprint, 504
DNA fragment, 129
DNA-intercalating dyes, 236, 239
DNA isolation method, 30
DNA laboratory, for molecular
authentication, 483–487
process requirements
handling of test items,
495–496
interlaboratory
comparison or
proficiency testing,
497
practices, 498
quality control plan, 497
record of test item, 495
sampling, 494–495
storage of test items,
495–496
test method and method
validation, 496–497

transferring materials among areas, 496
resource requirements, 487
amplification area, 489
BSC and PCR hood, 493
environmental conditions and facilities, 490–491
equipment, 492–494
facilities and environmental conditions, 487–491
location and placement of equipment, 492
nucleic acid extraction area, 488–489
performance and maintenance, 492
personnel, 494
pipette, 492–493
post-amplification area, 489
pre-PCR zone, ancillary facilities located in, 490
reagents, 493–494
sample receipt area, 488
sterilisation, 493
dnaLCW. *See de novo* assembly using low-coverage whole genome shotgun sequence (dnaLCW)
DNA sequencing, 17, 89, 279–281, 306, 502
forensically informative nucleotide sequencing, 288–290
DNA sequencing-based markers, 17–18
DNA technology, 501, 506
DNeasy plant pro kit, modified DNA extraction protocol using, 44–46
dominant polymorphism, 199–200
dual-labelled amplicons, 446

electric field, voltage of, 82
electropherograms, 97
electrophoresis
agarose gel electrophoresis, 77–79
cloning
E. coli, preparation of, 84–86
ligation and transformation of *E. coli*, 86–87
denaturing PAGE, 79–82
factors
concentration, 82
thickness, 82
voltage of electric field, 82
product purification, 83–84
temperature of, 83
Elongation factor 1-alpha (EF-1a), 440

enzyme immunoassay (EIA), 9
enzyme-linked immunosorbent assay (ELISA), 9
enzyme-specific sequence (ENZ), 154
Escherichia coli
  ligation and transformation of, 86–87
  preparation of, 84–86
ethidium bromide (EtBr), 16
European Nucleotide Archive under European Molecular Biology Laboratory (EMBL-DNA), 94

FastQC, 344
FINS. *See* forensically informative nucleotide sequencing (FINS)
fluorescence dyes, 16
fluorophore colour multiplexing, 239–240
forensically informative nucleotide sequencing (FINS), 270, 271
  DNA amplification and purification, 286–287
  DNA extraction, 283–286
  DNA sequencing, 288–290
  identification of commodities, 294–297
  molecular cloning, 287–288
  multiple sequence alignment, 290–294
  sample collection and preparation, 283
  steps in, 271–282
    DNA sequencing and sequence database analysis, 279–281
    loci selection and DNA amplification, 277–279
    phylogenetic analysis and identification, 281–282
    sample preparation and DNA isolation, 271–277
forward inner primer (FIP), 395, 428
Fourier transform infrared (FTIR) spectroscopy, 7
fragment size multiplexing, 223–235
fungal medicines, of DNA barcoding, 324–326

Gapcloser program, 368
genetically modified (GM) genes, 506
genetic variations, 17
genome-wide polymorphism, 269
genomic DNA amplification
  CITES-listed shark species, using loop-mediated isothermal amplification, 407–420
  DNA barcoding, 315–317

ginseng, 134, 137–139, 143–145, 506
ginsenoside Rb2, 6–7
global alignment, 101–102
Global Pharmacopoeia Genome Database (GPGD), 504–505
Good Manufacturing Practice (GMP), 18–19, 336
GPGD. *See* Global Pharmacopoeia Genome Database (GPGD)
guanghuoxiang, 134–136, 139–140, 145–146

HDA. *See* helicase-dependent amplification (HDA)
Hedyotis, 336
Hedyotis diffusa, 337
helicase-dependent amplification (HDA), 393, 394
hierarchical clustering tree (ML), 322
high-performance liquid chromatography (HPLC), 6
high-performance thin-layer chromatography (HPTLC), 6
high-resolution melting (HRM), 239, 458, 459
HPLC-evaporative light scattering detection (ELSD), 7
HRM. *See* high-resolution melting (HRM)
hybridisation-based markers, 14–15

integrated interspecific authentication system, 381–382
internal amplification control (IAC) DNA, 240
internal transcribed spacer (ITS), 457
International Plant Names Index (IPNI), 91
intraspecific plastome diversity, 373–376
isozyme polymorphism, 8

Kudidan, 133–134, 137–139, 141–143

lateral flow dipstick (LFD), 437–439, 448, 450–451
  Cordyceps, differentiation of, 451–453
  materials, 439–440
  methods
    PCR amplification, 444–449
    primer design, 443–444
    testing, 446–447
    total genomic preparation, 441–443
  pros and cons of, 453
  samples, 440–441
LFD. *See* lateral flow dipstick (LFD)
local alignment, 102–107

loop-mediated isothermal amplification (LAMP), 393–397, 409–420
amplification and optimisation, 426–427
primer, design of, 423–426
pros and cons of, 428–429

M23, 380
management system, 484
mass spectrometry (MS), 6
matK gene, 195
Maximum Likelihood (ML) model, 116
Maximum Parsimony (MP) model, 116
Max Score, 105
medicinal materials
authentication, 4–5
arbitrarily primed PCR, 137–139
data analysis, 140–141
ginseng, 134, 141–145
guanghuoxiang, 134–136, 145–146
Kudidan, 133–134, 141–143
materials and methods, 133–137
random amplified polymorphic DNA, 139–140
total genomic DNA preparation, 137
Yu-Ping-Feng San, 137, 146–148
organoleptic and histological analysis, 5–6
chemical analysis, 6–7
biochemical analysis, 7–9
DNA extraction for, 29–31
animal-derived CMMs, 46–52
CTAB extraction, 31–33
DNA yield and purity, 53–55
nucleic acid quantification, 52
PCR amplification and agarose gel electrophoresis, 52–53
PCR success rate, 55–60
plant-derived CMMs, 40–46
potassium acetate/SDS precipitation method, 33–35
RNase A digestion, 35–36
sample information and storage, 36–40
emerging DNA techniques, 18–19
molecular authentication markers for, 11–13
molecular marker technologies, 9–14

DNA sequencing-based markers, 17–18
hybridisation-based markers, 14–15
PCR-based markers, 15–17
monographs of, 90–91
substitutes and adulterants of, 4
Medicinal Materials DNA Barcode Database (MMDBD), 93–94, 109–114, 281
Medicinal Plant Names Services (MPNS), 91
MEGA program. *See* Molecular Evolutionary Genetics Analysis (MEGA) program
metabarcoding, authentication of medicinal products by, 333–337, 341–342
adaptor, design of, 354–355
adaptor trimming, 352
bioinformatics analysis, 344–349, 356–357
database construction, 351–352
data quality after, 351
DNA extraction, 337–340
DNA sample, adaptor assembly and pre-treatment of, 340–341
Hedyotis samples, 337
materials and methods, 337–351
next generation sequencing and, 343–344
NGS data, validation of identified species from, 353
read counting, 352–353
read mapping, 352
validation, 349–351
microsatellites, 15
Minicoanda, 345
minisatellite-region DNA polymorphism marker, 159–160
mitochondrial plastid DNA (MTPT), 376–379
MMDBD. *See* Medicinal Materials DNA Barcode Database (MMDBD)
modified CCDB/GCMTI spin column-based DNA extraction protocol, plant-derived CMMs, 42–44
modified CCDB spin column-based DNA extraction protocol, animal-derived CMMs, 48–50
modified DNA extraction protocol
animal-derived CMMs, 50–52
plant-derived CMMs, 44–46
using DNeasy plant pro kit, 44–46
molecular authentication, 87, 502
DNA laboratory for, 483–487
amplification area, 489
BSC and PCR hood, 493

environmental conditions
and facilities, 490–491
equipment, 492–494
facilities and
environmental
conditions, 487–491
handling of test items,
495–496
interlaboratory
comparison or
proficiency testing, 497
location and placement
of equipment, 492
nucleic acid extraction
area, 488–489
performance and
maintenance, 492
personnel, 494
pipette, 492–493
post-amplification area,
489
practices, 498
pre-PCR zone, ancillary
facilities located in, 490
quality control plan, 497
reagents, 493–494
record of test item, 495
sample receipt area, 488
sampling, 494–495
sterilisation, 493
storage of test items,
495–496
test method and method
validation, 496–497
transferring materials
among areas, 496
priority issues in, 504–506
pros and cons of, 501–504
molecular clock hypothesis, 116
Molecular Evolutionary Genetics
Analysis (MEGA) program,
116–117, 119, 120
molecular markers, uses of, 506
molecular marker technologies,
9–14
DNA sequencing-based
markers, 17–18
hybridisation-based markers,
14–15
PCR-based markers, 15–17
molecular technology, 19
monoclonal antibodies, 9
monographs, of medicinal
materials, 90–91
*Mse*I, 153
multidimensional
chromatography, 6
multiple sequence alignment,
forensically informative
nucleotide sequencing,
290–294
multiplex end-point
PCR-fragment size
multiplexing, 223–235

multiplex polymerase chain reaction, authentication of medicinal materials by, 219–221
adulteration detection, 249
application of, 248–250
ARMS-PCR for *P. ginseng* identification, 245–246
built-in internal control, 222–223
close species discrimination, 248
cost-effective tool, 222
cultivar identification, 250
definition of targets, 241
DNA-intercalating dyes, 236, 239
as fit-for-purpose, 221–225
genomic DNA extraction, 246–247
homologous sequence-based primer design, 241–243
limitations, 250–253
multi-component medicinal materials verification, 249–250
multiplex end-point PCR-fragment size multiplexing, 223–235
multiplex real-time PCR, 235–238
number of analytes per multiplex assay, limit on, 252–253
PCR product, visualisation of, 247–248
for *P. ginseng* identification and its adulteration detection, 245–248
precise species identification, 221
probes-fluorophore colour multiplexing, 239–240
random amplification sequence characterised amplification region marker-based primer design, 243–244
screening of candidate primers, optimisation and pooling, 244–245
types of, 223–235
uneven detection limit, 251–252
unknown targets remain unidentified, 250–251
workflow, 241–245
multiplex real-time PCR, 235–238

NanoDrop™ spectrophotometer, 69–70
Nanopore Sequencing, 19

National Centre for Biotechnology Information (NCBI), 92, 94–95
National Institutes of Health (NIH), 94
National Library of Medicine (NLM), 94
NCBI. *See* National Centre for Biotechnology Information (NCBI)
NCBI GenBank, 281
neighbour-joining (NJ) method, 116
neighbour-joining phylogenetic tree, 326–329
Next Generation Sequencing, 503
next generation sequencing (NGS), 18, 335, 336, 343–344
NGS. *See* next generation sequencing (NGS)
notoginsenoside R1, 7
nuclear magnetic resonance (NMR) spectroscopy, 7
nuclear ribosomal DNA, 379–380
super-barcoding of medicinal materials, 363–364
barcoding targets, genome information for, 364–366
genomics perspective of, 372–380
integrated interspecific authentication system, 381–382
intraspecific plastome diversity, 373–376
MTPT and DNA barcoding paradox, 376–379
nuclear ribosomal DNAs, 379–380
plastome diversity and database, 372–373
universal barcode primer, advantage and disadvantage of, 372
whole genome shotgun sequence, assembly of complete plastome using, 366–372
nucleotide variation, 372–373

Operational Taxonomic Units (OTU), 115
Ophiocordyceps sinensis, 439

PacBio Sequencing, 19
parallel sequencing, 279
parsley *(Petroselinum crispum)*, 240
PCR. *See* polymerase chain reaction (PCR)
PCR amplification, 444–449
DNA extraction, for medicinal materials, 52–53

PCR-based markers, 15–17
PCR-RFLP. *See* polymerase chain reaction-restriction fragment length polymorphism (PCR-RFLP)
PCR success rate, 55–60
phenol/chloroform extraction, 277
phylogeny, 117
plant-derived CMMs, 37–38
  equipment, apparatus and accessories, 40
  modified CCDB/GCMTI spin column-based DNA extraction protocol, 42–44
  modified DNA extraction protocol using DNeasy plant pro kit, 44–46
  reagents, 40–41
  sample preparation, 41–42
plant medicines, of DNA barcoding, 318–324
plastid genomes, super-barcoding of medicinal materials, 363–364
  barcoding targets, genome information for, 364–366
  genomics perspective of, 372–380
  integrated interspecific authentication system, 381–382
  intraspecific plastome diversity, 373–376
  MTPT and DNA barcoding paradox, 376–379
  nuclear ribosomal DNAs, 379–380
  plastome diversity and database, 372–373
  universal barcode primer, advantage and disadvantage of, 372
  whole genome shotgun sequence, assembly of complete plastome using, 366–372
plastome assembly, diverse methods for, 366
plastomes, 365
polyacrylamide gel electrophoresis (PAGE), 68
polymerase chain reaction (PCR), 9, 29, 70–72, 129, 153, 485, 502
  factors
    annealing temperature, 77
    reaction components, 75–76
  primer design, 74–75
  workflow of, 72–73
polymerase chain reaction-restriction fragment length polymorphism (PCR-RFLP), 171–172
  Beimu, 172, 174, 181–182, 192–193

choice of primers, 175, 181
Daihuang, 172, 175–179
total genomic DNA preparation, 175
potassium acetate/SDS precipitation method, 33–35
Primer3, 109, 110, 114
probes-fluorophore colour multiplexing, 239–240

quality control plan, DNA laboratory, 497
Qubit® fluorometer, 70–72
query sequence, 115

random amplified polymorphic DNA (RAPD), 130, 139–140, 243
randomly primed PCR (RP-PCR), 132
advantages of, 131
authentication of medicinal materials
arbitrarily primed PCR, 137–139
data analysis, 140–141
ginseng, 134, 141–145
guanghuoxiang, 134–136, 145–146
Kudidan, 133–134, 141–143
materials and methods, 133–137
random amplified polymorphic DNA, 139–140
total genomic DNA preparation, 137
Yu-Ping-Feng San, 137, 146–148
principle of, 130
taxonomic levels, molecular characteristics of, 133
RAPD. *See* random amplified polymorphic DNA (RAPD)
rare-cutter *Eco*RI, 153
raw data sequence pre-editing, 97–101
real-time amplification, CITES-listed shark species using loop-mediated isothermal amplification, 421, 422
Real-Time Analysis (RTA), 344
real-time PCR, bar-HRM analysis by, 467–469
recombinase polymerase amplification (RPA), 393
recombinase-primer complex, 394
restriction fragment length polymorphism (RFLP), 14, 153, 171
RFLP. *See* restriction fragment length polymorphism (RFLP)
RNase A digestion, 35–36

Sanger sequencing, 97
SCAR. *See* sequence characterised amplified region (SCAR)
second-generation sequencing, 19
sequence alignment, 101
sequence characterised amplified region (SCAR), 199–202
  authentication of medicinal materials by, 199–202
    materials, 202–203
    non-stringent amplification conditions, 210
    of *Panax ginseng* and *Panax quinquefolius*, 207
    primer SCAR.F1 and SCAR.R1, 210
    primers SCAR.F1 and SCAR.R1, 209
    primers SCAR.F2 and SCAR.R2, 208
    procedures, 204–207
    pros and cons of, 211–212
    RAPD markers and, 211
    RAPD reaction, 203–204
    total genomic DNA preparation, 203
sequence database analysis, 279–281
sequence-tagged sites (STS), 15
simple sequence repeat (SSR), 15
single nucleotide polymorphism (SNP), 318, 505
single-stranded DNA-binding protein (SSB), 393
SNP. *See* single nucleotide polymorphism (SNP)
sterilisation, DNA Laboratory, for molecular authentication, 493
strand displacement amplification (SDA), 393
super-barcoding of medicinal materials, plastid genomes and nuclear ribosomal DNA, 363–364
  barcoding targets, genome information for, 364–366
  genomics perspective of, 372–380
  integrated interspecific authentication system, 381–382
  intraspecific plastome diversity, 373–376
  MTPT and DNA barcoding paradox, 376–379
  nuclear ribosomal DNAs, 379–380

plastome diversity and database, 372–373
universal barcode primer, advantage and disadvantage of, 372
whole genome shotgun sequence, assembly of complete plastome using, 366–372

tandem repeats, 14–15
taxonomic identification, bioinformatics, 114–120
TCM. *See* traditional Chinese medicine (TCM)
thin-layer chromatography (TLC), 6
thin-layer polyacrylamide slab gels, 8
Tongil, 380
touch down PCR cycle, 166
traditional Chinese medicine (TCM), 3, 270, 505
tree-based method, 115, 116
tree-building algorithms, 115
Triphala, 249

ultra-high-pressure liquid chromatography (UHPLC), 6
ultraviolet (UV) spectrometer, 68
universal barcode primer, advantage and disadvantage of, 372
universal DNA barcoding, 363–364
Unweighted Pair-group Mean Analysis (UPGMA), 282
Unweighted Pair Group Method with Arithmetic Mean (UPGMA), 116
UV spectrophotometer, DNA concentration and purity measurement, 69

WGS. *See* whole genome shotgun sequence (WGS)
whole genome shotgun sequence (WGS), 366–372
de novo assembly using low-coverage whole genome shotgun sequence, 366–372
plastome assembly, diverse methods for, 366

Yu-Ping-Feng San, 137, 140, 146–148

Lightning Source UK Ltd.
Milton Keynes UK
UKHW020748241122
412764UK00002B/20

9 789811 261534